W9-AKU-960

PRAISE FOR
Anodea Judith's Chakra Yoga

Anodea's understanding and interpretation of the chakra system blew my mind and heart wide open and deeply influenced my personal yoga practice as well as my teaching. She is the teacher's teacher, the high priestess of sacred depth work, and a true pioneer in making these ancient practices accessible and meaningful in our contemporary world.—Seane Corn, founder of Off the Mat, Into the World

· · · · · · · · ·

Chakra Yoga is a wonderful embodied companion for Anodea Judith's pioneering decades of chakra books and teachings providing exploration through asana, pranayama, bandhas, mantra, and visualization as the yogic methods for liberating, transforming, and balancing our energetic body and life. A gift to the world.—Shiva Rea, founder of Prana Vinyasa and author of *Tending the Heart Fire*

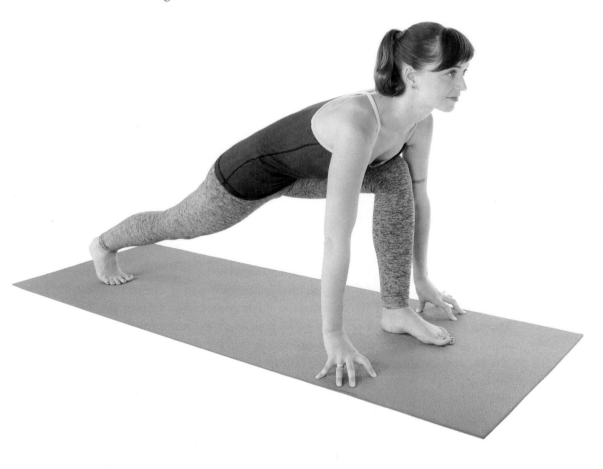

For decades I have been waiting, wishing, *longing* for such a book as *Anodea Judith's Chakra Yoga*. It is a multidimensional book, perfect for those who practice yoga but also for therapists who work with energy transformation through the chakras, Tantra teachers looking for the best information about the chakras, and those who want to heal their body and improve their meditation skills. The book is exquisitely presented, deep, practical, inspiring, easy to follow, contemporary: A MUST HAVE. Enjoy the ride!
—Margot Anand, author of *The Art of Everyday Ecstasy*

. . . .

Anodea Judith's Chakra Yoga makes a subject that has been mystical and mysterious—a subject whose time has come—accessible and usable in today's world. Exciting and practical, this is a book that I'm going to study!—Lilias Folan (Swami Kavitananda), PBS host of *Lilias, Yoga and You*

. . . .

Anodea Judith's Chakra Yoga masterfully presents and integrates the energetics and spiritual understanding of the chakras into the practice of asana. Judith offers us both a path and the means for attaining health, healing, well-being, and awakening to our essential nature, and she offers us beautifully designed practices that are easy to follow yet full of depth and inspiration that will motivate the reader for years to come.—Richard Miller, PhD, founder of iRest Meditation and author of *Yoga Nidra: The Meditative Heart of Yoga*

. . . .

Anodea Judith has created a masterly guide to practicing asana as a means to awaken and balance the chakras. Her deep knowledge and experience of the multiple dimensions of the yogic journey irradiates every page. *Anodea Judith's Chakra Yoga* is an indispensable guidebook for travelers on the inner path of yoga. Use it to help you open the doors that connect the physical and subtle worlds!—Sally Kempton, author of *Awakening Shakti* and *Meditation for the Love of It*

. . . .

Anodea Judith's Chakra Yoga is the culminating wisdom of Judith's forty-year journey through yoga and somatic psychotherapy, and it masterfully lays out the foundation of her posture-based bioenergetics system for balancing body, mind, and spirit. *Chakra Yoga* is a validating must-read for all of us awake to the transformative power of yoga, and it is the perfect gift for those who have not yet realized yoga's potential for mind-body healing.—Amy Weintraub, founder of the LifeForce Yoga Healing Institute and author of *Yoga for Depression* and *Yoga Skills for Therapists*

Anodea Judith has been at the forefront of chakra studies for over two decades, and her books have become the standard reference material both for students and teachers of yoga. *Anodea Judith's Chakra Yoga* is the most thorough and well researched available in this area and will also become a standard and a classic.—Joseph Le Page, founder and director of Integrative Yoga Therapy

· · · · · · · · ·

Anodea Judith's penetrating and exciting understanding of the body's chakra system is brought to life as she shows how specific yoga postures activate desired qualities that are associated with each of the body's energy centers. *Chakra Yoga* is a beautiful blend of the practice of yoga with the profound wisdom held in your chakras. This is a wonderful book.—Donna Eden, author of *Energy Medicine* and *The Energies of Love*

· · · · · · · · ·

For years students have been asking for a great book on yoga and the chakras. Finally, it is here! Anodea's masterful book is as beautifully illustrated as it is informative, giving a dynamic new depth to hatha yoga. It offers a clear understanding of the chakras in practice, presenting the skills to revitalize and balance our entire being. I wholeheartedly recommend this book; it is an essential guide to experiencing your own divine essence. An instant classic!—Nischala Joy Devi, teacher and author of *The Healing Path of Yoga* and *The Secret Power of Yoga*

· · · · · · · · ·

I loved reading *Anodea Judith's Chakra Yoga*, an offering that is profound in its content yet simple to read, practice, and understand. Anodea conveys the deeper meaning and power of yoga in a way that any level of yoga student or teacher can benefit from reading.—Desiree Rumbaugh, international yoga teacher, creator of the Wisdom Warriors classes, and author of the Yoga to the Rescue DVD series

· · · · · · · · ·

Anodea Judith's Chakra Yoga is a unique and beautiful contribution to the practice and integration of the chakras into the physical body. She interweaves the subtle chakras into the asanas in creative, clear, and effective ways beneficial to all levels of practitioners, beginner to advanced. This book is informative, inspiring, and well worth the read, especially for those who wish to develop a chakra yoga practice at home.—Todd Norian, founder of Ashaya Yoga and senior Kripalu yoga teacher

Anodea Judith's Chakra Yoga is an outstanding contribution to both yoga literature and yoga instruction. Anodea is the world's leading expert on the chakras, and she has brought her expertise to the daily practice of yoga. This book is well crafted, elegant, and instructive. Reading it is like being in a workshop with a delightful, caring teacher who wants only to help you bring out your very best qualities. If you're a yoga practitioner, teacher, or scholar, or merely yoga-curious, this book will be a gentle, comforting guide along your path.—Lion Goodman, Luminary Leadership Institute, co-author of *Creating On Purpose: The Spiritual Technology of Manifesting Through the Chakras*

. . . .

With utmost respect for the roots of classical yoga and yet with a clear Western psychological approach, Anodea brings another pearl to the string of knowledge proposed in her now-classic *Wheels of Life*. These are now the actual steps in the chakra roadmap to fullness that she so clearly delineates in her teachings. Thanks, Anodea!—Antonio Sausys, author of *Yoga for Grief Relief: Simple Practices to Transforming Your Grieving Mind and Body*

. . . .

Anodea Judith's Chakra Yoga is an excellent comprehensive guide to accessing and bringing into balance the subtle body energy chakra system through a hatha yoga practice. Anodea writes in a way that is extremely organized and clear: scholarly and astute for the seasoned yogi yet completely accessible for the new yoga practitioner. *Chakra Yoga* is outstanding, and anyone can apply the wisdom practices in this guide for their own body, mind, and soul renewal.—Benita J. Wolfe Galván, co-founder of the Anusara School of Hatha Yoga

. . . .

Anodea Judith's love and knowledge of the essence of the chakras and their practical application in our lives comes though clearly in this inspiring book. She has been a wealth of chakra and yogic knowledge for years, and this book, along with her others, are on the top of the must-read list for my training and programs. Congratulations on a wonderful, uplifting work.—Jeff Migdow, holistic MD, prana yoga teacher training director

ANODEA JUDITH'S
CHAKRA YOGA

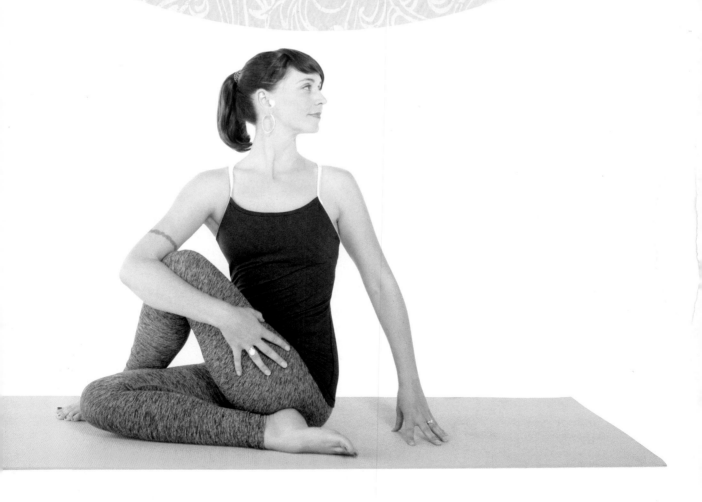

About the Author

Anodea Judith, PhD, is the founder and director of Sacred Centers, a teaching organization that promotes sacred knowledge for the transformation of individuals and cultures (www.SacredCenters.com). A groundbreaking thinker, writer, and worldwide spiritual teacher, her passion for the realization of untapped human potential matches her concern for humanity's impending crises— her fervent wish is that we wake up in time. She holds masters and doctoral degrees in psychology and human health, with advanced certification in yoga and lifelong studies of mind-body medicine, mythology, history, psychology, systems theory, and mystic spirituality.

Anodea is considered the country's foremost expert on the chakras and therapeutic issues. She teaches worldwide, with workshops and trainings offered across the United States, Canada, Europe, Asia, and Central America.

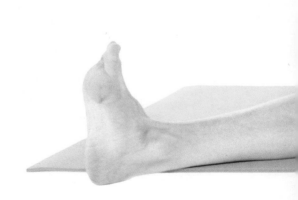

ANODEA JUDITH'S
CHAKRA YOGA

Llewellyn Publications
WOODBURY, MINNESOTA

Anodea Judith's Chakra Yoga © 2015 by Anodea Judith. All rights reserved. No part of this book may be used or reproduced in any manner whatsoever, including Internet usage, without written permission from Llewellyn Publications, except in the case of brief quotations embodied in critical articles and reviews.

FIRST EDITION
First Printing, 2015

Book design by Rebecca Zins
Cover design by Kevin R. Brown
Cover images: www.shutterstock.com/119040046/119040043/119040037/
119040040/119040055/119040052/119040049©sita ram;
www.shutterstock.com/62384575/©Zvonimir Atletic;
iStockphoto.com/28187954/©szefei
Anatomical illustrations on pages 324 and 367 by Mary Ann Zapalac
Interior pattern: iStockphoto.com/29651788/©alexmakarova
Photography by Yuzu Studios

Llewellyn Publications is a registered trademark of Llewellyn Worldwide Ltd.

Cover model used for illustrative purposes only and
may not endorse or represent the book's subject.

Library of Congress Cataloging-in-Publication Data
Judith, Anodea, 1952–
   Anodea Judith's Chakra yoga / Anodea Judith.—First edition.
       pages cm
   Includes index.
   ISBN 978-0-7387-4444-5
   1. Hatha yoga. 2. Chakras. I. Title. II. Title: Chakra yoga.
   RA781.7.J83 2015
   613.7'046—dc23

                                                                    2015018123

Llewellyn Worldwide does not participate in, endorse, or have any authority or responsibility concerning private business transactions between our authors and the public.

   All mail addressed to the author is forwarded but the publisher cannot, unless specifically instructed by the author, give out an address or phone number.

   Any Internet references contained in this work are current at publication time, but the publisher cannot guarantee that a specific location will continue to be maintained. Please refer to the publisher's website for links to authors' websites and other sources.

Llewellyn Publications
A Division of Llewellyn Worldwide Ltd.
2143 Wooddale Drive
Woodbury, MN 55125-2989
www.llewellyn.com

Printed in the United States of America

Disclaimer

This book contains suggested yoga practices and is not intended to replace necessary medical attention from a qualified healthcare provider. Consult your physician before engaging in any new exercise program. Not every exercise is recommended for every person or condition, and caution should be used in engaging with any physical practice that is unfamiliar.

If you are new to yoga, the postures within these pages are best learned from a live class with a qualified instructor. Do not continue anything that causes pain or aggravates a current condition. No guarantees are made for any results from this program, and no liability is assumed for any direct or indirect damages that may result. The information in this book is to be used carefully and at your own risk.

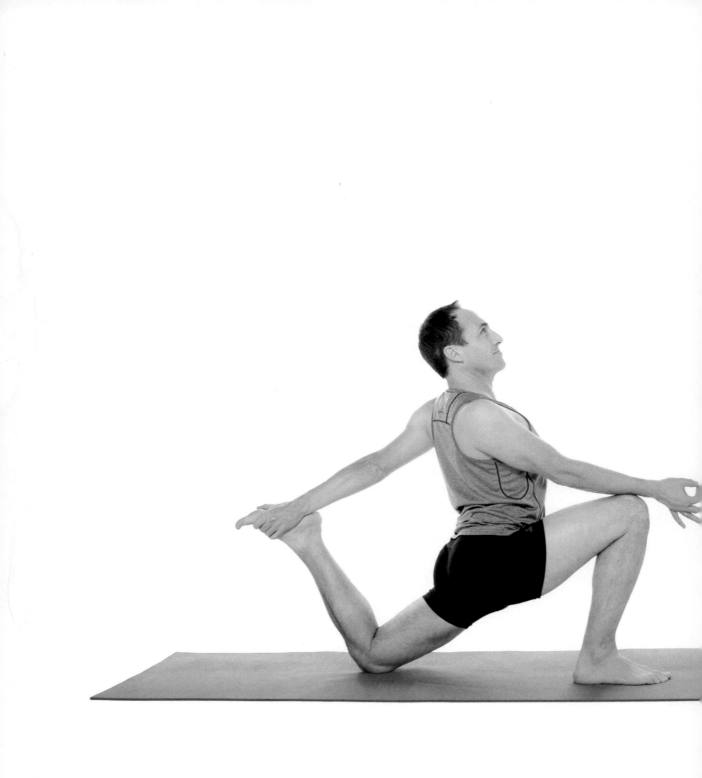

Contents

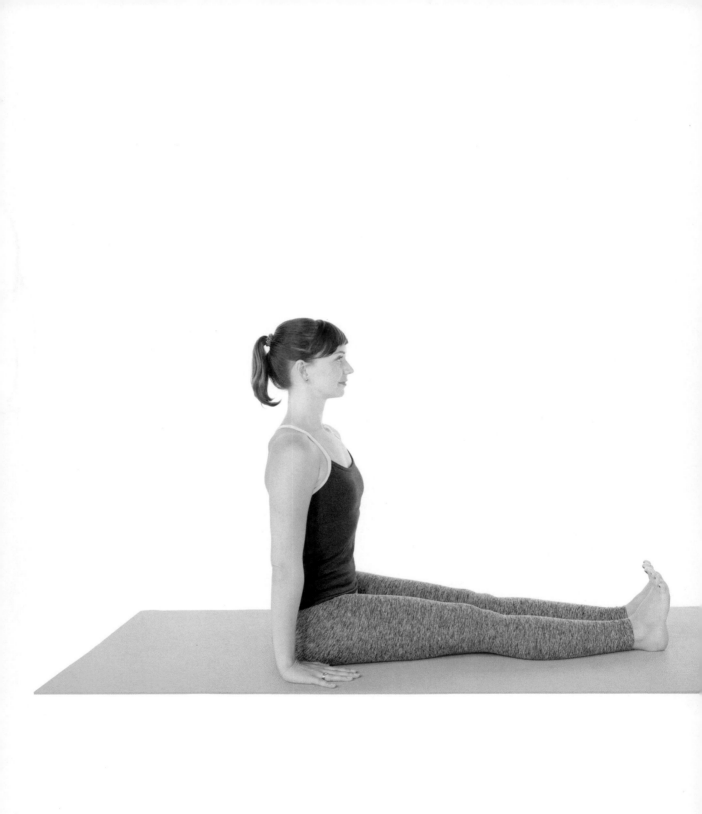

Postures by Chakra

Chakra One

Chakra Two

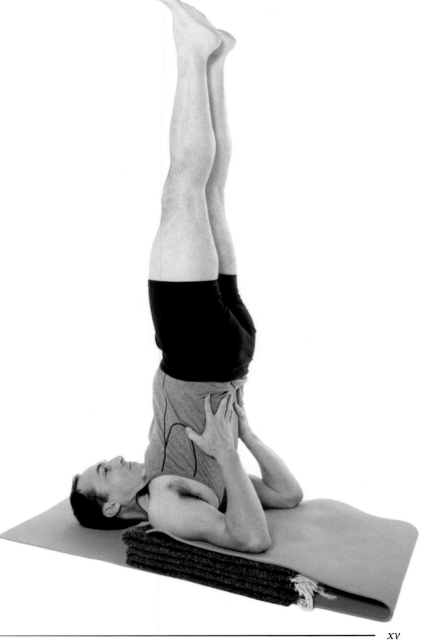

Chakra Three

Chakra Four

Chakra Five

Chakra Six

Chakra Seven

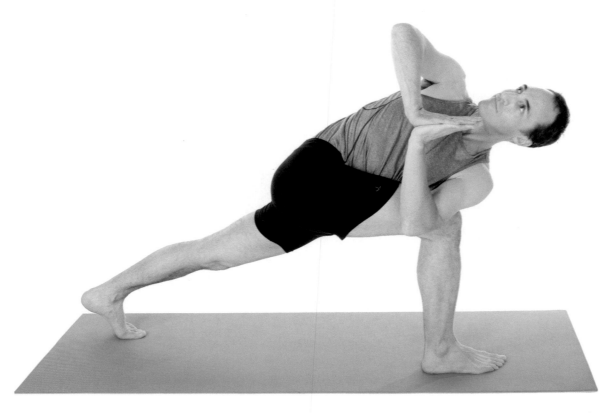

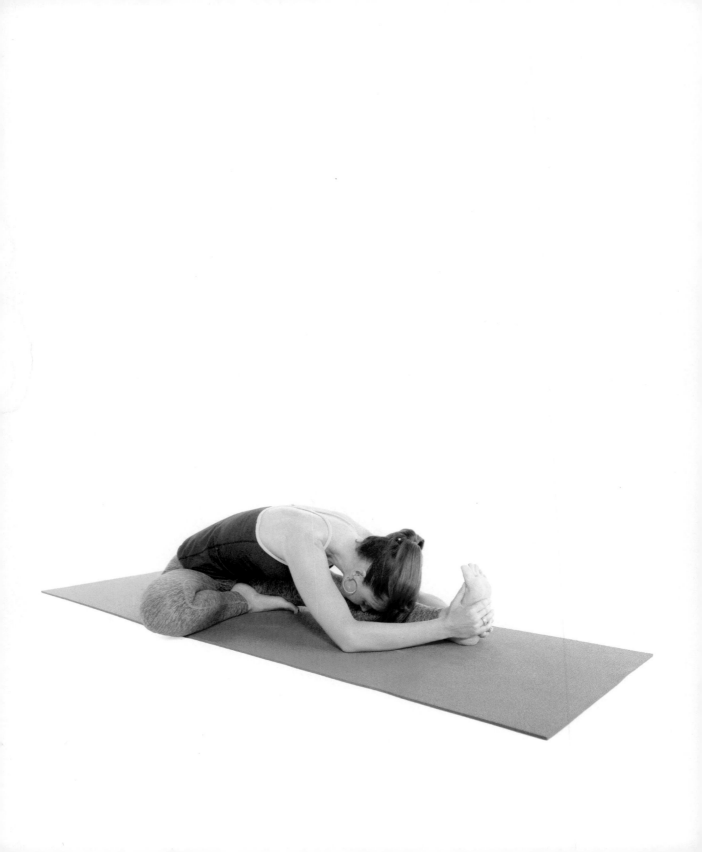

Acknowledgments

It is an illusion that yoga is something you do alone on your mat. In truth, everything that we learn has come down to us through a long line of teachers and students, from Patanjali's first lectures over two thousand years ago to the creative license teachers take today as they refine poses and create new traditions. I have never subscribed to any one form of yoga, nor any one teacher, but have taken the attitude that I can learn something from everyone, even a new teacher freshly out of her teacher training. However, there are a few leading teachers that stand out and need mention.

I would like to acknowledge Swami Satchidananda and his book *Integral Yoga Hatha* for my very first start in yoga back in 1975. Joseph Le Page introduced me to yoga therapy and gave me my first certification in that discipline. When the going got tough and my health challenges would have kept me off the mat, John Friend kept me inspired, practicing, and learning, as did many of the wonderful teachers in the Anusara lineage, such as Sianna Sherman, Jonas Westring, Todd Norian, Martin Kirk, and BJ Galvan. Seane Corn and Shiva Rea continue to raise the bar of what yoga can be and do for the world, for which I am grateful and continually inspired. Rodney Yee has shown me what exquisite teaching is like. Matthew Sanford puts to shame anyone who allows themselves to be limited by disabilities and keeps me transcending my own. Bikram and Sumits yoga have allowed me to sweat out the years of antibiotics and toxins that have helped my healing. Kripalu Yoga Center has been a consistent home for my teachings for nearly two decades, and I have studied with many excellent teachers there.

In the creation of this book, I would like to first acknowledge Bobbi Lance of Yuzu Studios and Larry Martinez, her assistant, for the professional photography work and Bobbi's patience with sorting through thousands of images. I have only the highest praise for the models, Sarah Jenness and Mark Silva, who held difficult poses under bright, hot lights, hour after hour, refining and repeating, showing up in spite of other challenges (like being in the middle of moving!) and keeping us all laughing and having fun with yoga.

I couldn't do any of this without my trusty assistants: Shanon Dean, who manages everything in the Sacred Centers office so that I can spend time writing and teaching, and Gianna Perada, who helped with some of the fastidious tasks of formatting and other office details. My partner, Ramone Yaciuk, put up with me while I turned the living room into a photo studio and buried myself in my office writing. Thanks to Nini Gridley, who handles the Sacred Centers Certification Program and keeps me dancing along the rainbow bridge.

I would like to give heartfelt appreciation to Carl Weschcke for publishing my first book, *Wheels of Life*, back in 1987. Carl, this book is my "thank you" for believing in me back when I was a nobody and for helping to put the chakras on the worldwide map of conscious awakening. Also at Llewellyn, I would like to thank Angela Wix and Becky Zins for editing and layout, and Bill Krause for pestering me for another book long enough to get me to write this one. Thanks also to publicist Kat Sanborn, who gave me such wonderful support in getting this book out.

I would like to thank all the studios and retreat centers that have sponsored my teachings, as the workshops allow me to continually refine this work, and last, but certainly not least, the thousands of students who have studied with me, investing their time, money, and energy in learning about the chakras, and who have, in turn, taught me so much.

It takes far more than a village to create a body of work, and I am deeply grateful for all who have graced my path of the chakras along the way.

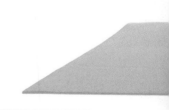

Welcome to the Journey

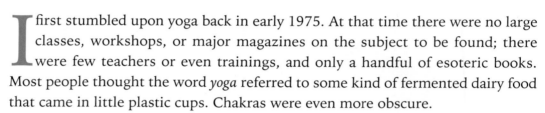

The practice of yoga brings us face to face with the extraordinary complexity of our own being. ~ SRI AUROBINDO

I first stumbled upon yoga back in early 1975. At that time there were no large classes, workshops, or major magazines on the subject to be found; there were few teachers or even trainings, and only a handful of esoteric books. Most people thought the word *yoga* referred to some kind of fermented dairy food that came in little plastic cups. Chakras were even more obscure.

Classes for six to eight students were held in people's living rooms. We wore baggy white pants and T-shirts. Rather than mats, we stretched out on towels. Poses were simple and held for a long time, accompanied by slow, deep breaths. I remember how the teacher burned incense and chanted something in a language I didn't understand, but it all sounded lovely and left me with a feeling of having just been to church. I was hooked.

I bought what books I could find and spread them out in my attic apartment, trying to copy the poses as best I could—so I know well what it's like to study yoga from a book. I was lucky if I could even get into one of those pretzel-like configurations, never mind whether I was doing it right, with all the subtle cues taught today. But I practiced and breathed, chanted and meditated daily until it began to transform me.

I felt so good and couldn't understand why everyone wasn't doing yoga. I quickly became one of those insufferable converts who could talk of nothing else. It wasn't long before people asked me to show them what I was doing—to demonstrate some poses. Intrigued, my friends asked me to teach a class. At that time I knew nothing of teacher trainings or even of proper alignment techniques, but, naively, I started teaching what I knew.

I was reading everything I could on consciousness, psychology, metaphysics, mysticism, and spirituality. It was in a classic book by Ram Dass, *The Only Dance There Is*, that I first read the word *chakra*. It was like a shot of energy ran through my whole body. Somehow I knew in that moment that I had found a profound key that simultaneously unlocked and tied together just about everything. I couldn't stop thinking about it.

I was also doing a lot of meditation at the time, having been initiated into Transcendental Meditation (TM) back in 1972, sleeping only about four hours a night because I was meditating so much. One day, while meditating, I had my one and only out-of-body experience: I saw myself sitting in full lotus position with a book in my lap. It was on the chakra system, and it had my name on it. I knew then that the chakra system was to become my life's work.

At the time I was making my living as an artist (if you could call it a living), painting large interior murals of visionary landscapes. I discovered that my state of consciousness affected the clarity of my painting, so I began a systematic purification of my diet, eliminating coffee, meat, and—much as I hate to admit I ever used them—cigarettes. I had an application all filled out to go to art school in New York City, but I threw it in the trash after my vision of the chakra book and abruptly changed course in my life.

I started teaching yoga along the lines of the chakra system, creating a seven-week series that focused on each chakra in turn. People were transforming before my eyes! Four decades later, the chakra system has led me to studying and teaching all over the world and writing a number of best-selling books, starting with *Wheels of Life*, published in 1987, and culminating in the book you now hold in your hands. The chakra system has become my archetype of wholeness and my holy grail.

Today yoga centers are popping up everywhere, the way churches did in the first few centuries of Christianity. Mats line up wall to wall, with little space to spare in classes of hundreds. A 2012 study conducted by *Yoga Journal*[1] showed that 20.4 million Americans practice yoga, spending over $10 billion a year on classes, workshops, products, and media. Some find it merely a means to a healthier, sleeker body. Others use yoga as a method of stress reduction. Some, I'm sure, find it the trendy thing to do. Yet regardless of what drives a person to their mat,

1 http://www.yogajournal.com/press/yoga_in_america

the deeper gifts of yoga eventually reveal themselves. A healthier body produces a more refined state of awareness and greater sensitivity. Flexibility allows a new kind of freedom, not only in your body but in your life. Strength helps you get through tough situations. Subtle energies become less subtle, inviting curiosity about our deeper nature. Consciousness emerges as a new frontier. Yoga philosophy creeps into your viewpoint on life. More than just a physical practice, yoga begins to emerge as a life path—an entire tapestry of philosophy, practices, behavior guidelines, and insights—and a doorway into another world.

My personal path in yoga has been neither easy nor straightforward. About ten years after I began to practice, I was struck down by a severe case of Lyme disease that went undiagnosed for five years and had me on the way to a wheelchair, though it never got quite that bad. My tissues were so sensitive that I couldn't rest my forearms on the edge of a table or clap my hands together, let alone hold a Downward Dog because of the pain in my hands and elbows. My joints were painful with every move, and everything having to do with yoga was affected: flexibility, balance, strength, mental clarity, and the ability to endure pressure on any part of my body. Even kneeling on a mat was painful. It took fifteen years to rebuild my body and strength again, and even longer to accept that I would never be able to touch my feet to the back of my head, walk across the room on my hands, or grace the cover of *Yoga Journal* in a fancy pose. Yet I believe yoga is one of the reasons I have been less debilitated than many who suffer from Lyme disease, and for that I am immensely grateful.

Now, in my sixties, I see what a blessing this has been, for it has forced me to discover a deeper level of yoga—the yoga of the subtle body and the discovery of the inner world of awakening, rather than the outer world of performance. Working with a compromised body, I was forced to listen intently to the inner teaching of each pose. I've learned to use the postures to move and enhance the flow of my subtle energy more than perfecting the outer form of the pose.

Often too shy to go to classes where I would be expected to perform beyond my capability, I went deeper into my own practice at home, finding my cues from within. Not that I didn't study with teachers—as I got healthier, I studied everything from Anusara to Zen—but my own body was the fundamental laboratory. My inner guru became my best teacher as I experimented on the mat, coming up with my own discoveries.

In addition, I trained as a somatic psychotherapist with a focus on bioenergetics and trauma work, marrying my love of psychology with the workings of the body and eventually getting my doctorate with a focus on mind-body medicine. Bioenergetics, which was grandfathered by Wilhelm Reich and his students John Pierrakos and Alexander Lowen, is a therapeutic approach to the human psyche that works through the energetic processes of the body. Bioenergetics seeks to dissolve psychological defenses and body armor through freeing up the life force of the body, which in yoga is called *prana*. Through my studies and private practice as a somatic therapist, I found ways of moving the subtle energy through my clients and students, then took these techniques into a workshop format to share with others.

What emerged was my unique style of chakra-based yoga combined with bioenergetic techniques, which I have taught for over two decades of traveling the world as a workshop presenter. This yoga is more about the inner world than the outer. It is focused more on the subtle energy than on the mechanics of a pose. It embraces the chakras as a profound path to divine awakening within your own inner temple, which is what yoga has always been.

This book is my tribute to the royal road of yoga and all that it has taught me. It is my humble offering of the map I have used to navigate the chakra path. Using this map, you can rise to heights or nestle into delicious depths, blaze forth in power or open your heart in softest intimacy. Once you understand this map, you can use it for the rest of your life to go wherever you want to go. You can diagnose and address your imbalances by using techniques and postures that transform you—not instantaneously but systematically over time.

I am honored to offer this guidebook for the inner journey along the mythical rainbow bridge that represents the seven chakras and connects heaven and earth through the center of each person. I believe that our task as humans is to learn to create heaven *on* earth, and learning the stepping-stones of the chakras is a template for the transformation of individuals and the cultures we live in. This map tells you how to do it. May your travels take you on a glorious journey.

Namaste.

The Yoke of Yoga

Yoga is the spiritual language through which we poetically dance with the Divine. ~ ANODEA JUDITH

The word *yoga* means yoke or union. Yoga is a set of principles, beliefs, and practices for yoking matter to spirit, body to mind, personal to universal, and mortal to immortal. It is a path for aligning and opening more deeply to the Divine, not only for liberation and transcendence but also for manifestation and immanence. Yoga has always been a path to higher states of consciousness, but it is simultaneously a path for bringing divine energy down into us, to shine out through us and radiate out into the world. Ultimately this path dissolves separation between self and Divine until we realize there really is no difference. Inner and outer worlds are one inseparable, ecstatic emanation of the Divine. We are that.

If yoga means yoke—what hitches one thing to another—then the chakra system is the architecture of that yoke, providing a comprehensive map to the way the mortal and the Divine yoke together. Much as anatomy texts describe the architecture of the body through the bones, muscles, and organs, the chakra system describes the architecture of the soul through seven subtle energy centers shining out from our core. The elegant arrangement and meaning of these centers provide a map for the journey to divine realization and an evolutionary map for our civilization's next awakening. When you open up these sacred centers within yourself, you awaken the Divine within your own inner temple.

As a yoke, the chakra system is a bridge between polarities: heaven and earth, inner and outer, above and below, matter and consciousness, mind and body. This bridge is made from stepping-stones of energy centers arranged along a vertical channel running through the central core of each one of us. In yoga, this vertical channel is called the *sushumna*. It is one of many energetic pathways, called *nadis*, that carry the flow of our vital life force.

The stepping-stones of the chakras form a ladder upon which we can travel up and down our central axis, climbing up to heaven or getting down to earth, reaching up toward liberation and transcendence or stepping down into manifestation and immanence. The goal of the chakra system is not some otherworldly or disembodied enlightenment but rather wholeness and integration, spanning the full spectrum of human possibility. In this way, the chakra system provides both a ladder for liberation and a map for manifestation.[2] It is simultaneously a template for transformation and a profound formula for wholeness.

The purpose of chakra-based yoga is to create vibrant health and spiritual awakening through contact with the divine energy of Shakti moving freely through your core and activating all of your chakras. Shakti is the name of the Hindu goddess of primordial energy. She is what everything is made of—the basic life force within and around you. It is said that Shakti is always seeking Shiva, her divine partner, who represents pure consciousness. In her search, Shakti rises up the spine, piercing and awakening each chakra in turn. In this way, she becomes Kundalini-Shakti—the vital energy that awakens the chakras. Chakra-based yoga is a way to prepare the body for the emergence of your spiritual fire.

Let this book be a travel guide for your journey to sacred places. Decide what part of the temple you want to explore and use the keys revealed in these pages to open that sacred chamber in your inner palace. Take good care of yourself while you travel, listening deeply to your own body and the still, small voice within. Enjoy the process of each chakra as you Enter, Align, Activate, Soften, Attune, Illuminate, and finally Awaken the Divine Presence within you. From this awakening, shed light for others. Shine the way along the rainbow path, and help the world come into wholeness once again.

---

2 For more on the downward current, see *Creating On Purpose: The Spiritual Technology of Manifesting Through the Chakras* by Anodea Judith and Lion Goodman (Sounds True, 2012).

How to Use This Book

This book is about how to focus your yoga practice on the chakras and how to use yoga to access your subtle energy by using postures, *pranayama* (breath control), mantras, imagery, and meditation. It is written for anyone who wants to explore the chakras through specific practices, for beginning and intermediate yoga practitioners, and especially for yoga teachers who want to bring this material to their students. Even advanced yogis, while not finding new poses herein, may find new ways of understanding these poses from a chakra perspective.

While most yoga books organize their postures by sitting, standing, backbending, or inversions, I have cataloged the postures and other practices according to the chakras. At the end of each chapter, a suggested sequence, or flow, is listed if you want to focus on one chakra at a time. In general, there are fewer poses specifically for the upper three chakras, as practice for these chakras has more to do with chanting, visualizing, and meditating. Therefore, sequences for the upper chakras involve repeating postures given in previous chakras but with the slightly different focus of linking movements from the base chakra upward. This book does not contain a lot of complex or advanced poses, as I believe these are better learned in a live setting from a qualified teacher.

Dividing the classic postures into their various chakras is not cut and dried, however. Many postures, if not most, influence several chakras at once. Other postures influence one chakra or another depending upon your focus or even your variation of the pose. Postures for one chakra may be useful for opening another. Forming a solid foundation in chakra one will support the expansion of the heart, or the activation of the power center. A posture whose focal point is in the heart, for example, may be very useful in opening the throat or third eye center. Using your third eye to visualize a lower chakra will help send the energy to that part of the body. For this reason, some of the basic poses will appear in more than one chakra.

Each chakra chapter opens with a chart of basic principles, properties, and purposes of each chakra, along with a keyword—which, as its name implies, is a kind of spiritual key that unlocks that particular chakra when put into practice. The chapter then talks about the basic concepts of each chakra in more detail before going into specific practices to implement them. Then follows a meditation on sensing the subtle energy of each chakra before going on to the more physical practices. This meditation is a nice way to focus your practice—or, if you are teaching a series of classes on the chakras, these meditations can be a good way to start your class. Each chapter concludes with a different focus for Savasana, or Corpse Pose, usually done at the end of a yoga class. At the very end of each chapter, the poses are listed as a posture flow for that chakra, with thumbnail pictures put in a logical sequence.

Following the Instructions

There is no substitute for a skilled teacher. Reading instructions in a book while holding yourself upside down or looking at a picture while trying to sort out right leg from left is very cumbersome. I know because I checked out a lot of books as I worked on this manuscript!

For this reason, I have kept the initial instructions very basic: first do this, then do that. These instructions are numbered 1, 2, 3, etc. Do them in order, and do not skip a step. If you find yourself at your limit in one step, stay there; do not go on to the next step until you are ready.

I find that new students who are just trying to get their feet and hands in the right place are overwhelmed with too many subtle instructions, and those who already know the basic shape of the pose are only interested in the subtler alignment cues. Therefore, I have followed the basic numbered instructions with bulleted guidelines. In general, the order here is less important. These refer to the subtler movements within a pose, such as hugging into your core, rooting down into your legs, rotating your thighs, lifting your crown, etc. They may also include variations for beginners to make the pose easier and the use of props. Since the nature of injuries and limitations vary greatly, I have listed common contraindications as "avoid or use caution" because, in some cases, a condition may be mild enough to still do the pose, but caution is still necessary. Pregnancy is often a contraindication in many poses, depending on how far along you are in that process. If you are pregnant, get an experienced prenatal teacher to help you with the poses appropriate to your stage of pregnancy and level of ability.

In referencing the poses, I give the name both in Sanskrit (the language of ancient India) and in English whenever possible, though Americans have ways of creating poses that were never known in Sanskrit. In referring to poses, when they are mentioned elsewhere, I use the phrasing you will find in most yoga classes. Tadasana (Standing Mountain Pose) and Uttanasana (Standing Forward Fold), for example, will be referenced in their Sanskrit names. Downward Facing Dog (Adho Mukha Svanasana) or Table Position (Bharmanasana) are referred to in English, since fewer people are familiar with their Sanskrit names.

Humanity is now being asked to play together
in a grand symphony of creation. But as any
musician can tell you, to play in a symphony
you have to practice, practice, practice.

. . . .

ANODEA JUDITH

Practice

If you were to enter a temple, a church, a synagogue, or any other holy place, you would hopefully pause at the threshold and take a moment to adjust your focus from the mundane to the sacred. You would know you were entering a special place, one that required focused attention, an attitude of reverence, or at least respect. You would prepare yourself for encountering the Divine.

Getting on your mat is no different. While yoga is a cultivation of attitude that occurs throughout your day, your mat becomes the sacred classroom you enter whenever you practice. Therefore, your mat becomes like an outer temple, a place to step onto with reverence and intention, to hold you in grace as you open your inner temple.

So each day before you step onto your mat, think about your intention. Why are you practicing? What do you hope to accomplish today? Perhaps you want to dedicate your practice toward some purpose—the healing of a friend, the contribution to a peaceful world, or the resolution of a difficulty. Perhaps you want to calm your mind, heal your own body, purify, or develop strength. Set your intention first, then step consciously onto your mat.

When I teach, I ask students to tape a string lengthwise right down the middle of their mat. They can put a little tape at the top and bottom, or some like to take

The Yoke of Yoga

markers and simply draw a line on their mat. This emphasizes the center line, which in turn emphasizes the center line within the body. As we rise and fall in our various postures on the mat, we continually align our central channel, the sushumna, with the center line down the mat. We can also orient the four corners of our body to the corners of the mat, and in chakra one we will look more deeply at grounding the four corners of the body and limbs in our practice.

I also like to arrange my mat precisely on the floor, whether I practice at home or in a class, meaning that I place it with regard to the orientation of the room or to the other mats around me. Putting your mat down helter-skelter doesn't contribute to your alignment, whereas proper orientation to your surroundings, fellow students, floorboards, furniture, windows, or scenery can enhance your body's relationship to physical space.

Yoga is not about touching your toes or standing on
your head or folding yourself into a lotus pretzel.
It's about how you do what you do and how you live
your daily life on a moment-to-moment basis.

ERICH SCHIFFMANN

Creating Your Own Practice

Yoga is fundamentally a practice. While there are many texts that can teach you its philosophy, guidelines, and principles, you learn yoga from the laboratory of your own body. Your awareness is the inner guru that will teach you. Your practice is the place where you enter the crucible, heat up your body, and alchemize lead into gold. Through trial and error, effort and surrender, learning and teaching, you gradually discover what yoga is and does. It is through cumulative practice that you learn yoga.

If you made an appointment for a massage or to get your teeth cleaned, you would likely show up for your appointment on time and not do anything else during that hour. If you actually schedule your practice with the same integrity as if you were going to a class or having an appointment, you are more likely to keep at it.

Find a time that works for you. Practicing in the morning gets your body energized, open, and balanced for the day. Practicing in the afternoon is great since your body won't feel as stiff as it does first thing in the morning. Practicing in the evening is a nice way to let go of stress from the day, but it's not a good time for vigorous or energizing poses.

Taking a longer yoga retreat by enrolling in one of the many workshops offered by qualified teachers all over the world is a good way to boost your yoga to a new level. Practicing for several hours at a time, several days in a row, gives you something beyond the effects of an occasional class or even a daily practice. You don't have time to slip back to your old ways. Muscles develop, flexibility opens, and you have new skills (as well as friends) to guide you on your path. You are guaranteed to end up in a different place than where you started.

Ultimately your practice is like a relationship. It requires time and attention. It must be cultivated with good communication, intimacy, and respect. And like a relationship, you may need occasional therapy! Engaging a skilled yoga instructor for a private session can be very helpful, especially if you have injuries or chronic pain and need some individualized variations on the poses. Yoga therapy can help you understand the subtleties of alignment in your own body by addressing your own innate tendencies. It can help you understand the "issues in your tissues" with someone who can adjust postures to your individual needs.

There is more in this book than anyone can do in a single session. Therefore, you will want to have a way of creating your own practice that keeps you in balance. You may want to focus on a particular chakra, or you may want to do a few poses from each chakra to have a full-spectrum experience. Always let your body and your needs be your guide, but be mindful that most of us favor what's easy and avoid what is difficult. Make sure you balance your strenuous poses with relaxation and vice versa. Over time, balance your upper-chakra focus with lower-chakra grounding and movement, your forward bends with backbends, and your strength poses with postures of surrender. Find the poses that bring you the most benefit and that work your stiffest places and your weakest chakras.

The Yoke of Yoga

You must savor the fragrance of a posture. Until
you are relaxed, you cannot savor the fragrance.

. . . .

B.K.S. IYENGAR

How Long Do You Hold a Pose?

In general, I avoid giving instructions for how long to hold a pose in a written book. This is for several reasons.

In my opinion, most yoga classes move through poses far too quickly and do not allow the student to really "find" the pose. This makes for slower progress in the long run, as speed can allow bad habits to form and you can miss the "aha" that comes when alignment falls into place. Muscles and connective tissue take time to release. In your home practice, take as much time as you need to find your center and develop your ease in the pose. Often that takes longer than you think, so err on the side of holding the pose longer. If possible, wait until you feel the pose happening by itself—an internal letting go that takes you to a deeper level. If you are in too much discomfort to remain in the pose for more than a few moments, then back off a bit and take it to a milder level. Deep, effortless breathing is a good sign that you are there. As a former piano teacher once said to me, "Practice slow before you try to play it fast."

Everyone's body and abilities are different. Just as it is in a yoga class, what may be too short a time for one person to hold a pose is already way too long for another. The idea of yoga is to find *your* center, *your* stability, and *your* grace. Pushing yourself to hold a pose when you are suffering or pushing yourself to move too fast to really feel the pose negates the deeper purpose of yoga. That purpose is not performance but increased body consciousness.

Our world is full of people who tell you how to look, move, have sex, and be. This means you shape yourself by outer instruction rather than inner guidance. While good yoga instruction is important, it is more empowering to find out what your body needs from the inside. Having too many external commands takes you out of your inner temple rather than deeper within it. The ultimate point is to deeply feel your own body and breath within each pose. Ask your body how long to hold the pose. Follow your own inner timing.

It is unlikely you will hold a pose for too long unless you are in pain, straining a muscle or injury, pushing too hard, or "spacing out" in the pose. In a home practice, it is much more likely that you will rush through a pose and not hold it long enough. As you continue your practice and gain skill at the postures, try holding the pose a little longer each time. For balance and strength poses, this will increase your endurance. For poses of surrender, you will find a deeper letting go.

Yoga is not about self-improvement;
it's about self-acceptance.

. . . .

GURMUKH KAUR KHALSA

Finding Your Edge

Yoga happens whenever your consciousness pays close attention to what you are doing, whether you are reaching for the peanut butter jar on a top shelf or holding a posture. Yoga happens when you bring breath to your body, attention to a feeling, or whenever you penetrate that space between your thoughts and enter a deeper presence in the moment. Yoga happens when your actions are conscious, deliberate, and aligned with your values and virtues. It happens whenever you are connected to grace.

In practicing on your mat, however, yoga happens at your edge. Many poses have beginning, intermediate, and more advanced positions or variations. There are also a wide variety of possibilities as to how far you move into a pose. For instance, a standing forward bend like Uttanasana is the same pose whether your hands come all the way down to the floor or you can only reach your knees. In fact, there is a lot more happening for the person who can only reach their knees than the one who has already opened up their hamstrings to full flexibility. Where the important "happening" takes place is right at your edge.

How *do* you find your edge?

In each pose, there is a delicate place between your comfort zone—that place where you can move easily, without undue effort, strain, pain, or resistance—and where the efforts become more intense or the natural pain and resistance of your body makes itself apparent. Often pushing into pain will make the body go into contraction, and the whole process of opening will take even longer.

Yet to progress in yoga, you do want to gently push your edge. If you only stay in your comfort zone, you will not deepen your yoga. The idea is not to jump over your comfort zone but to *expand* your comfort zone. As you continue to practice yoga, your comfort zone naturally expands—not only in your body but also in your life. You become less reactive, more centered, and more able to handle the stress of outer situations. Expanding your comfort zone means that you can move more deeply into a pose and still be without pain, connected with your breath, and enjoy the pose.

Your edge is there for a reason. It was put there at one time to keep you safe. It may contain unfelt emotions, repressed memories, or physical injuries from which you are still healing. If you can bring your consciousness precisely to that edge and feel what is happening there, your body-mind can begin to process what you are holding and release it. Be curious about what is going on at your edge. Explore exactly where you are holding, and feel into it deeply. Breathe into it and let the breath do the work of opening your body, rather than pushing.

Being curious doesn't mean you have to identify the source of the discomfort, as in the event from your childhood that taught you to contract. That is helpful, but it doesn't always shift the body. What shifts the body is conscious acknowledgment of what is locked and saying inside, "It's okay—you can relax just a little. You don't have to hold on like that anymore."

For instance, if I am bending forward in an open-leg forward bend, I will feel my resistance at some point in my inner thighs. If I have a curiosity about what muscles are holding, where I am contracting, or what I am feeling, I can gently begin to relax and let go, little by little, without pushing. My progress may be a quarter of an inch at a time, but over time that amounts to a lot of progress, and it occurs without injury. Understanding your edge gives you a greater sensitivity to your body and its boundaries, and it serves you well in other situations.

Let the breath be the thread that weaves
your mind and body together.

. . . .

RODNEY YEE

Utilizing the Breath

Additionally, you can use the breath to work your edge. When you find a tight spot, imagine that you can breathe right into that spot, fill it with air, and then allow it to release as you exhale. Repeat this many times in each place where you feel resistance.

The breath is the link between consciousness and unconsciousness and between body and mind. While we normally breathe unconsciously, we can bring consciousness to the breath when we desire to do so. We can focus the breath on a particular chakra, on a body part, or on a thought, emotion, or shape. We can hold the breath full or we can hold it empty, but most of all we can use the breath to create space and expansion in the body. We create energy or relaxation depending on how we breathe. This book will contain many breathing practices for the chakras, from bandhas that hold and lock the breath into various parts of the body to rapid Kundalini breaths designed to energize the different chakras. A more detailed exploration of the breath is included in the chapter on the fourth chakra, whose element is air.

The Yoke of Yoga

That's exactly how it is in yoga. The places where you
have the most resistance are actually the places that
are going to be the areas of the greatest liberation.

. . . .

RODNEY YEE

Paradoxical Stretching

Holding patterns come from past experiences in which we contracted, braced, or shut down. Often they become stuck in the body because they did not get to finish their expression and have since become frozen in that unfinished state. This is especially true in the cases of trauma and post-traumatic stress disorders (PTSD).

Your contraction occurred slowly over time and may be the result of years or decades of holding yourself in a certain way. That means it will unravel slowly as well. For the brain-body interface to really process this unraveling, it must be done very gradually, carefully following the body with your consciousness.

One way to work with this is by allowing the contraction, or the tightness, to first exaggerate and then release, slowly going back and forth several times like an accordion.

Here's a way to try this right now, using the shoulders as an example since most people carry at least some tension there.[3]

1. Bring your attention to your shoulders and notice any tension or discomfort that might be there. Simply feel it and acknowledge it.

2. Notice what you are doing muscularly or energetically to create that tension. Are you drawing your shoulders slightly upward toward your ears or in toward your neck? Are you subtly holding your breath, tilting your head forward, or tightening your arms?

---

3   This is an adaptation of the Accordion Exercise by Stanley Keleman.

3. Whatever you can identify that you are unconsciously doing, make it conscious by doing it on purpose and exaggerating it, making it larger. If you are unconsciously lifting your shoulders toward your ears just slightly, do it even more. If you are subtly holding your breath, do it even more. Exaggerate what you are doing so that you can fully feel it.

4. When you can't go any further in the direction of doing it more, slowly begin to do it less, or "undo" what you are doing, following the body as it unravels itself from that habitual response. It's important to move very slowly as you unravel your habitual response, and simply follow your body as it moves to a new place. Stay with it until the unraveling feels complete, and take a moment to sense this new place without moving.

5. When your undoing comes to a natural resting place, simply let yourself be. See if something new has emerged. Experience that newness and give it a moment to anchor in your awareness.

Granthis

The word *granthi* is Sanskrit for knot and refers to the stuck places in your chakras—places where the sushumna, or central axis, gets knotted up and does not allow the prana to pass through. I believe that knots can occur in any chakra, though classic sources vary, stating that they occur in the first, fourth, and sixth chakras, while others say they occur in the fourth, fifth, and sixth chakras. It is said that the fiery energy of Kundalini pierces these knots the way a heated rod pushes through the knots in a bamboo stick. To free the energy that travels up and down the spine, we need to untie the knots in the chakras.

I like to think of these knots as places where we are "not"—places where we will not or cannot or do not go inside ourselves. Opening the knots is about turning a chronic no into a flowing yes or at least a choice. Untying these knots can sometimes create an intense flow of energy, such as the rush of Kundalini, and must be done slowly and carefully, opening all the chakras and keeping a good sense of your ground.

Bandhas

The word *bandha* means lock—not in the sense of a locked door, but more like a channel lock in a waterway, designed to hold energy. In the same way that the previous accordion exercise re-creates the pattern of our chronic holding in order to release that holding, the practice of using bandhas is like creating knots on purpose in order to help the prana flow into new places. When the knots are held, the prana builds up; when the knots are released, the prana flows.

Imagine a big tube of water with sides flexible enough to squeeze. If you pinch the tube at the bottom, the water will rise toward the top—but as soon as you release your pressure, the water will fall right back down again. If you had a way to bind the tube at a certain height, the water could stay near the top. Bandhas are a way of consciously creating locks in the central channel for the purpose of sending energy into various chakras. They are an essential tool in the practice of postures and breathing practices, as they direct the subtle energy.

The three classic bandhas we will refer to in this book are

- Mula bandha, the root lock, related to chakra one
- Uddiyana bandha, or abdominal lock, related to chakra three
- Jalandhara bandha, or chin lock, related to chakra five

Using a bandha at one chakra can stimulate chakras above and below it depending on your intention, what posture you're in, and whether you are holding the breath when it's full or empty. Instructions for practicing bandhas will be described in their respective chakras listed above.

Basic Posture Starting Points

There are three postures that are referred to again and again as starting points for doing other postures. These postures are Tadasana, or Standing Mountain Pose; Dandasana, or Staff Pose; and Table Position (technically called Bharmanasana but rarely referred to by that name).

Tadasana: Standing Mountain Pose

This pose forms the central pillar of your yoga practice, as it is the simplest upright pose there is. The whole body is like a pillar from earth to heaven. Your core is vertically aligned, with all your chakras stacked on top of each other. (This is also true for handstand and headstand, but they are more difficult, whereas anyone who can stand up straight can do Tadasana.) I have even heard it said that if you do Tadasana properly and can hold it steady for one hour, you don't need to do any other postures that day. Despite its simplicity, this pose has a lot going on. While many teachers give a lot of anatomical commands for creating Tadasana, I prefer to let students find it through their chakras and subtle energy. Build your Tadasana from the ground up, chakra by chakra.

1. **Establish chakra one.** Stand with your feet parallel, hip-width apart. Feel the floor beneath your feet and root into it, lifting the toes, spreading them widely, then deliberately placing them on the floor. Distribute your weight evenly on both feet, perhaps rocking slightly back and forth from one foot to another to find your center of gravity. When you do find this center, lock it into place by simultaneously pressing downward and outward with your feet, as if you were trying to widen your yoga mat. Hug the muscles of your legs into your bones, slightly lifting your kneecaps. Point your tailbone down to the center of the square formed by your feet. (Tadasana can also be done with feet together. This makes for a smaller base and more difficulty grounding but places more emphasis on the core.)

2. **Establish chakra two.** Allow your pelvis and hips to sway gently forward and back, making smaller and smaller movements as you sense your center, aligning your second chakra over your base. It should feel like something clicks into place. Gently rotate your inner thighs toward the back, hollowing out the groin area in the front of your hips. Slightly increase the curve of your sacrum, then extend the tip of your tailbone down toward the earth. Firm your abdominal muscles by pulling the navel in toward the spine.

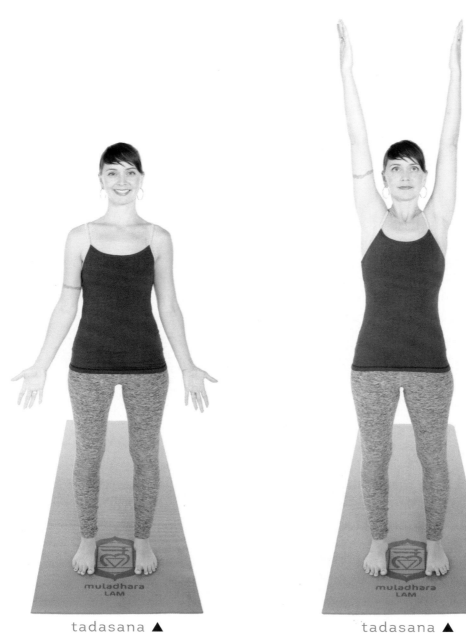

tadasana ▲

standing mountain pose,
position a

tadasana ▲

standing mountain pose,
position b

3. **Establish your third chakra.** Lift your ribs up out of your hips without puffing them forward, opening the kidneys slightly toward the back body. Lengthen the sides of your body between your hips and your armpits, being careful not to lift your shoulders toward your ears. Firm up your belly and fire up your third chakra by hugging into the midline.

4. **Open your fourth chakra.** Lift your sternum, rotating the upper arms toward the back body and pointing the shoulder blades down the back. Imagine your third and fourth chakras can move independently. Open your heart and soften your chest.

5. **Align your fifth chakra.** Draw upward from your clavicles toward the base of your skull, bringing the top of your neck back and up. Lower your shoulders away from your ears. Soften your jaw and lips. Relax your tongue.

6. **Focus on the sixth chakra.** Pick a focal point a few feet in front of you. Draw your attention backward into the center of your head at brow level. Soften your gaze or even close your eyes.

7. **Lift the crown chakra.** Extend up toward your crown chakra at the midpoint of the top of your head and align your upper chakras with your heart. Imagine the thousand-petaled lotus blossoming out from your crown as your attention stays calmly in the exact center of your lotus.

8. **Align from the inside.** Close your eyes and imagine that you are dropping a plumb line down from the center of your seventh chakra. See if it feels like all your chakras align through your innermost core.

9. Bring your hands to prayer position over your heart, fingers pointing upward, aligning your inner palms with your sacred core.

10. Take a deep breath. As you exhale, draw the corners of your mouth upward toward your ears!

The Yoke of Yoga

Guidelines

- Press evenly into the four corners of the feet and imagine the first chakra symbol on the floor forming your foundation (more on this in chapter 1). Feel the solidity of the floor supporting you.

- Bend and straighten your knees a few times to energize the legs.

- Build the pose from the ground upward. Press down and slightly outward with your feet to create stability through your hips.

- Do not lock the knees or hyperextend. Find the core of each leg. Hug your leg muscles in toward the bones and draw the kneecaps up slightly.

- Firm the muscles on the front of your belly without hardening.

- Imagine your chakras clicking into place, each one on top of the one below it, aligned from base to crown.

- Find the ease in the pose and allow your whole body to expand with the breath.

Dandasana: Staff Pose

This pose is good for launching seated postures, forward bends, and some backbends. It calls for both lifting and rootedness as well as awareness of your legs and your core.

1. Sit upright on the floor with your legs extended out in front of you.

2. Make an L shape with your body, lifting your crown.

3. Flex your feet, extend into your heels, and press the back of your knees toward the floor while drawing the legs together.

4. Press the tailbone toward the back, firm up the belly, lift the ribs, take the shoulders back, and lift into your crown.

5. Press your hands into the ground alongside your hips, fingertips pointing forward.

The Yoke of Yoga

Guidelines

- If your legs or back are too tight to make an L shape, lift your hips by sitting on a folded blanket or block. Avoid rounding your back.

- You can check your alignment by practicing with your back against a wall. Press your shoulders and buttocks into the wall but notice how the back of your neck and the curve of your low back should not be touching the wall.

- Sit toward the front of your sitting bones, drawing your tailbone back. Rotate your inner thighs toward the floor. See if you can push enough energy into your legs to lift your heels slightly off the floor.

- Keep your chin and eyes level with the horizon.

- If desired, lay sandbags on the top of your thighs to ground them deeper into the earth.

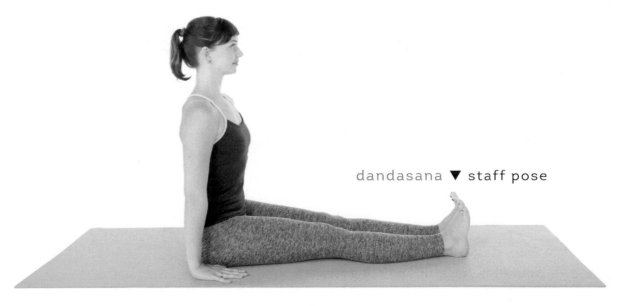

dandasana ▼ staff pose

Bharmanasana: Table Pose

This is probably the first yoga pose that any of us ever did, back when we were infants just learning to crawl. Therefore, it taps into a younger part of the self as well as an ancient part of our mammalian brain. If your knees are sensitive or if you're on a hard surface, fold a blanket under your knees.

1. Come onto all fours, with your knees directly below your hips and your wrists below your shoulders.

2. Allow your spine to be neutral, meaning that it is neither flexed nor extended but relatively flat, like a table.

3. Extend from the tip of your tailbone to the center of your crown, keeping your head level.

Guidelines

- Spread your fingers wide, with your middle fingers parallel to each other and your wrist crease parallel to the front of the mat.

- Firm your belly into your core.

- Open the heart by softening the place between your shoulder blades without collapsing the chest. Press into your palms to draw the ears away from the shoulders.

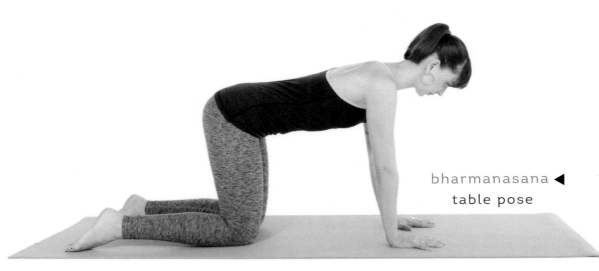

bharmanasana ◀
table pose

Opening the Inner Temple

*Grace is the power of the Absolute
in its infinitely loving emanation
of being.* ~ ANODEA JUDITH

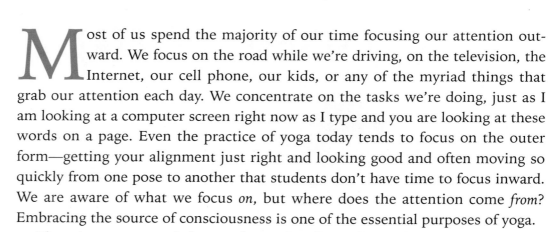

Most of us spend the majority of our time focusing our attention outward. We focus on the road while we're driving, on the television, the Internet, our cell phone, our kids, or any of the myriad things that grab our attention each day. We concentrate on the tasks we're doing, just as I am looking at a computer screen right now as I type and you are looking at these words on a page. Even the practice of yoga today tends to focus on the outer form—getting your alignment just right and looking good and often moving so quickly from one pose to another that students don't have time to focus inward. We are aware of what we focus *on*, but where does the attention come *from*? Embracing the source of consciousness is one of the essential purposes of yoga.

There is a very sacred place at the center of you that I call the inner temple. It is a palace of splendor and illumination, a refuge of exquisite peace and tranquility, the sacred residence of the Divine within. The body is the outer form of this temple. Keeping the body healthy and vibrant is essential for maintaining the inner temple. But yoga, as the connecting yoke between the worlds, serves both the physical temple and the spiritual reality within.

The chakras can be seen as chambers in the temple of the body. By opening these chambers, you gain access to the inside of this temple and give the god Shiva (who represents pure consciousness) and the goddess Shakti (who represents the energy of life) a place to join together. Of course the inner temple is not a literal space; if you dissected someone, you would not find an empty space inside the body. But it does give you a sense of spaciousness when the subtle

Opening the Inner Temple

energy of the chakras opens up and allows you room to dwell within the temple of your own being.

In addition, the chakras are portals between the inner and outer worlds, connection points between mind and body, acting as resistors and capacitors in the flow of life energy. As portals, they filter or distill energy from the outside, as well as limit or enhance what gets expressed from inside. Because chakras are the gateways through which this exchange takes place between inner and outer, it is essential that you come to understand how to care for them.

The purpose of chakra-based yoga is to discover the keys to opening each chamber in your inner temple and awaken the Divine within. The body is the vehicle you take to get there. Your consciousness is the driver that will guide the way. The practices contained herein are the keys. Yoga provides the path. The chakra system is the map.

What Are the Chakras?

If you are new to studying the chakra system or if you are a teacher who wants to teach this subject to your students, you will need to be able to explain the chakra system in basic terms. I find the best way to do that is through direct experience of your own subtle energy. In yoga, that subtle energy is called *prana*, a word that means first unit. Prana is the basic energy of life. It exists in everything—sunlight, air, food, and the energetic exchanges you have with other people and the environment. The body handles prana within the cells, through various channels called nadis, and through the chakras.

Here's a simple exercise that helps people have a tangible experience of how it feels to open a chakra and experience the subtle energy. It involves opening the minor chakras that exist in the hands. Because the hands are relatively unencumbered by the psychological baggage that our major chakras pick up along the way, they are much easier to open and experience, so this tends to work with almost anyone. I like to start with this exercise before I give the more intellectual knowledge.

Your hand opens and closes and opens and closes.
If it were always a fist or always stretched open,
you would be paralyzed. Your deepest presence is in
every small contracting and expanding, the two as
beautifully balanced and coordinated as bird wings.

RUMI

Opening the Hand Chakras

1. Extend both arms out in front of you with elbows straight,
   preferably with one hand up and one hand down as in position B.

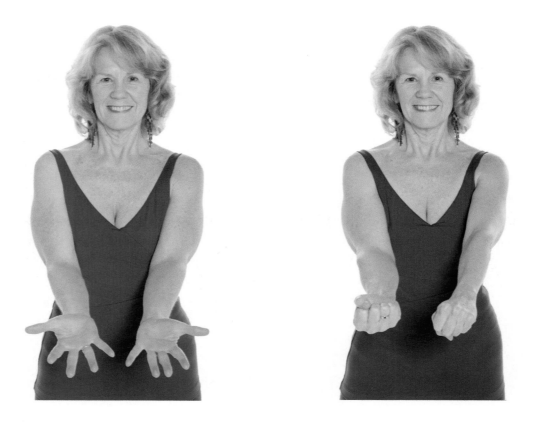

Opening the Inner Temple

2. Open and close your palms rapidly, moving many times from fully open to fully closed. Make sure you really stretch your fingers all the way open and then make a complete fist (positions A and B). Do this until your hands start to feel tired.

3. Then separate your hands as wide as your shoulders and, with relaxed palms, very slowly bring your open palms toward each other (position C).

4. As your palms come within a few inches of each other, you may experience a subtle field of energy between your hands, almost like a magnetic field. If you tune in very closely, you might even feel it as a spinning vortex of energy.

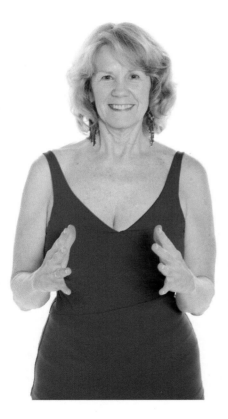

positions from far left ◄
a, hands open wide
b, hands in fists, and
c, palms 8 inches apart

This is what a chakra feels like—a spinning vortex of subtle energy, reflecting the Sanskrit meaning of the word *chakra* as wheel. The hand chakras are very simple to open. Once activated, they not only have more energy, but they become more sensitive, so this is an easy way to experience what is meant by subtle energy. Some people have trouble feeling this energy because it is so subtle. Don't expect it to feel like plugging into a socket. It's called "subtle energy" for a reason!

This exercise also reflects a basic principle in yoga. You activated your hand chakras through a process of expansion and contraction—reflecting the basic pulsation of life, which in yoga is called *spanda*. Your lungs do this every time you breathe; your heart, every time it beats. You activate the chakras in your body in a similar way—it's just that it becomes a bit more complicated when it comes to the torso and the major chakras at the core. This is the purpose of yoga *asanas,* or postures, which use expansion and contraction in a way that moves *prana,* or energy, into different parts of the body.

So now that you've had a direct experience of feeling the energy generated between your hands, repeat the exercise again and see if you can feel the energy of the chakra itself *in* your hands.

What does it feel like when your hand generates a field of energy through the flesh of your palm and fingers? Do you feel a subtle vibration or perhaps a warmth or tingling? Can you feel that your hand chakra not only generates energy but is a living center of energy itself? Can you feel a difference between your two hands? Is one of them more open than the other? What happens when you put your activated hand on your heart or some other place on your body?

Defining the Chakras

Now let's develop a deeper understanding of what a chakra is and what it does. It is an energy center, yes, but even more, it is a center that coordinates energy for the system as a whole, much like an office coordinates energy for a business. In this way, a fuller definition of a chakra is "a chamber in the temple of the body that receives, assimilates, and transmits life force energy." To open your inner temple and gain access to its resplendent interior, you must be able to enter and dwell in each chamber and operate effectively from each chakra's center.

*A chakra is a chamber in the temple of the body that
receives, assimilates, and transmits life force energy.*

· · · · · · · · · · · · · · · ·

Let's look at the parallel between the chakras in your body and the chambers in your home. Most likely your home has a kitchen—a place where you receive, process, and deliver food. You sleep in the bedroom and shower in the bathroom. When guests come to visit, you probably entertain in the living room, which is designed for that experience.

Each chamber is optimally set up for receiving, assimilating, and transmitting a particular kind of energy. You want each chamber to have what it needs to perform that function: a refrigerator, stove, and countertop in the kitchen, places to sit in the living room, and a soft place to sleep in the bedroom. You also want each chamber to be clean enough to perform its function—not too big or too small to be comfortable. You want each chamber to have a doorway and light from both outside (through windows) and inside (for when it's dark), as well as good air circulation. You can definitely have a chamber that isn't well equipped with these things, but you wouldn't want to spend much time there.

In the same way, your chakras need the necessary internal structures to handle the type of energy that is related to their function. For example: to handle earth energy in the first chakra, you need to be able to eat, digest, and eliminate food. To have a healthy relationship (fourth chakra), you need good self-esteem, some basic relationship skills, and an open heart. The second chakra needs to be able to receive, accept, and express sexual and emotional energy. The third chakra handles power, the fifth chakra processes communication, the sixth chakra receives intuition and turns it into insight, and the seventh chakra represents consciousness itself.

Each chakra needs to be able to receive energy from outside, to assimilate that energy into the body-mind complex, and to express, or discharge, energy. This means that each chakra has a kind of gateway where energy enters and leaves the chamber, as well as a core center where energy is assimilated and distributed through the body.

Balancing Excess and Deficiency in the Chakras

To keep a chakra in balance, it needs to be able to do all three of these functions—receiving, assimilating, and expressing—at its appropriate level. Receiving more than we can assimilate is like eating more than we can digest: we get indigestion and can't process all the material. The chakra becomes too full, or what I call excessive, and it doesn't function as well. Eventually, overeating turns into excess body weight—energy that becomes dense and stagnant because we haven't been able to assimilate the input. You could say we have too much of the first chakra's element of earth. We get heavy.

An excessive chakra results from a defensive pattern in life that is trying to compensate for something we didn't get enough of, such as safety, pleasure, attention, power, or love. We become overly attached, fixated at that level, still trying to obtain fulfillment or healing.

However, if we release or express more energy than we take in, we become depleted, which results in a deficient chakra. If the first chakra becomes deficient, for example, then we tend to be underweight and ungrounded, and we have trouble feeling like we matter. Deficiency can happen through any chakra—through the inability to receive or the habit of releasing too much. For instance, too much activity (an excessive third chakra) will eventually make us feel tired, and the resulting low energy is characteristic of a deficient third chakra. Being unable to receive love (or even perceive that it's there) results in a deficient heart chakra. That deficiency then makes it more difficult to receive because the chakra closes up like a flower and it's harder for love to get through the defensive wall.

A deficient chakra results from an avoidance strategy, avoiding something we might not have the tools or desire to deal with, while an excessive chakra is a compensating strategy. We can avoid taking our power and feel like a victim (third chakra deficiency), or we can compensate for feeling powerless by being a bully (third chakra excess). We can avoid our emotions by numbing out or compensate by focusing on them too much. Both attachment and avoidance are two of the *kleshas,* or afflictions, that create obstacles on the path in yoga.[4]

An unbalanced chakra influences other chakras and the rest of your energy system. Poor grounding makes it hard to be powerful. Lack of power makes it

---

4 Classically, there are five *kleshas* described in the *Yoga Sutras*: (1) ignorance, or *avidya*; (2) ego, or *asmita*; (3) attachment, or *raga*; (4) aversion, or *dvesha*; and (5) fear of death, or *abhinivesha*.

hard to express yourself. Eventually problems show up, either externally in jobs or relationships, or they manifest in your internal world through illness, limiting beliefs, or difficult emotional states. Excess and deficient characteristics of the chakras are included in the chart of chakra correspondences shown on the following page. More information about the psychological causes of these imbalances can be found in my previous book *Eastern Body, Western Mind*,[5] while this book focuses specifically on using yoga practices to awaken and balance the chakras.

Like a chamber, chakras have gates through which energy enters and leaves each center. Those gates serve to keep energy in as well as to keep energy out, according to what is needed. A child may defend against a parent's toxic energy by trying to keep that energy out of their chakras. Or a child may get the message that their inner emotions are not acceptable, and then use these gates to inhibit their own vital energy from expressing itself. These defensive strategies, which are formed unconsciously, become like sentry guards who monitor the gates of the chakras and check everything that enters or exits. This slows down the flow of vital energy between the inner and outer worlds. To heal these unconscious strategies requires becoming conscious of them.

Energetically, a deficient chakra needs to charge itself up—to receive and assimilate more energy and learn to expand. This requires increased focus and attention, perhaps directing energy from other places that are more excessive. An excessive chakra, by contrast, needs to release energy, or discharge, and even contract. We need to make that aspect of ourselves a little less important and let go of our attachments in that area.

While a chakra can become unbalanced within itself, the chakras also try to balance each other out. Someone who is not very grounded in their lower chakras may live in their head or try to balance their disembodiment with excessive spirituality. Someone who is emotionally insecure may be excessive in their throat chakra and talk too much. In some cases, we can exhibit excessive and deficient characteristics in the same chakra. These are just more complex defenses that have been trying to create balance by emphasizing some parts of the chakra but avoiding others. A person whose second chakra has a high sexual charge and a

5 Anodea Judith, *Eastern Body, Western Mind: Psychology and the Chakra System as a Path to the Self* (Berkeley: Celestial Arts, 1997). See also Anodea Judith, *Chakra Balancing: A Complete Course in Diagnosis and Healing* (Boulder, CO: Sounds True, 2001).

Chakra Correspondences

Chakra	Name: Meaning	Location	Element	Central Focus	Goals	Identity	Demon	Excessive Characteristics	Deficient Characteristics	Bija Mantra
7	Sahasrara: Infinitely Unfolding	Top of head, cerebral cortex	Conscious-ness	Awareness	Awakening, union, realization, emptiness	Universal (Self-Knowledge)	Attachment	Overly intellectual, spiritual addiction, dissociation from body	Learning difficulties, spiritual cynicism, disconnection, depression	None
6	Ajña: Perceive and Command	Brow	Light	Intuition, imagination	Insight, intuition, stillness, wisdom	Archetypal (Self-Reflection)	Illusion	Delusional, difficulty concentrating	Poor memory, poor vision, denial	Om or Ksham
5	Vissudha: Purification	Throat	Sound	Communi-cation	Truth, resonance, communication, creativity	Creative (Self-Expression)	Lies	Loud, overly talkative, inability to listen	Fear of speaking or making noise	Ham
4	Anahata: Unstruck Sound	Heart	Air	Love, relationships	Love, compassion, radiance, expansion	Social (Self-Acceptance)	Grief	Needy, co-dependent, narcissistic	Shy, lonely, isolated, bitter	Yam
3	Manipura: Lustrous Gem	Solar Plexus	Fire	Power, will	Power, will, energy	Ego (Self-Definition)	Shame	Dominating, controlling, aggressive, anxious	Poor self-esteem, passive, powerless, tired	Ram
2	Svadhisthana: One's Own Abode	Sacral area	Water	Sexuality, emotions	Fluidity, flexibility, feeling	Emotional (Self-Gratification)	Guilt	Indulgent, emotional, addictive	Rigid, joyless, numb	Vam
1	Muladhara: Root Support	Base of spine	Earth	Survival, grounding	Stability, grounding health, steadiness, solidity	Physical (Self-Preservation)	Fear	Heavy, sluggish, dense, overweight	Underweight, spacey, ungrounded, fearful	Lam

low emotional charge or someone who is powerful at work but powerless at home is exhibiting both excessive and deficient characteristics in the same chakra.

There are many possibilities in how you arrange energy throughout your chakras; it all depends on which strategies worked for you in the past and which ones didn't. Over time you adopted the "successful" strategies and discarded the ones that got you in trouble. However, the strategies you adopted as a child often work against you in adulthood. The defenses later become blockages, fixating your life force, inhibiting the flow of energy into and out of your chakras, and keeping you from fully occupying your inner temple. They become hard-wired into your physical structure as body armor in the form of muscular tension, excess weight, numbness, or disease. Yoga is a good way to combat body armor, not only because it stretches and conditions the body, but because it increases awareness and distributes energy into places that have been shut off from consciousness.

You gain access through your inner axis.

· · · · · · · · · · · · · · ·

ANODEA JUDITH

Accessing the Core

Everything in life has a core: every blade of grass, every tree trunk, every leaf on the tree, every cell, and every person. Even concepts have a core, as do homes, planets, and stars. The core is what everything, living and non-living, has in common. For this reason, I think of the core as the divine center from which everything originates—the source of all creation. The core is God/Goddess, or whatever name you prefer for the Divine.

I like to think of CORE as standing for Consciousness Organized in Relation to Energy. Your consciousness developed as you encountered both positive and negative experiences in your life. If you're reading these words, then you survived those experiences. But you survived because you learned to deal with them in some way. You probably closed down some aspects of yourself, while ramping up other traits. You moved toward or away from things, either compensating or avoiding or some combination of both. In this way, you formed the shape of your

Opening the Inner Temple

core by how you dealt with life. This happens first in your energy body, then in the structures and tissues of your physical body, then in your behaviors, which are further reinforced by experience.

If the chakras represent the seven chambers of the inner temple, then accessing your deepest core is the master key that unlocks these chambers. By *core* I don't mean the mid-torso muscle strength that has become the focus in exercise classes these days. Instead, I am referring to the vertical channel running between your crown and your base through the deepest center of you, called your *sushumna*, or central axis. When your chakras are aligned, the core is an open and expanding tube of prana in which energy flows easily both upward and downward, through all the chakras, into the body, and in exchange with the world. Think of the sushumna as a pranic tube that distills the subtle energy from its coarsest form to its finest. It is also your most direct connection between heaven and earth, and your deepest access to Source.

The chakras can be thought of as energetic pouches in the pranic tube for storing energy that moves up and down the core. In addition to receiving, assimilating, and transmitting energy, they also store energy at a particular level for use in your life, much the way the stomach stores food to digest slowly and release energy. If you get a nice feeling in your heart from sharing love with someone, it's beneficial to be able to keep that energy there when you feel lonely or scared. Expanding your chambers allows you to store more energy in your chakras.

To access your core is to access the Divine within, but that Divine is bigger, deeper, and higher than most of us can allow within our core. In fact, with the restrictions most of us have, it is even difficult to withstand the full force of divine prana, should we be lucky enough to experience it. For that reason, we need to open the chakras. If the body is the vehicle and the chakras are the map, the core is the master key that unlocks everything.

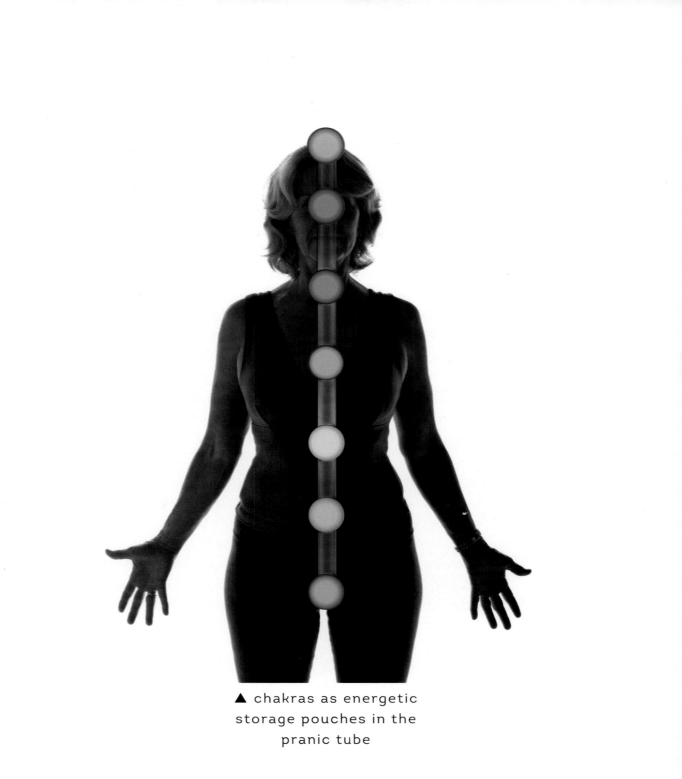

▲ chakras as energetic
storage pouches in the
pranic tube

*The fulfillment of your highest potential
is directly proportional to your ability to
function as a clean and efficient channel.*

. . . .

ERICH SCHIFFMANN

Clearing the Nadis

In yoga terminology, energy, or *prana*, travels through us via subtle pathways called *nadis*, a Sanskrit word that means movement or flow. Nadis come in all shapes and sizes, from major highways like the sushumna going right up the center to well-established routes like the *ida* and *pingala* making figure eights around the chakras (see figure) to minor nadis flowing through each cell. Just as our major highways in the outer world serve to transport food and goods to cities, stores, and homes, the nadis distribute prana to the various chakras and throughout the body.

The chakras are places where many nadis meet, much like a city is an intersection of highways, phone lines, plumbing, and people. There is more activity and energy in a city than along the back roads, but those back roads are still important.

Yoga is a practice that clears the nadis for the distribution and full experience of prana, or life force. Prana brings vitality and health to the body. It brings consciousness and presence in the here and now. As the nadis are cleared through the practice of yoga *asanas* (postures), *pranayama* (breathing practices), right action (karma), and meditation, the chakras are cleared and energized. They begin to shine like polished jewels emanating a light from within. You experience more spaciousness inside your body and have greater access to your inner temple.

Opening the Inner Temple

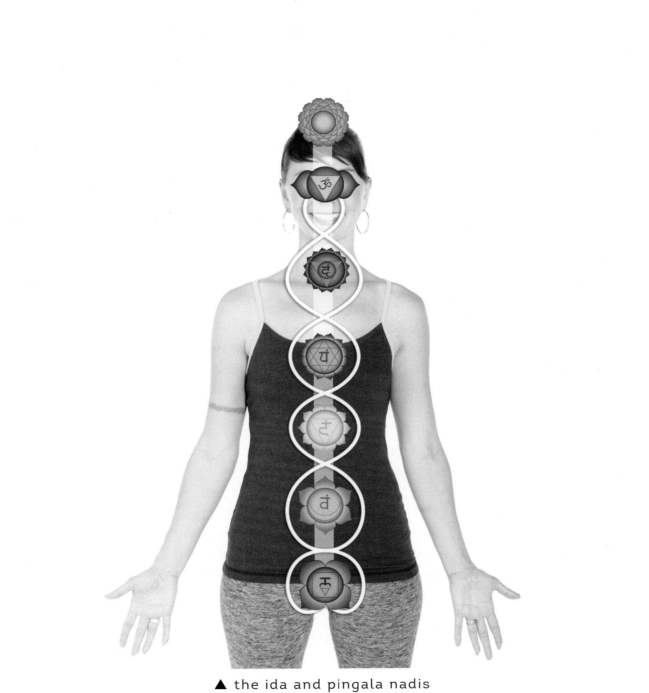

▲ the ida and pingala nadis
flowing around the chakras

Opening the Inner Temple

At such times I felt instinctively that a life and death struggle was going on inside me in which I, the owner of the body, was entirely powerless to take part, forced to lie quietly and watch as a spectator to the weird drama unfolding in my own flesh.

. . . .

GOPI KRISHNA

Kundalini

No discussion of the chakras would be complete without discussing Kundalini, the underlying spiritual force of chakra awakening. Often misunderstood and always mysterious, this serpentlike goddess of the chakras is the form that Shakti sometimes takes as she rises up the spine. As Kundalini-Shakti, she rises in search of her eternal lover and counterpart, Shiva.

Kundalini is a force that lies latent within each person. Latent, there is little drive toward awakening or perhaps the drive is scattered or sporadic. Spirituality may well exist, practices may be beneficial, but the underlying force that activates these practices may be absent. Many people have said to me over the years, "Oh, I've tried meditation (or yoga or pranayama or…) and it just didn't do much for me." I've never met anyone with a Kundalini experience who would say that.

Kundalini is like the electricity that runs through a string of Christmas lights. The lights are there, and they may even have pretty ornaments hanging from them, but until the energy shoots through the wire, there is nothing special about them. Once lit up, they provide a whole new experience. When Kundalini energizes the chakras, they are no longer an intellectual concept but a direct experience.

Kundalini is an archetypal force that needs to be understood symbolically, if not experientially. Symbolically, she is said to lie coiled three and one-half times around the root chakra, perhaps holding matter together. (*Kundala* means coiled.) When she awakens, she journeys up the spine, piercing and activating each chakra in turn. Her final goal is to reach the crown chakra and merge with Shiva, then reside with him in eternal union in the heart.

When Kundalini energizes the chakras, they are no longer an intellectual concept but a direct experience.

. . . .

Experientially, Kundalini is an electrifying spiritual force that runs through the body, shaking you to your core. Her power and presence can be invited through prayers and practices, but she is only activated through grace. Whether that grace comes from a qualified guru giving *shaktipat* (direct transmission), from years of yoga or meditation, from stress that breaks down defenses, or even from drugs or fasting, once Kundalini awakens she is an autonomous healing force that moves within you of her own accord.

Most people can neither start nor stop Kundalini with their will. She may appear briefly for moments, intermittently for years, or become a constant presence that changes your entire perspective on life. Always she is a teacher, seeking to dissolve illusion and blockages in order to reveal the true spiritual nature of creation.

As such, Kundalini is a tricky force to play with. My many years of traveling and teaching have exposed me to countless people telling me about their Kundalini experiences—all of them profound but not all of them pleasant. Awakening is not always gentle. Some have had trouble sleeping, eating, having sex, or doing many of the mundane things previously taken for granted. Some have been visited by visions, twisted into postures by spontaneous movements called *kriyas*, or heard sounds or voices in their head. Some thought they were going crazy, as Kundalini can sometimes resemble psychosis. Some were completely rearranged by the experience, generally for the better, as if the central organizing principle within their body and their life had suddenly taken charge and pulled everything together in a more cohesive form. Inevitably, Kundalini pushes up against our blocks. Until those blocks are dissolved, the experience can be very uncomfortable.

Because Kundalini's spontaneous movements, or kriyas, are often wavelike or trembling, she is equated with the movement of a serpent slithering up the spine. Kriyas often resemble yoga postures and may be the origin of some of the asanas, or yoga postures, that we practice today. Practicing the asanas consciously is a good way to prepare the body to tolerate and handle the intense pranic rush of

Kundalini. This is why people are advised to engage in years of practice and study under a true master before engaging the Kundalini force.

For these reasons, this is not a book on Kundalini per se, but rather a book on opening the chakras themselves and making the way smoother for Kundalini, should she grace you with her presence. As you open your inner temple, she has a larger place to reside and may visit more peacefully, not having any walls to knock down. If so, ground yourself, meet her with openness and gratitude, and rely on your practices. Above all, she should be respected and honored as the divine queen of the evolutionary life force that runs through us all.

The attainment of wholeness requires one to stake one's whole being. Nothing less will do. There can be no easier conditions, no substitutes, no compromises.

· · · · · · · · · · · · ·

C. G. JUNG

Formula for Wholeness

Carl Jung said that everyone needs an archetype of wholeness to guide their life. As a totality, the chakra system describes a profound formula for wholeness, spanning the full spectrum of human experience—from your physical body to your highest spiritual aspirations—and leaving nothing out. It encompasses your physical and emotional self, your egoic self, your relational and creative self, your intuitive self, your highest self, and your deepest interior soul.

The chakras map onto levels of being that occur both internally and externally, through the archetypal elements that are deeply associated with the chakras: earth, water, fire, air, sound, light, and consciousness.[6] These elements exist within us through the solid, liquid, gaseous, or vibratory elements of our bodies and all around us through the manifestation of these elements in our world—the earth we walk upon, the air we breathe, the light we see through our eyes.

6 Classically, there are only five elements associated with the chakras; from bottom to top: earth, water, fire, air, and ether, with no elements given for the upper two. The seven-element system is my own formulation, now widely accepted.

Opening the Inner Temple

In this way, the chakras are portals between the inner and outer worlds—portals through which we access these elements and bring them into balance. In the external world, many of these elements are severely threatened. Our earth has extreme environmental issues; water imbalances show up as droughts or floods. Power is misused while appropriate use of energy is crucial to our environment. The atmosphere is polluted. We live in a cacophony of conflicting vibrations, where truth, light, and consciousness are often obscured.

It is no wonder that these elements get scrambled inside ourselves as well. But according to the spiritual maxim *as within, so without,* we bring these elements into balance in our world as we balance them within ourselves. The reverse is also true. As we clean up our environment, as we insist on healthy food choices or make our voices heard on the airways, we simultaneously create an environment more conducive to our spiritual growth.

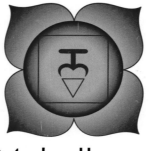

Muladhara
ROOT SUPPORT

Element	Earth
Principles	Gravity, solidity
Purposes	Foundation, support, stability
Properties	Grounded, solid, steadfast
Body parts	Legs, feet, bones, large intestine
Practices	Grounding, widening the base, opening the leg channels, strengthening the legs, cultivating stillness, solidity, and stability
Actions	Pushing downward, extending roots, surrendering to gravity
Poses	The base of every pose but especially relevant to standing poses
Masculine	Roots penetrating earth, pushing energy into matter
Feminine	Drawing nutrients up from the roots, drawing energy from matter
Deficient	Scattered, ungrounded, ephemeral, underweight
Excessive	Heavy, lethargic, overweight
Balanced	Stability, beautiful form

chakra one

Enter...

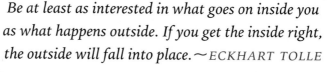

Be at least as interested in what goes on inside you as what happens outside. If you get the inside right, the outside will fall into place. ~ ECKHART TOLLE

The first step to opening your inner temple is to step across the threshold and truly enter the realm of your body. You must fully occupy your temple to open its gateway to the Divine.

Your body is the vehicle in which you take the journey and the physical aspect of your temple. You are only given one vehicle per lifetime, so it's important to care for it. It's the only thing you know you will have for as long as you live. Like any other vehicle, you have to climb inside before you can take a journey. You have to learn where the controls are and how to accelerate, steer, and brake, as well as keep the vehicle running smoothly. This is the task of embodiment. It is something you learn from the inside.

The key to entering the body is to embrace the first chakra element, which is earth. This element represents everything solid—not only the dirt beneath your feet but all material substance, especially the flesh and bones of your body. As matter, or *mater*, it represents the mother principle, the original matrix. It is the place we all come from—our roots and origin. Here, the goddess Kundalini-Shakti lies asleep, tightly coiled around the first chakra, awaiting her sacred journey up the spine.

The essential properties of the earth element are gravity and solidity, and they make an important pair. Gravity pulls your body down toward the earth while solidity holds you up. The more solid something is, the greater its gravity. Think of how the earth's mass makes the gravitational pull greater here on earth than on the moon. Gravity is always pulling you toward the floor in a yoga pose while the solid floor beneath you, as well as the solidity of your muscles and bones, are what hold you up.

The earth plane is where gravity and solidity meet—usually the surface of the ground or the floor. You can't go below the earth plane because it's solid, and most of the time you can't rise above it either because of gravity. All movement originates from this basic plane. All movements dance with gravity meeting this solidity. This is an important concept to understand in establishing the foundation of your temple. It will play out in nearly every posture.

Solidity gives you something to push into. You push into the solidity of the earth with your legs or arms, and the energy expended turns around and fills your body. You can try this right now by simply pushing one hand into the floor (or anything solid, like a wall or a desk) and noticing how the muscles in the arm wake up. The more you push, the more energy you generate. The root chakra uses the principles of gravity and solidity as the starting point for filling the body with prana.

This is best expressed by the first chakra paradox: *push down to rise up*. Consider what your body does in order to jump. First you have to bend your knees, then push downward into the earth. You can't jump very high if you don't bend your knees and lower yourself closer to the ground. It is this pushing into the earth that allows you to lift upward into a jump. The stronger you push into the earth, the higher you can jump. Jumping is easier if the ground is hard and solid than if the ground is soft, like a beach. In the same way, the more you push your legs as roots into the ground, the higher you can climb.

You form the foundation of all your yoga poses by pushing down into the earth. Because the earth is solid and not easily penetrated, the energy used to push downward turns around and fills up the part of the body that is pushing. When you walk or run, pushing into the earth energizes your legs. When you push into the floor or a wall with your hands, you energize the arms. If you use this principle wisely, you can fill the whole body with energy, spilling over into each chakra sequentially. In this way, you also push down to *wake* up.

Many spiritual traditions see the material world as a trap and resist the density of the body. There's no doubt that the physical world is less expansive than the limitless realms of the upper chakras, yet this density is precisely what keeps us grounded, connected to our bodies and the earth, focused, disciplined, and dynamically present. Without some weight to ground us, we can feel flighty, spacey, nervous, and fearful—in short, ungrounded. With too much weight, however, we feel sluggish and dull.

Many people unconsciously gain weight as an attempt to stay grounded when their normal grounding channels are not connected to the earth. While additional weight does slow you down and make you feel earthy, it can dominate the rest of the chakras. By contrast, those who have very light and skinny bodies may find it more difficult to ground. There is simply not enough tissue, or mass, to settle all the energies that affect the body daily.

The body is a container for the subtle energy—a storage battery for prana, or charge. A small body has less storage space and charges up more quickly, while a large body can hold more charge, yet has a harder time mobilizing that energy. The body works best with a balanced amount of charge—too much can make us feel anxious or scattered, while too little can feel lethargic or depressed. Since the first chakra represents your foundation, it can affect all the other chakras when it's out of balance.

The first chakra represents your most primal level of consciousness: your survival instincts. Designed to keep you alive so that you may continue the journey, survival instincts are hardwired into the body, mostly operating below the level of conscious awareness. Bringing your body into harmony with these instincts is essential for health and embodiment. Dynamic presence and radiant health are the gifts that result.

Muladhara: The Root Chakra

The Sanskrit name of this chakra, *Muladhara*, means root support or foundation. Just as you plug in your television to receive various channels, you plug your roots into the earth to activate and receive each of your chakra "channels," or frequencies. But roots need to be held by the earth. The clay pot around a houseplant holds the dirt firmly around the plant's roots, creating enough solidity for the plant to grow. It holds in the water and nutrients so the plant can sustain itself. If you were to break the pot, the dirt would become loose and the plant would fall over and die.

In the same way, there is an energetic holding, essential for the root chakra, that draws inward, toward the core. It hugs the muscles to the bones, solidifies the body, and creates edges and boundaries. It consolidates things, which means it makes you solid.

At the center of this holding are your roots and your trunk. They provide the structure that supports everything you do, but they are dynamically alive, channeling energy to and from the earth. The plant is free to branch out and blossom when the roots are secure. Roots need to be strong enough to support the plant, to feed and nourish it and to dig down into the earth. Eventually, it's the roots that hold the dirt together rather than the other way around, as any gardener can tell you. If you resist structure in your life, you are resisting the support necessary for manifestation. A structured base, rooted in solidity, allows for freedom above.

Since the first chakra is situated at the base of the torso, the legs become your roots. You can even think of the spine as extending all the way to the ground, except that it divides in two for the legs. In a pose like Downward Facing Dog or a handstand, your arms also become roots. Every pose has an orientation to the earth plane.

Roots have both masculine and feminine qualities; both aspects need to be activated, regardless of your gender. The masculine aspect pushes out from the seed, penetrating the soil. Here, you push downward from your first chakra, through your legs, then outward with your feet, spreading a wide base. The feminine aspect receives nourishment and moisture, drawing it upward through the roots—from the ground into the plant. This draws earth energy up the legs to nourish the rest of the body.

Grounding is not the antithesis of spiritual experience; it is literally the root of it. Just as a plant must have deep roots in order to grow taller, your ability to root down into the ground will allow you to reach higher toward the upper chakras. Establishing a firm foundation in the solidity of the earth begins the whole process of rising up the spine.

Forming Your Foundation in Tadasana, Standing Mountain Pose

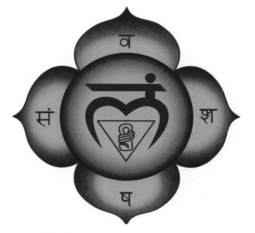

▲ first chakra symbol

The first chakra symbol is a four-petaled lotus that often contains a square, a downward-pointing triangle, and the Shiva lingam pointing upward, wrapped three and a half times around by the serpent Kundalini. Let's look at how you can incorporate those symbols into the way you stand in Tadasana.

Imagine the entire first chakra symbol on your mat. Place your feet so that the linear core of each foot—from the center of the heel to the second toe—forms the right and left sides of the square. Imagine drawing a line across your toes and behind your heels; here, you have the top and bottom of the square. You don't want this to be a rectangle or a trapezoid but a solid and deliberate square.

Then find the midline of your body, midway between front and back (the coronal plane). Locate the place where that plane intersects your hips and imagine that these points form the upper corners of the downward-facing triangle (see figure). Your perineum, which is the center of the pelvic floor, midway between the anus and genitals, also intersects the coronal plane and forms the base of the triangle. Imagine pointing the base of your triangle downward to the center of the square between your feet.

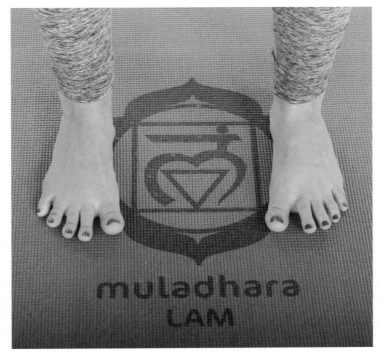

▲ standing on your first chakra

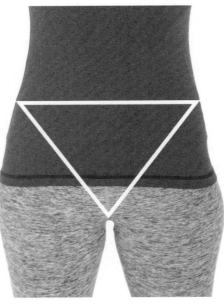

▲ downward-pointing triangle

In the middle of the square, the Shiva lingam represents the uprising energy of the sushumna, the central channel of the body, your core. The coiled serpent of Kundalini-Shakti represents the containment of our life-force energy, condensing it into solid matter in the first chakra. In honor of this symbol, you hug into your core, condensing yourself into solidity, and root down to rise up.

The four petals of the chakra then represent the four directions—your body's orientation in physical space. This takes you from "embodiment" to "emplacement." It puts you in the world, oriented from your ground and from your core. Think of this as a "mudra of the feet" that establishes your foundation on the sacred space of your mat.

The Sanskrit letter within the square is the seed sound of the first chakra, which is *lam*. You can now seal your foundation by repeating the seed sound a few times rhythmically. Speak it first aloud, then softer and softer, until you hear it only on the inside. Plant that seed in the middle of your first chakra. (For more on the bija mantras, see page 323.)

First Chakra Subtle Energy

Mula Bandha, or Root Lock

This bandha is an inward and upward contraction of the perineum, where the first chakra is located. Mula bandha tones the muscles around the first chakra and can definitely help you become more aware of your base chakra. I do not find, however, that it helps with grounding, as it closes off the pelvic floor from its natural downward flow. In fact, the general use of mula bandha is for closing off the first chakra for the purpose of raising energy up the spine. However, for an excessive first chakra, this bandha can help you consolidate your energy and draw it inward. For a deficient first chakra, I do not recommend mula bandha.

Because it is internal, it can't be shown in a picture.

1. Sit upright on the floor in a seated position, legs crossed, with your right heel pressing gently against your perineum. Widen your base by pressing your tailbone toward the back and rotating your inner thighs slightly downward.

2. Inhale, drawing breath and prana up your core.

3. Hold the breath for a count of five while forming
   mula bandha, contracting inward and upward
   with the muscles around your perineum.

4. Continue to hold mula bandha as you release the breath
   slowly and completely for a count of five or more.

5. When the exhalation is complete, take a moment to hold
   the breath empty as you release mula bandha.

6. Then inhale once again. Keep the perineum open as you inhale,
   then engage mula bandha as you hold the breath and exhale.

7. Repeat 5–10 times. Then relax and breathe
   normally, noticing the effects.

First Chakra Practice and Postures

Grounding the Four Corners

A square, with its flat bottom, sits solidly on the ground. It has a parallel surface on top that is capable of holding solid things. So a square, with its four corners, is the perfect image for the first chakra. It is, in fact, the only square present in any of the chakra symbols from the old texts—all the rest have triangles or curves.

In yoga, we talk about how the feet and the hands, as well as the torso itself, have four corners. To be properly grounded, all four corners of the feet move downward toward the earth equally, as do the hands if they are touching the ground. I like to think of the four corners of the torso as being like the corners of a fitted sheet that we pull down over the mattress. When lying on your back in a pose like Apanasana, Knees to Chest Pose (see page 62), pull the shoulders and the hips down toward the floor as if you were pulling the corners of the sheet over a bed, grounding the torso into the earth and thus offering support and greater opening to the front of the body. When standing in a basic standing pose like Tadasana, Standing Mountain Pose, you will want to pull your shoulders back and

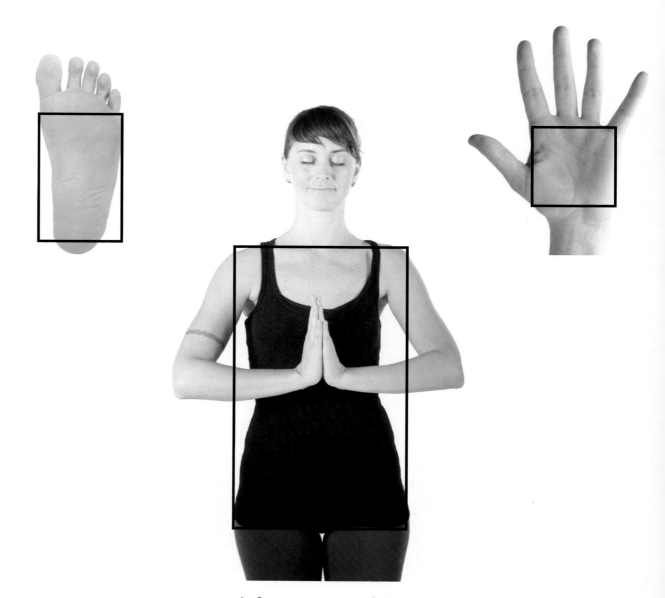

▲ four corners of the
foot, torso, and hand

ground into your hips as well as consciously place the four corners of your feet on the mat.

Basic Bioenergetic Grounding

To energize the roots, begin with a basic bioenergetic grounding exercise to open your leg channels. Use it at the start of your practice to wake up your roots and energize your legs. Part A gives you your basic grounding while standing, and part B shows you how to energize the legs by utilizing the principle of pushing down to wake up.

Part A: Firming Your Ground

1. Stand with your feet shoulder-width apart, pressing the four corners of each foot into the mat. Allow your heels to be slightly wider than your toes, making your feet just a little bit pigeon-toed.

2. Bend your knees just slightly over your second toe, so that you can look down at your feet and spot your big toe on the inside of your kneecap.

3. Press your feet downward as well as outward into the earth, as if trying to widen your sticky mat. Notice how your feet and legs become firm and grab onto the ground, giving your whole body a feeling of solidity. Keep the four corners of both feet grounded equally into the mat.

4. This is your basic bioenergetic grounding stance, which you can practice anytime you need to ground. Next, we will bring more prana, or charge, into the legs by using the principle of pushing down to wake up.

Part B: Energizing Your Ground

1. Begin with your basic stance above. Inhale and slowly bend your knees, keeping your shoulders directly over your hips.

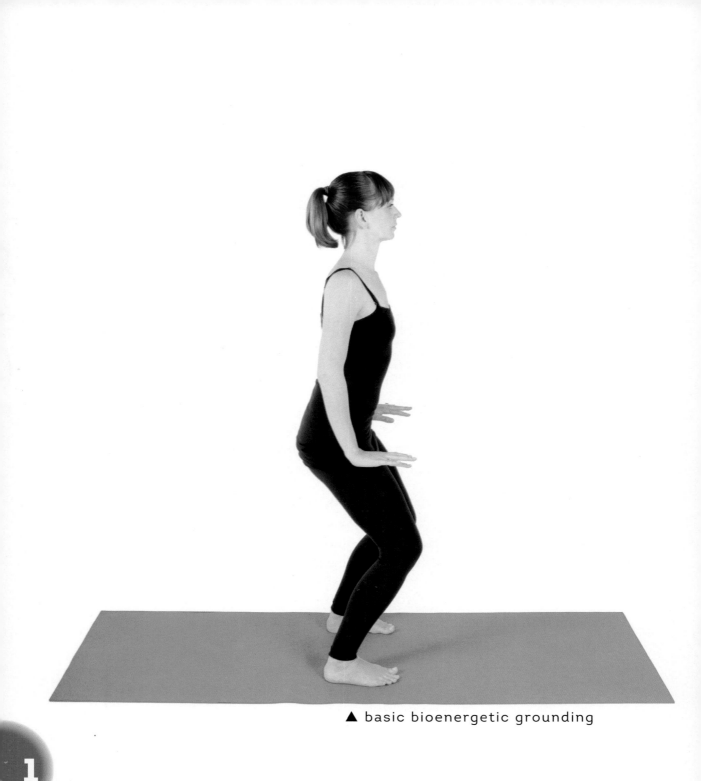

▲ basic bioenergetic grounding

2. Exhale and slowly push through the core of each leg, pushing simultaneously downward and outward as you did above, imagining you are penetrating the earth with your roots. As you push down and out through your legs, they will naturally begin to straighten. Be sure to do this slowly, and only let them straighten about 90 percent of the way. Never lock your knees in this particular exercise, as it shuts off the charge you are trying to build.

3. Repeat slowly for several minutes, bending the knees as you inhale and extending the legs as you exhale, taking a long, full breath with each movement.

4. Soon you will start to feel a mild trembling in your legs. The time it takes for this to happen varies greatly from one person to another, but it can be anywhere from ten seconds to a full minute.

5. As the trembling begins, observe what makes it increase: Where, on the journey between up and down, does it tremble the most? How can you find just the right amount of relaxation and muscular energy to maximize the trembling? Can you surrender to the trembling and allow it to enter your first chakra?

Guidelines

- *Important!* Locking your knees will shut off the charge you are trying to build up. Do not straighten your legs all the way as you push into the earth—only straighten them about 90 percent, keeping a soft bend in the knee.

- Make sure all four corners of both feet remain equally grounded.

- Pressing outward as well as downward with your feet makes dynamic contact with the ground and gives you stability.

- Keep your shoulders directly above the hips as you bend your knees. Do not lean forward.

- Inhale when bending, exhale when straightening.

1

- Be patient and allow the trembling to occur. Slow down. If you move too quickly, it is less likely to happen. The trembling will increase in intensity the longer you do the exercise.

- If your legs become tired, rest. If you feel overcharged, simply run in place, kick, or stomp your feet to discharge.

- As your legs straighten, imagine your roots are penetrating the earth, reflecting the masculine energy of the first chakra.

- As your knees bend, imagine you are drawing earth energy up your legs into your first chakra, reflecting the feminine. Notice which one—masculine or feminine—is easier for you.

- Allow your legs to tremble. Find the movement that creates the most trembling, focus your attention there, and let it happen. Let your tissues absorb the energy, and enjoy the activation of your root chakra!

Benefits
- Energizes a deficient first chakra

- Gets sluggish energy moving in an excessive first chakra

- Stimulates Kundalini

Avoid or Use Caution
- High anxiety (as it increases energetic charge)

- Knee injuries

Apanasana: Knees to Chest Pose

The first chakra includes the base of the spine, the legs, and the place where the legs meet the torso around the top of the thigh. This exercise helps you feel your lower spine and become aware of the legs meeting the torso. *Apana vayu* is the movement of energy downward, so this exercise emphasizes the release of the downward current. It is good for both excess and deficiency in the first chakra.

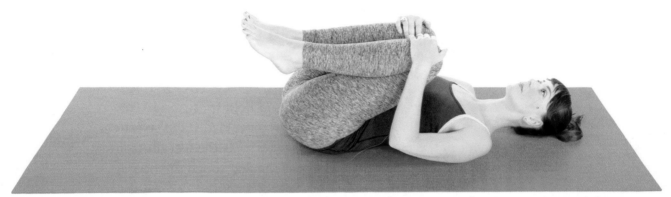

apanasana ▲ knees to chest pose, position a

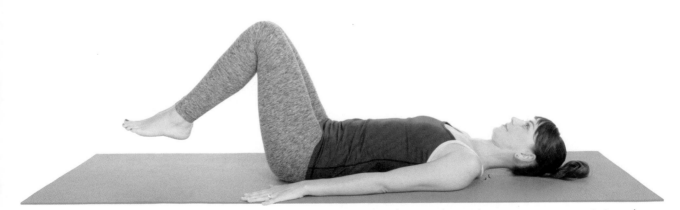

apanasana ▲ knees to chest pose, position b

63

1. Lie on your back with your legs extended. Slowly bend your knees while moving them toward your chest. Feel the difference in the back of your sacrum (the lower curve of your back) as your feet lift off the ground. Notice how the tip of the tailbone lifts off as well.

2. As the knees come in closer to the chest, wrap your arms around the top of your shins, pulling your knees in deeper toward your chest (position A). Take a few breaths here, emphasizing a long exhalation.

3. Release by slowly bringing your feet back to the floor. Notice what happens in your lower spine when the feet touch the floor. Can you feel something release?

4. Pick your feet up a few inches off the floor and hold (position B), then place your feet on the floor again, comparing these two states. Notice the engagement of the muscles in the lower torso as the feet lift from the floor, then the relaxation that occurs as the feet touch the floor.

Guidelines

- Pull all four corners of the torso down to the earth like a fitted sheet. Feel how this grounds you deeper into your body.

- Energetically bring your tailbone down toward the mat even as your legs are lifting it upward.

- Align your core from base to crown.

- Take time to feel the floor massaging your lower spine as you draw your knees in and out.

Benefits

- Opens and releases first chakra excess

- Improves digestion by massaging internal organs

- Good for constipation and menstrual cramps

- Relieves low back pain

- Good warm-up for deeper hip-openers

- Relieves stress

Avoid or Use Caution

- Knee injuries

- Hernia

Opening the Leg Channels

In this bioenergetics exercise, you use the resistance of a strap to energize the legs. The strap represents the ground by forming a limitation to push against. This opens the channels in the legs and builds up energy. Practice it slowly and mindfully, and allow the charge to build in the form of involuntary trembling in your raised leg.

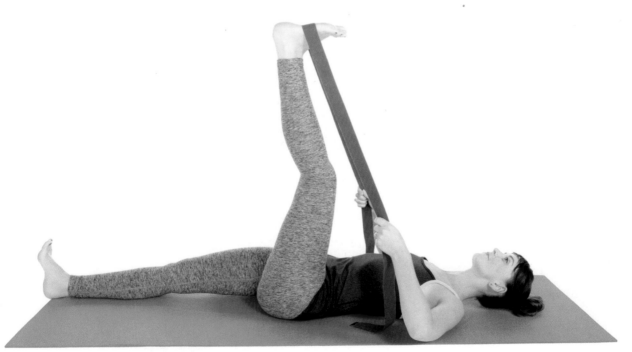

opening the leg channels ▲ position a

1. Bend your left knee into the chest, allowing your right leg to lie straight on the floor, toes pointing upward. Extend your tailbone down toward the floor even as the left leg lifts the coccyx (the lower tip of the spine) slightly upward.

2. Place a strap over the arch of your left foot and lift your foot upward, directly over the hip, knees just slightly bent (position A). (**Note:** flexible yogi types have a strong tendency to misalign in this exercise by moving their foot toward their face. The proper alignment for this exercise is with the foot directly above the hip.)

opening the leg channels ▲ position b

3. Hold one end of the strap in each of your two hands like a triangle and slide the strap back and forth across your foot several times, moving from heel to toe, creating some heat on the sole of your foot. See if you can discern the foot chakra in the arch of the foot—the place where the sensation is the strongest. Let your strap settle over the arch, bending your knee slightly. (If you are very stiff in your hamstrings, you may need to bend your knee even more. If necessary, bend the right leg as well.)

4. As you inhale, bend your lifted knee in toward your chest while keeping the bottom of the foot parallel to the ceiling (position B). This means that you are moving your thigh inward but keeping your calf pointing straight upward, with the foot flexed at the ankle.

5. As you exhale, push your foot upward into the strap, creating resistance by holding the strap tight. You should create enough resistance that your leg has to make considerable effort to move your foot upward, yet not so much resistance that your leg cannot move at all.

6. Continue back and forth, inhaling as you bend your knee, exhaling as you push your foot into the strap, doing so slowly and steadily, with long, full breaths. When pushing upward, take the leg into 90 percent of its full extension but not all the way. Do go the full 90 percent, however, as most of the charge opens up between 80 and 90 percent.

7. After a few rounds of inhaling and bending, exhaling and extending, you may notice a slight trembling in your raised leg. Congratulations! That means you are doing the exercise correctly and that prana is flooding into the roots of your legs. Notice how much pushing and resistance creates the most trembling. Allow your leg to surrender to this movement of prana. As you continue, the tremblings will gradually become more pronounced until they become involuntary movements of the legs. Allow this to happen.

8. Continue to Supta Padangusthasana, described on page 68, before moving to the other side.

Guidelines

- Place the strap over the arch of the foot and hold one end of the strap in each hand. Push through the core of the leg. Use the resistance of the strap to generate muscular energy in your leg.

- Keep your foot parallel to the ceiling. Do not bend the calf down but take the thigh toward your chest.

- When extended, the foot should be directly over the hip, with the leg perpendicular to the floor. Do not pull the foot toward the face. Do not lock your knee.

- This exercise brings charge, or prana, into the legs. If this is uncomfortable and you want to experience a discharge, bend both knees and pound your feet into the floor, one after the other, like a child having a tantrum. When tired, straighten your legs along the floor and take a few moments to feel the tingling in your legs and feet.

Benefits

- Strengthens the legs

- Increases grounding and aliveness

- Relieves tension and low back pain

- Opens channels for energy to enter and leave the first chakra

Avoid or Use Caution

- Knee injuries

Supta Padangusthasana: Reclining Hand to Big Toe Pose

When you buy a fruit tree at a nursery, the roots are all bound up in a sack. Before planting, you must get them to spread out and put them in a big enough hole in the earth for them to do so. This pose helps the roots spread out to the sides. Imagine opening the root ball at the base of your spine.

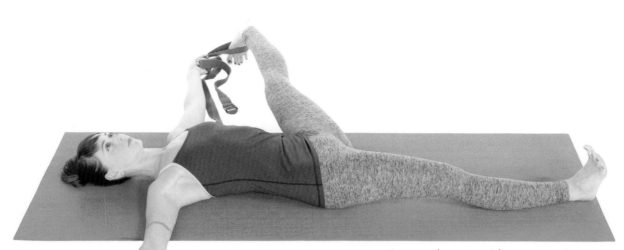

supta padangusthasana ▲
reclining hand to big toe pose,
position a

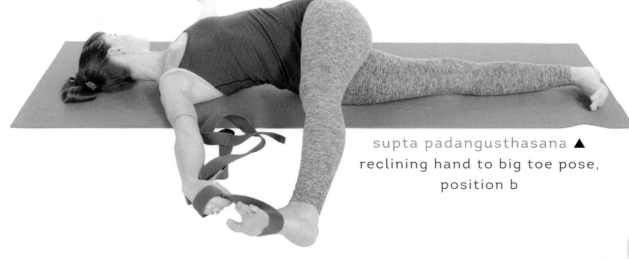

supta padangusthasana ▲
reclining hand to big toe pose,
position b

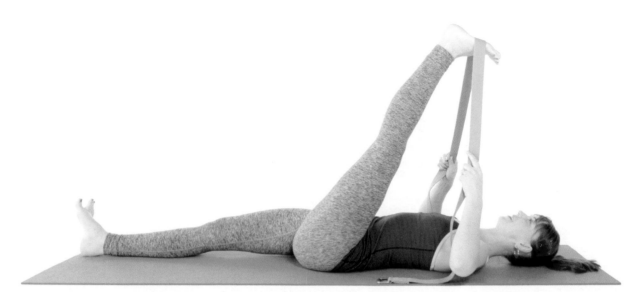

supta padangusthasana ▲ reclining hand to big toe pose,
position c, hamstring stretch

1. Once you have a good amount of trembling in your left
   leg, hold both ends of the strap in your left hand.

2. As you extend outward into both heels, slowly move your extended
   leg outward to the left until you meet the natural resistance of your
   flexibility, trying to keep your right buttock on the floor (position
   A). Hold and breathe until you feel a settling in your root chakra.

3. Lift your left leg back toward center. Switch the strap to your right hand
   and take your left leg across the body to the right side, endeavoring to
   keep your left shoulder on the floor as much as possible (position B).

4. Move your left hip away from your armpit, toward the bottom of
   your mat. Extend the tip of your tailbone toward the back body.

5. Release and move the left leg upward again. With a little
   tension on the strap, slowly pull your left leg in toward
   your face for a hamstring stretch (position C).

6. Slowly lower your left leg down to the floor, releasing the strap as your leg touches down.

7. When your left leg returns to the ground, compare your two legs and experience the difference between them. Does one feel longer, lighter, or heavier? Which feels more open?

8. Repeat the whole sequence on the other side, including the previous exercise of pushing into the strap, followed by taking the other leg to the right and left. Then compare your two legs once again.

Guidelines

• Keep the four corners of the torso pressed down toward the mat.

• Feel for the core of each leg and imagine you are pushing energy through it. Imagine your roots are flowing simultaneously from your hips to your feet in each leg.

• Keep the leg that's on the floor actively engaged by flexing the foot, pushing into the heel, straightening the knee, and hugging the muscles to the bones.

Benefits

• Stretches the hamstrings, psoas (hip flexors), and inner thighs

• Promotes grounding and openness in the hips

• Promotes deeper relaxation and opening of the entire lower body

Avoid or Use Caution

• Hip surgeries or hip replacements

Setu Bandha Sarvangasana: Bridge Pose

If you are going to build a bridge between heaven and earth, it must start with a solid foundation. This pose sets the foundation for your bridge and stimulates the legs and first chakra, as well as chakras three, four, and five. It is a good preparation for the deeper back-bending of the upper chakras. It strengthens the buttocks and opens the groin area in front of the hips.

1. Now that your legs are energized, lie on your back with your hands alongside your body, knees bent, feet hip-width apart, and heels toward the tips of your fingertips.

2. Pushing through the core of each leg, press your feet into the floor, feeling how the soles of the feet make deeper contact with the mat and the solidity beneath you. Feel how your legs are energized by this action even before lifting your hips.

3. Continue pushing your legs into the floor to slowly lift your hips up off the mat.

4. Hold for as long as is comfortable, with the option of rolling your shoulders toward each other and clasping your hands beneath your body.

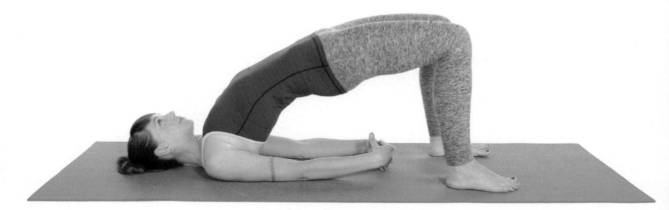

setu bandha sarvangasana ▲
bridge pose

Guidelines

- The action in the legs lifts the hips, not the belly muscles. Think of pressing the floor away rather than lifting the hips. Use the floor to push your hips higher.

- Press your midback toward the ceiling and your tailbone toward your knees.

- Draw the knees toward each other and rotate the thighs inward. Try holding a block between your thighs to accentuate this action.

- To press evenly into the four corners of each foot, press more deeply on the inner edges of your feet, as the feet tend to roll to the sides.

- As you press your heels down, draw them toward your shoulders to engage the hamstrings. To widen and activate the bridge, press your feet away from your shoulders. Roll slightly side to side to wiggle onto the outer edge of your upper arms, hugging your shoulder blades toward each other. Interlace your fingers with straight arms beneath your body.

- Press your arms into the floor to create more lift in the chest.

Benefits

- Strengthens the legs

- Improves shoulder flexibility

- Stimulates the nervous system and combats fatigue

- Aids digestion

Avoid or Use Caution

- Neck or shoulder injury

- Low back injury

Salabhasana: Locust and Half Locust Pose

When the front of the chakras are facedown on the ground, they can release into the earth. Take a moment to empty out before starting this pose. This exercise tones the area at the base of the spine and energizes the back of the legs.

1. Lie on your belly, arms alongside your body, palms facing downward. If possible, bring your arms beneath your body so that your palms press into the floor and the backs of your hands press against your upper thighs. Turn your face to the mat, resting your forehead on the floor.

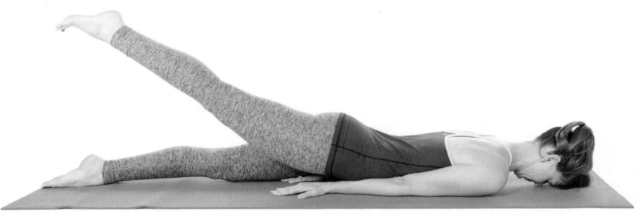

salabhasana ▲ half locust, position a

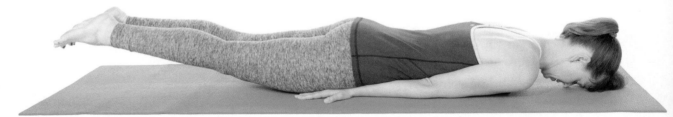

salabhasana ▲ full locust, position b

2. Extend energetically into your right leg, all the way down to your toes (position A). Keeping your knee straight, imagine that you are extending so much energy into your right leg that it lifts off the ground.

3. Hold for a few breaths, then exhale and lower the right leg slowly, staying in control.

4. Repeat steps 2 and 3 on the other side.

5. Once you have warmed up with one leg at a time, you can lift both legs, drawing your legs and feet together like a single tail of the Kundalini serpent (position B).

6. On an exhalation, release back down to the ground slowly, staying in control.

Guidelines

- Draw into the core of each leg while extending to the toes.

- Point the toes, keeping the knees straight.

- Press your palms into the floor.

- Keep your face centered on the mat.

- Stay in control as you lower your legs on an exhalation.

Benefits

- Strengthens and tones the first chakra

- Strengthens the legs

- Aids digestion

Avoid or Use Caution

- Pregnancy

- High blood pressure

- Headaches

1

Bhujangasana: Cobra Pose

When you were an infant, long before you could walk you began to lift yourself off the floor and look around. This begins the curiosity that stimulates the desire to move forward, which leads to creeping, crawling, and walking. Cobra begins to strengthen your spine while rooting down into your pelvis. It accesses the primal part of your brain known as the reptilian brain, which is oriented to survival, the psychological aspect of the first chakra.

1. Begin facedown on your belly, with elbows bent and hands placed alongside your shoulders, fingertips in line with the tops of the shoulders (position A).

2. Draw your legs together as if you were making them into a single tail of the cobra. Firm up your belly, pulling the abdominal muscles inward. Hug into your core.

3. Inhale and lift the head and chest off the floor, rolling the shoulders back (position B). For Baby Cobra, use your back muscles only, lifting your hands off the floor a few inches.

4. For Full Cobra, push down through the core of each arm to raise your chest higher (position C).

5. Hold for several breaths.

6. Come out of the pose on an exhalation. Turn your head to one side, place your arms by your sides, and relax.

Guidelines

- From your root chakra, extend through the core of your pelvis, up through the heart, and to the top of your crown.

- Outwardly rotate the upper arms and keep the elbows in close to your sides.

- Press your shoulder blades toward each other, pointing the tips of the shoulder blades down the back. Lower your shoulders away from your ears.

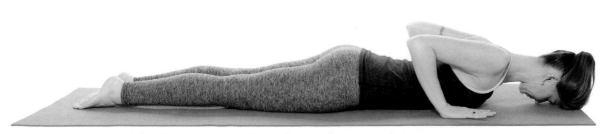

bhujangasana ▲ cobra prep, position a

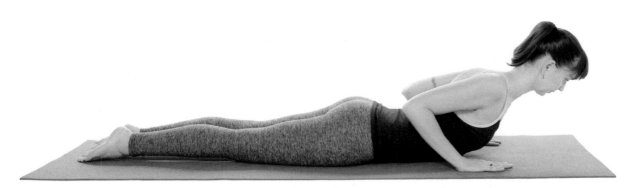

bhujangasana ▲ baby cobra, position b

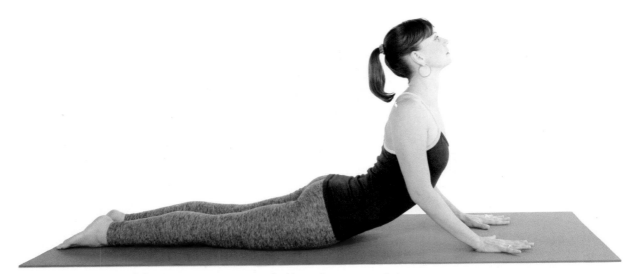

bhujangasana ▲ full cobra, position c

- Lift and lower your upper body a few times slowly, coordinating the movement with your breath, exercising the muscles of the back.

- If you cannot keep your shoulders down as you straighten your arms, bend the arms a little more and soften the pose.

- Use the resistance of the ground to deepen the pose by drawing the heels of your hands toward your hips.

Benefits

- Grounds the pelvis

- Opens the heart and clears the mind

- Increases spinal flexibility

- Stimulates circulatory and lymphatic systems

Avoid or Use Caution

- Pregnancy

- Spinal injury

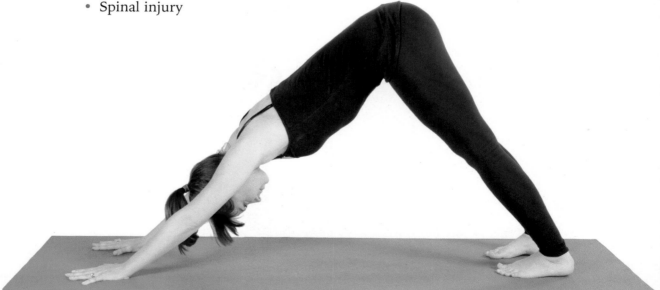

adho mukha svanasana ▲ downward facing dog

Adho Mukha Svanasana: Downward Facing Dog Pose

People who walk their dogs in the morning start their day by getting outside and walking upon the earth. In this quintessential yoga pose, both your arms and legs become roots. You also accentuate the four corners of the torso, squaring it up firmly by pressing into the four corners of each foot and hand. By pushing both hands and feet firmly into the ground, you can truly experience how pushing down will wake you up. This pose is good for balancing and integrating upper and lower chakras, as the inversion aspect brings prana to the upper chakras, while rooting down through the legs and heels grounds the lower chakras. I often call the pose Downward Facing God and think of the divine intelligence looking down over the earth, holding the planet in compassion.

1. Begin in Table Pose. Place your palms firmly on the mat, fingers spread wide, first fingers parallel to each other, wrist creases parallel to the front of the mat.

2. Engage your legs by tucking your toes into the mat and pushing your feet and hands into the floor. Firm up your shoulder blades, drawing them downward. Feel this engagement with the ground before you lift your hips.

3. From that engagement, lift your hips until your body forms a triangle, with the floor as the base.

4. You may wish to alternately bend and straighten your knees a few times as you "walk your dog" and wiggle your way into the pose.

5. With feet hip-width apart, press your heels down toward the mat. Don't worry if your heels don't touch; it may take years of practice to get your heels all the way down.

Guidelines

- Energize the pose by pressing both hands and feet more firmly into the floor, as if you were trying to lengthen your mat from top to bottom, distributing your weight evenly among the four corners of this pose: your two hands and two feet. Notice how this rooting action energizes the body.

1

- **Legs:** Hug your muscles in toward the bones, lifting your kneecaps. Press the front of your thighs toward the back, with a slight rotation of the inner thighs toward the back, creating more space in the pelvic floor and widening the back of the sacrum.

- **Arms:** The fleshy part of the hand between the thumb and first finger contains a point in Chinese medicine used for grounding. Pressing this part firmly into the ground will give you a slight inner rotation of your forearms. Simultaneously outwardly rotate your upper arms, opening the shoulders and chest. Soften the heart as you extend from the heart to your wrists and from the heart to your pelvis.

- Be wary of hyperflexion in the shoulders. Ideally, there should be a straight line from your hips to your wrists.

- Experiment with bending and straightening your knees, rising up on your toes and lowering your heels, and bending and straightening your arms to experience different dynamics in the pose.

Benefits

- Grounds the whole body

- Creates core strength and increases steadfastness

- Opens the arms and shoulders, stretches the hamstrings, and loosens the hips

- Improves digestion

- Energizes the body

Avoid or Use Caution

- Late-term pregnancy

- Carpal tunnel syndrome

- High blood pressure

- Headaches

Uttanasana: Standing Forward Fold

This is an essential and rudimentary pose that should be part of any practice. It stretches the entire backside of body, especially the legs and lower back, and it massages the internal organs and helps detoxify the liver, spleen, and kidneys. It allows the torso to let go, increasing the upper back's flexibility as well as stretching the hamstrings. It also brings blood to the head and is a good pose if you feel dizzy; it's also a good counterbalance to backbends. Uttanasana is excellent for both excess and deficiency in the first chakra, as it both opens and releases.

1. Begin in Tadasana, with feet hip-distant apart and parallel to each other. Consider the first chakra symbol between your legs, with your feet making a square (see page 55). Ground the four corners of your feet.

2. Extend your roots down and lift your crown up, aligning between heaven and earth through your core.

3. Open your arms out to the sides and keep the spine lengthened as you fold forward into the pose on an exhalation.

4. Ideally, your legs are straight but your knees are not hyperextended or locked. If your knees need to bend a little, you can gently push them back over time, being careful not to push farther than the natural limits of your body.

5. Rise up out of the pose on an inhalation, softening the knees.

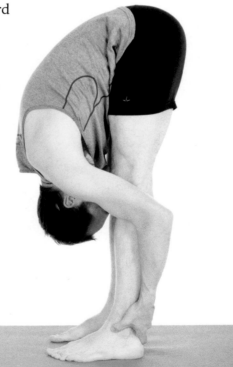

uttanasana ▶
standing forward fold,
position a

1

Guidelines

- Rotate the inner thighs toward the back, widening the pelvic floor and the back of the sacrum while lifting the sitting bones.

- Allow your legs to be strong, like posts, while letting your torso soften and let go. This letting go takes time and breath, so linger in this pose while you allow your torso to gradually release. Imagine space opening up between your vertebrae.

Variations

1. **Ardha Uttanasana:** Lift up to a flat back, hands on your knees, and extend from root to crown (position B). Inhale, then exhale and lower back down.

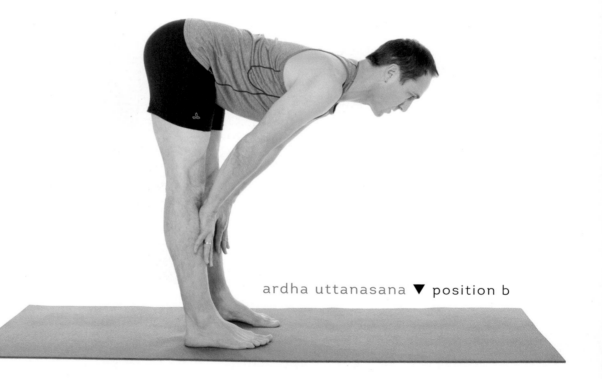

ardha uttanasana ▼ position b

2. Place your fingers under the front of your feet (position C).

3. Bend and straighten your legs, inhaling as you bend and exhaling as you straighten.

4. Place one hand on the floor between your feet and lift the other arm up into the air (position D).

5. For a deeper relaxation, bring a hand to each elbow and swing side to side (position E).

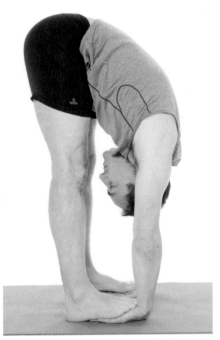

uttanasana ▲ position c

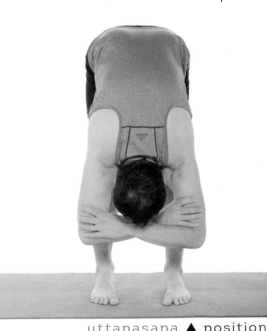

uttanasana ▲ position e

uttanasana ◀ position d

83

Benefits

- Stretches the hamstrings and calves

- Opens the hips

- Improves digestion and eases menstruation

- Releases back tension

- Calms the nervous system

- Cools excess heat

Avoid or Use Caution

- Advanced pregnancy

- Low blood pressure (you might be dizzy coming back up)

- Low back injury

- Hamstring injuries

High Lunge Pose

Lunges strengthen the legs and help develop steadiness in your practice. Holding a lunge is a good way to draw earth energy into your first chakra. Bending and straightening the front leg a few times energizes the legs, much like the previous exercise of opening the leg channels.

1. Begin in Tadasana, then bow forward into Uttanasana.

2. On an inhalation, step your left foot back about four feet, keeping your right knee directly above the right ankle.

3. Keep your back leg firm and strong. Beginners may choose to lower their back knee to the floor.

4. Move to reverse lunge, described below, then repeat both on the other side.

Guidelines

- Keep your feet hip-distance apart. Press both feet into the floor and energetically draw your feet toward each other. Feel your legs becoming more solid.

- Hug the muscles to the bones, making the back leg straight and strong.

- Energetically pull the hip of the straight leg slightly forward and the hip of the bent knee slightly backward. Lift up from the inner left thigh, moving the thigh bones toward the back of the leg.

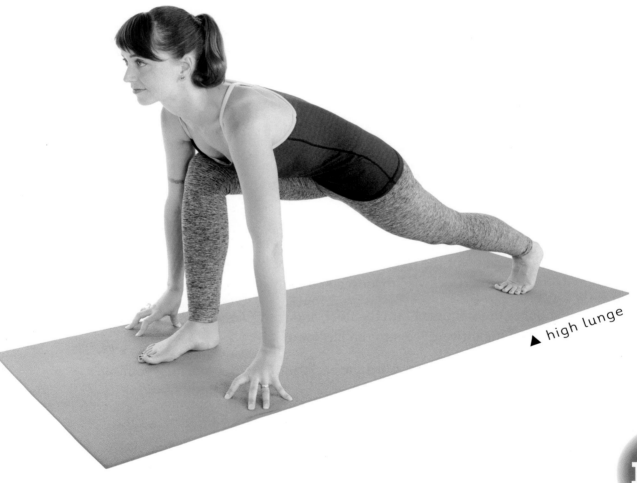

▲ high lunge

- Lift your eyes and gaze straight ahead, spreading wide the four corners of the torso.

- Align the central axis of your body with the midline of the mat, extending from base to crown.

Ardha Hanumanasana: Reverse Lunge

Reverse lunges help pull the roots out of the base of the spine and down the back of the leg. They are a way to humble our upper chakras by bring them down over the leg. As you bend forward, honor the legs that carry you on your journey.

1. From the lunge position above, lower your left knee to the floor.

2. Push through the core of the right leg, engaging the muscles to create some resistance as you slowly straighten your right leg, bringing your hips over your back knee and sliding your hands back accordingly.

3. Extend your crown away from your base as you inhale, lengthening the spine.

4. As you exhale, stretch the midline of the torso over your extended leg. Hold for several deep breaths.

5. Inhale and lift the head to come out of the pose. Repeat on the other side.

Guidelines

- Flex and point the toes of your front foot. Rotate the foot clockwise and counterclockwise to loosen and lubricate the ankle joint.

- Press the front heel into the floor, and muscularly draw the forward leg into the hip socket.

- Press your tailbone toward the back, and imagine widening your hips.

- Align with your core as you extend upward before bowing. Keep the length in your spine as you bend forward.

- Beginners may wish to use blocks placed beside each hip.

Benefits

- Opens a contracted first chakra

- Stretches your hips, hamstrings, calves, and low back

- Good for restless leg syndrome

- Lubricates ankle, toe, and knee joints

- Good warm-up for full splits

- Calming, soothing, and cooling

Avoid or Use Caution

- Advanced pregnancy

- Hamstring injuries

- Hip or low back injuries

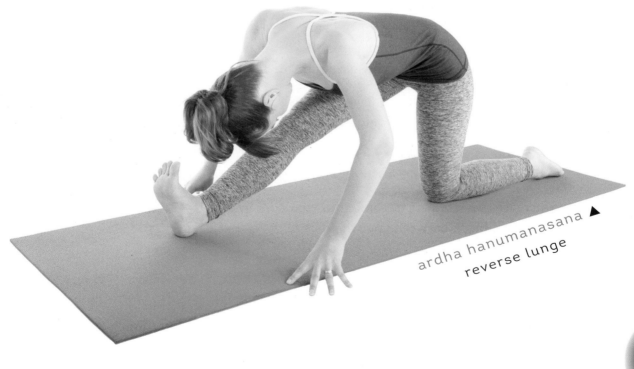

ardha hanumanasana ▶
reverse lunge

1

Utkatasana: Awkward Chair Pose

This pose helps strengthen the legs and develop a sense of the core. Bring it into your daily life by holding it for a moment each time you are about to sit down! Utkatasana is excellent for deficient first chakras, as it develops more connection to the earth.

1. Stand with your feet hip-width apart. Press down and out with your feet as you inhale and raise your arms up overhead. Take a full breath here, connecting heaven and earth through your core.

2. On the next inhalation, bend your knees, pressing your tailbone toward the back, and lift your chest, creating a slight curve in the spine.

Guidelines

• Hug into the core. Accentuate the natural curve of your lower back while drawing in your belly.

• Avoid bending your torso forward. Lift your shoulders and keep your shoulder blades moving down your back.

• Lengthen through the crown and gaze up toward your hands. Let your eyes guide the movement of your neck. If your neck is strained, then simply gaze forward at eye level.

• Deepen the pose by bending your knees farther and sinking your hips lower while still keeping your torso extending upward.

• For more challenge, repeat with feet and knees together (position B), pressing the palms into each other overhead, hands in steeple position.

• Increase the action of hugging into your core by placing a block between your thighs.

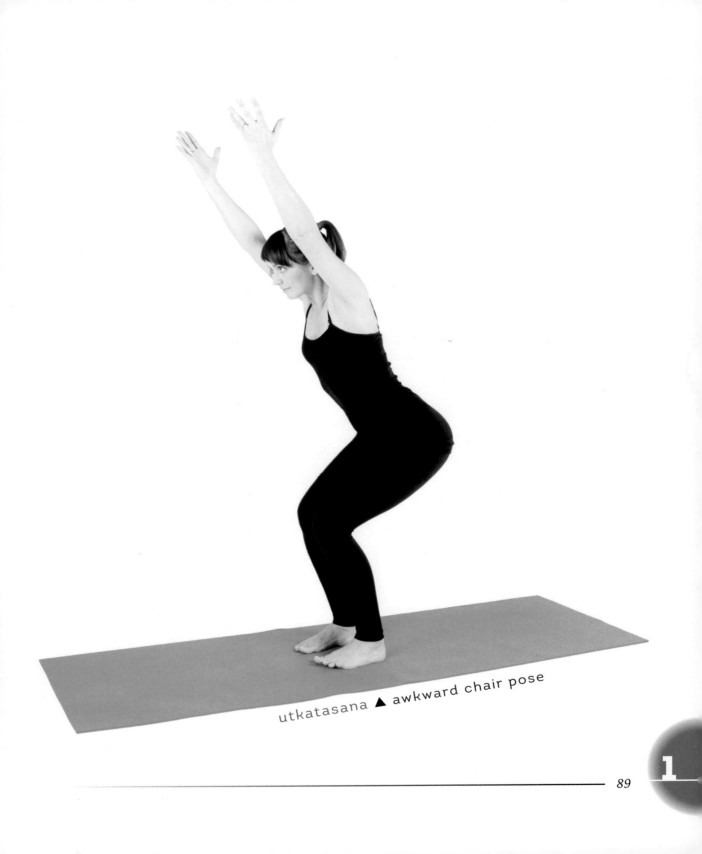

utkatasana ▲ awkward chair pose

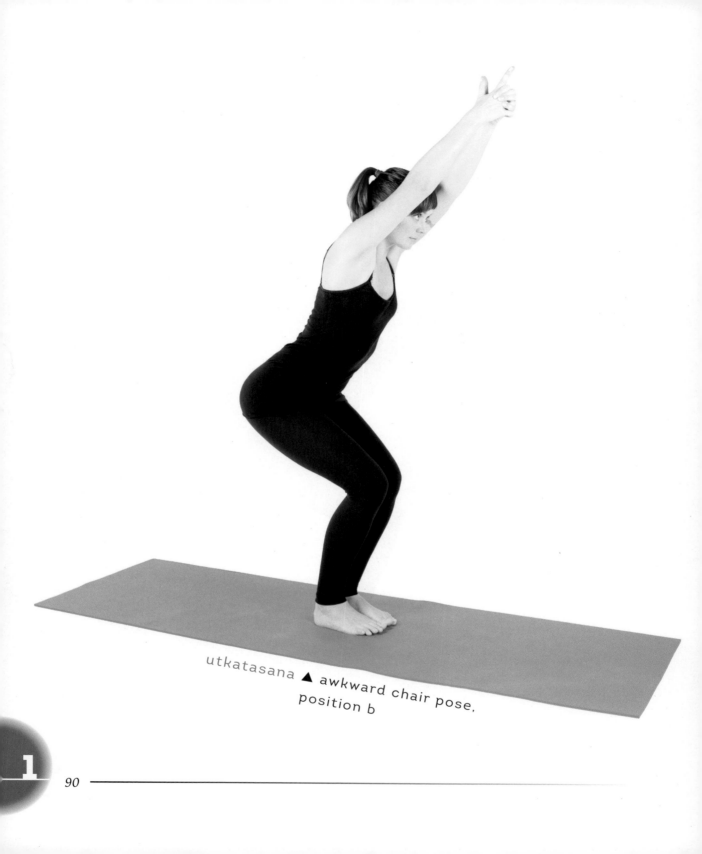

utkatasana ▲ awkward chair pose,
position b

Benefits

- Increases strength and stamina

- Builds energy and focus

- Strengthens the legs

- Stimulates digestive and reproductive systems

Avoid or Use Caution

- Low blood pressure

- Insomnia

- Knee injuries

Utkata Konasana: Goddess Squat

While the masculine gods are often associated with disembodied spirit, the Goddess is more often earthy, fleshy, and physical. Here, the Goddess fully owns her earthly power by claiming a large base and lowering her roots to the earth.

1. With elbows bent, lift your hands, palms facing forward, elbows nearing shoulder height.

2. Spread your feet about as wide as your elbows, toes pointing to the corners of your mat.

3. On an inhalation, bend your knees, lowering your roots.

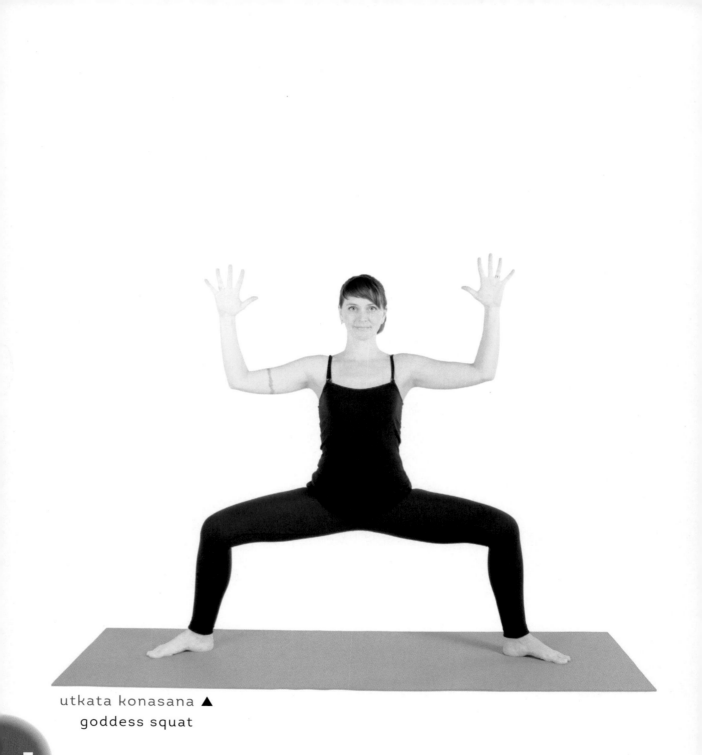

utkata konasana ▲
goddess squat

Guidelines

- Practice working your thighs toward being parallel to the floor, but don't force it.

- Press your feet down and out to energize the legs. Keep your heels on the ground, spreading your legs wide enough to do so easily.

- Be careful of your knees. Keep them moving in the same direction as the feet. Stop when the knees are over the ankles.

- Imagine widening the base, tailbone slightly toward the back, drawing the belly firmly into the core.

- Keep your spine vertical and draw upward toward the crown, hugging into your core.

- Bring the corners of your mouth gently toward your ears, imagining the power and benevolence of the Goddess flowing through you.

- Alternate arm positions are with hands folded over the heart in prayer position or arms lifted high overhead. See where you feel the most power in the pose.

Benefits

- Strengthens the legs

- Opens pelvic floor

- Builds energy, power, and confidence

Avoid or Use Caution

- Knee injuries

Vrksasana: Tree Pose

Another quintessential grounding pose, Tree Pose invites you to be rooted into your ground, solid in your trunk, and expansive as you branch out above. This pose shows how the root chakra supports the solidity in your core and the freedom in the upper chakras.

1. Begin in Tadasana. Stand tall and straight, finding your core and rooting into both legs. Imagine standing upon your first chakra square described on page 55.

2. Shift your weight to the left leg while lifting your right foot just slightly off the floor. Solidify your balance before moving farther.

3. Place your right foot against the inside of your left leg. It's okay to use your hands to do this if you need to. Beginners may place the foot lower, on the ankle or the inner shin. Avoid pressing against the knee.

4. Bring your palms together in prayer position, over the heart (position A). Hug into your core and lift your crown while rooting downward and extending your tailbone down toward the center of the square beneath you.

5. When you are stable, you may wish to raise your arms and extend your branches (position B).

Guidelines

- Move slowly, keeping your balance at each stage. Fix your gaze at a focal point a few feet in front you to help with balance.

- Push your foot firmly into the thigh to stabilize by hugging into your core.

- Try closing your eyes and see if you can keep your balance by truly feeling your core.

- For a variation and deeper hip opening, place the outside of your right foot against the top of your left thigh (position C). Point the knee toward the ground.

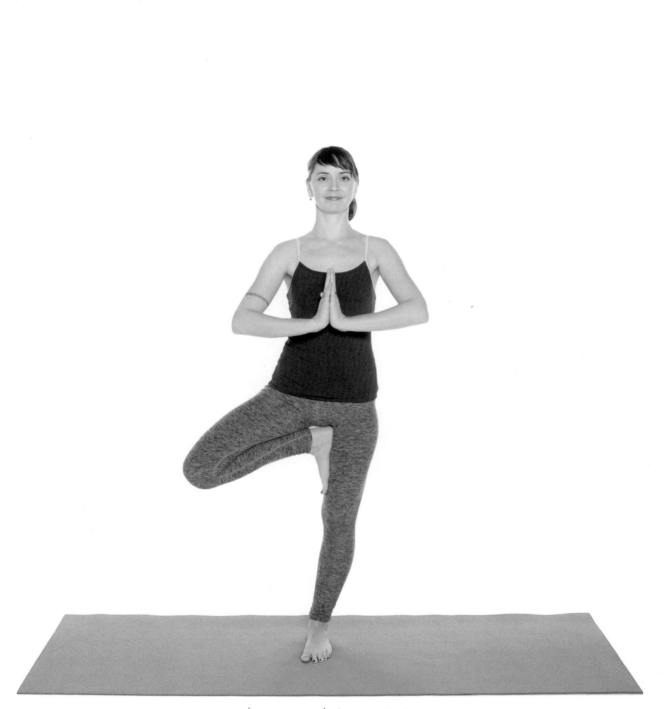

vrksasana ▲ tree pose,
position a

1

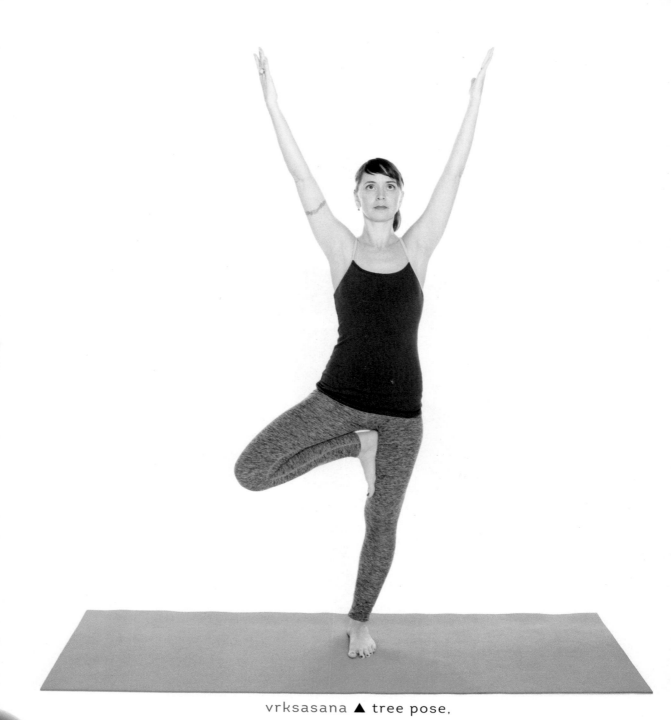

vrksasana ▲ tree pose,
position b

Benefits

- Develops balance and focus

- Establishes grounding and self-reliance

- Strengthens the feet, ankles, calves, and thighs

- Remedies flat feet

- Increases awareness of the core

vrksasana ▲ tree pose, position c

Utthita Hasta Padangusthasana: Extended Hand to Toe Pose

Balance poses require rooting down into the standing leg and hugging into the core. This pose can be taken in stages, mastering each one before proceeding to the next. Move slowly and carefully. It is easier to keep your balance as you go than to regain it once you start to fall out of the pose.

1. Begin in Tadasana, drawing into your core. Bend your right knee and interlace your fingers below the knee, drawing it into the chest (position A). Regain your balance and solidity.

2. If you are steady here, interlace your hands underneath your right foot (position B). Practice here until you feel stable.

3. If you are balanced here, wrap your first two fingers around your big toe and extend your right leg forward (position C).

4. Rooting into your standing leg and extending into your lifted leg, slowly move your right foot and leg out to the right side (position D).

Guidelines

• Move slowly, establishing your balance and steadfastness at each step. Do not proceed if you do not feel steady.

• Keep your standing leg firm but do not lock your knee. Lift up on your kneecap and draw the muscles to the bones, extending through the core of the leg. Pull the front of the standing thigh back so that your hip is directly over your knee.

• Keep the hips square to the front of the mat.

• Make sure your torso stays lifted, drawing the shoulders back, with your crown over your base.

Benefits

• Improves balance

• Strengthens the legs and all parts of the feet

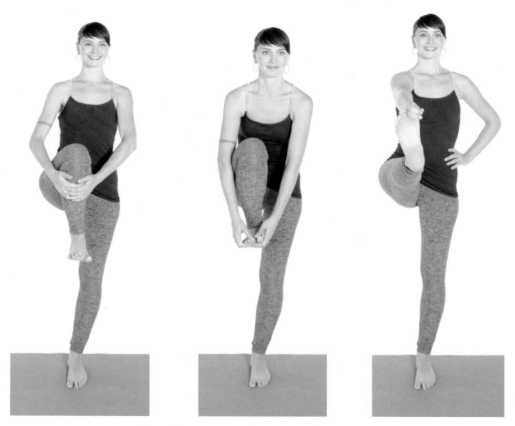

utthita hasta padangusthasana ▲
extended hand to toe pose; from left,
positions a, b & c

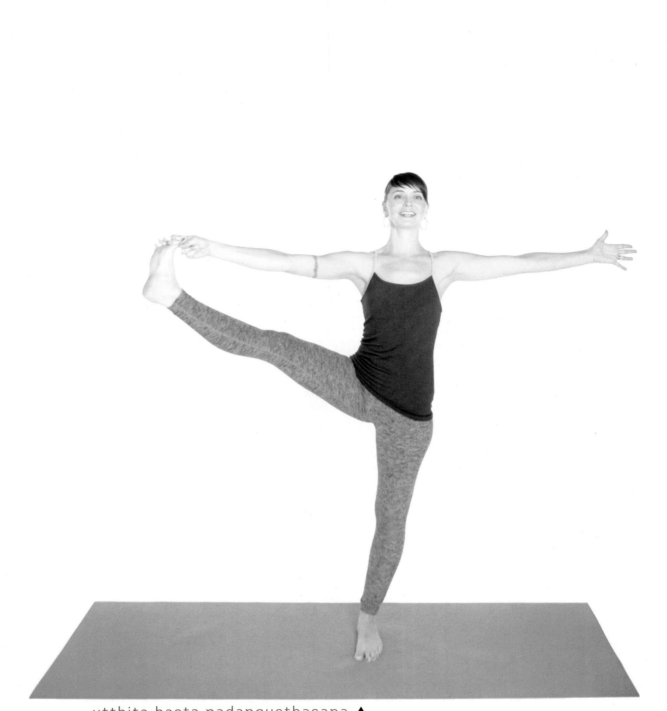

utthita hasta padangusthasana ▲
extended hand to toe pose, position d

- Stretches the hamstrings

- Builds concentration, steadiness, and focus

- Increases awareness of the core

Avoid or Use Caution
- Hernia

- Knee, ankle, or hip injury

Virasana & Supta Virasana: Seated & Reclining Hero Pose

This pose gives a good stretch to the quadriceps and hip flexors, and it opens the groin area while stimulating the root of the spine. It is a nice counterstretch to all this work on the legs and allows the body to sink into gravity.

1. Begin in a kneeling position, knees hip-width apart. Spread your feet slightly wider than your knees.

2. With your hands, roll the flesh of your calves slightly outward, toward the sides.

3. Lower your buttocks down to the floor, sliding your butt between your heels. Point your toes straight back, with your heels just on the outside of your hips (position A).

4. If you are comfortable here, without strain on the knees, then reach back with your hands and lower onto your elbows as you slowly lower your back to the floor.

5. If you are comfortable reclining, raise your arms overhead and hold opposite elbows (position B).

6. To come out of the pose, lead with the heart, first using your elbows, then your hands, for support, with your head coming up last.

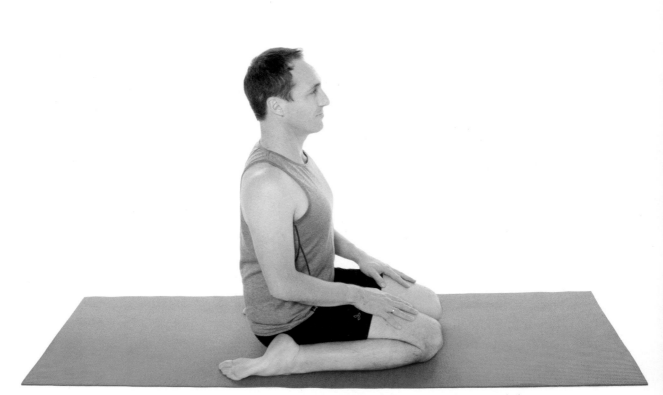

virasana ▲ seated hero pose, position a

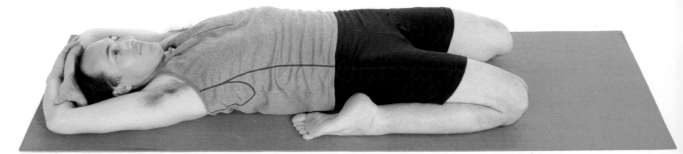

supta virasana ▲ seated hero pose, position b

Guidelines

- You may place a block or bolster under your buttocks for additional support to lift your hips higher.

- Point your tailbone toward your knees while pressing the kneecaps down toward the earth.

- Avoid allowing the knees to spread wider than your hips. This can strain the hips and lower back.

- This is an intermediate pose. Do not expect instant results.

Benefits

- Stimulates tailbone

- Stretches the quadriceps and psoas muscles

- Opens the lower back

Avoid or Use Caution

- Knee, ankle, or hip injury—avoid any pain

Siddhasana: Baby Cradle Pose

For plants to grow, the roots must be nourished. Cradling your leg like a baby is a good way to nurture yourself and honor the lower legs while opening up your hips at the same time.

1. Sit in an easy cross-legged pose.

2. Grab the foot and knee of your right shin with both hands, keeping your left shin in its cross-legged position.

3. Draw the right shin up toward the chest and slide your right knee into the crook of your right elbow and the right foot into your left elbow. If possible, interlace your fingers along your shin (position A).

4. Press the four corners of your torso toward the back.

5. Gently rock your shin back and forth like a baby, slowly working it toward your torso.

6. Repeat with the other leg.

Guidelines

- A more preliminary stage of this pose is to take both hands under the shins (position B).

- Be careful not to round the spine; keep it upright and extended. Press your tailbone down into the earth.

- Be gentle with your leg, as you would with a baby.

- Keep the sole of your lifted foot flexed, strong, and engaged.

Benefits

- Opens the hips

- Improves digestion

- Stimulates colon, liver, and kidneys

Avoid or Use Caution

- Knee or hip injury

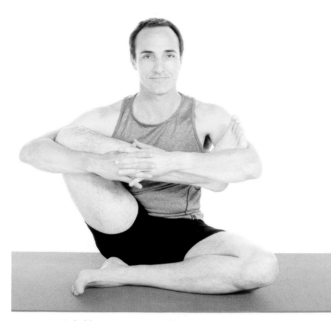

siddhasana ▲ baby cradle pose,
position a

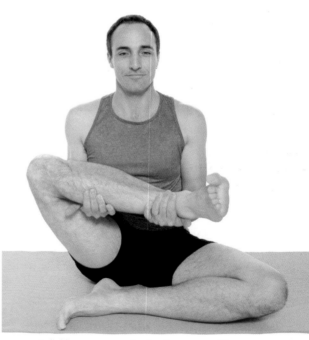

siddhasana ▲ baby cradle pose,
position b

Janu Sirsasana: Head to Knee Forward Bend

The next two poses lengthen the entire spine and pull your roots down the back of your legs while gently massaging the internal organs. Use for cooling down toward the end of your practice, before Savasana. These are great for excessive first chakras to learn to let go and trust the ground.

1. Sit in Dandasana, or Staff Pose. Press the backs of your legs firmly into the floor, extending your tailbone toward the back and your spine upward to your crown. If you cannot keep the natural curves of your spine in this position, raise your hips on a folded blanket.

2. Bend your left knee and draw the left foot up toward your perineum, the sole of your left foot pressing against your right inner thigh.

3. Inhale and draw your arms upward, flexing your right foot and extending into your right heel. Lengthen your spine upward.

4. Exhale and bow forward over your right leg, keeping the spine lengthened and avoiding rounding the back.

5. Reach for your toes and clasp your hands beneath the sole of your foot. If you do not have the flexibility to reach your toes, allow yourself to find your edge, then place your hands on whatever you can reach comfortably: your ankle, shin, knee, or the floor on either side of your leg.

6. Rest here for several deep, full breaths, allowing a little more release with each exhale.

7. To come out of the pose, inhale and lift your head, then massage up your legs as you return to a seated pose.

8. Change legs, and repeat on the other side.

Guidelines

• Beginners or those with tight hamstrings may wish to use a strap over the foot.

- Align your midline with the core of the extended leg.

- Spread your elbows wide to deepen the pose, bringing your forehead to your knee or shin. Press your tailbone out behind you.

- It is better to keep the spine lengthened, even if it means your forehead does not come down as far toward your legs.

Benefits

- Stretches the hamstrings and lengthens the spine

- Improves digestion as it massages the lower organs

- Stimulates liver and kidneys

- Cooling and calming

- Opens the hips

- Opens the root line of the legs

Avoid or Use Caution

- Knee injury

- Diarrhea

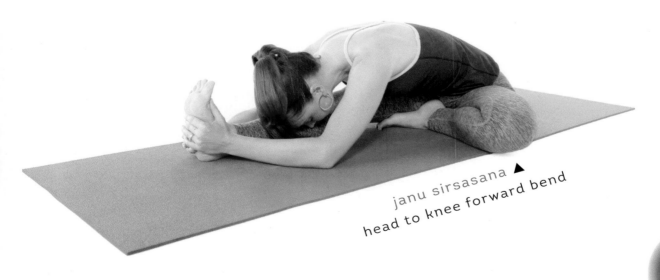

janu sirsasana ▲
head to knee forward bend

Paschimottanasana: Seated Forward Bend

1. Begin as above in Dandasana, Staff Pose, with legs out in front, adjusting the height of your hips with a folded blanket if necessary.

2. Flex your feet and extend through the core of each leg into your heels, pressing the backs of your knees into the floor. Slightly rotate your upper thighs inward, even using your hands to do so.

3. Press your tailbone toward the back body and draw up your midline into your crown.

4. Inhale and lift your arms overhead, lifting your ribs and drawing your shoulder blades down the back.

5. Keep that lift as you exhale and bow forward over both legs. If this strains your back, allow your arms to rest on your knees and slide them forward toward your feet as you bow forward.

6. Reach for your toes or interlace your hands beneath the soles of your feet. If that is not possible, grab whatever you can reach: your toes, ankles, shins, or knees. Find your edge first, then see where your hands fall naturally.

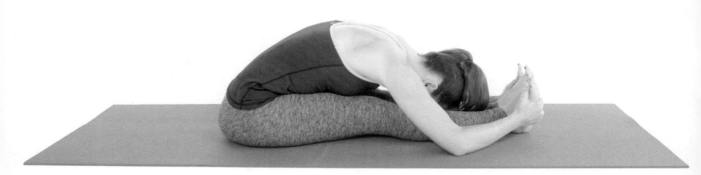

paschimottanasana ▲ seated forward bend

Guidelines

- Bend the elbows outward, drawing the chest forward.

- Lengthen the spine rather than rounding it over the legs.

- Press the inner thighs toward the floor, widening
  the space between the thigh bones.

- Do not push past your edge into pain. Release a little with each exhale.

- Hold for a minute or more, and surrender to the pose.

Benefits

- Lengthens entire spine

- Stretches hamstrings

- Promotes hip flexibility

- Cooling and calming

- Opens the root line of the legs

Avoid or Use Caution

- Back injury

- Advanced pregnancy

Balasana: Child's Pose

This is one of the most grounding poses you can do. If you feel tired during practice and need to rest, or if you feel jittery from too much energy, simply allow yourself to return to this simple pose that resembles the time before birth when you were held safely in the womb.

1. Turning your heels slightly outward, separate your knees about 12–18 inches and lower your buttocks onto the bottoms of your feet.

2. Raise your arms upward and reach for the sky, extending the spine as you inhale.

3. Continue to lengthen from base to crown as you bow forward over your legs.

4. You can choose to extend your arms, bring them alongside the body, or fold your hands to make a pillow under your forehead.

Guidelines

- This should be a comfortable resting pose. If it is difficult, you may wish to use a pillow or a blanket behind your knees or under your forehead, or substitute with Apanasana, Knees to Chest Pose (page 62).

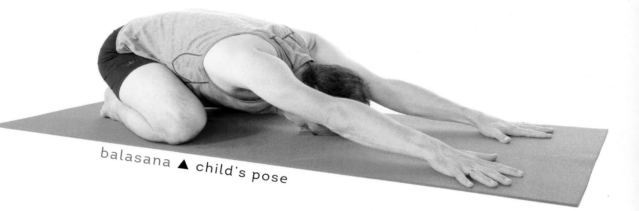

balasana ▲ child's pose

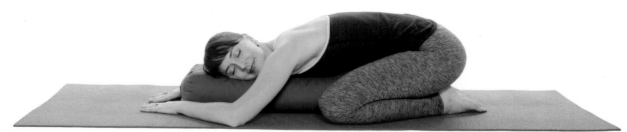

balasana ▲ restorative child's pose, position b

- Settle in deeply, slowing your breath. Imagine the simplicity of being a baby, where all you have to do is just be.

- If your shoulders pinch when extending your arms, widen the distance between your hands until you are comfortable.

- To make it even more restful, widen your knees and place a bolster under your chest (position B).

Benefits

- Promotes digestion and massages lower organs

- Calms and quiets the nervous system

- Cools the body down from practice

- Brings deep connection with Self

Avoid or Use Caution

- Advanced pregnancy

- Knee, ankle, or hip injury

Savasana: Corpse Pose

While nearly all practice should end in Savasana, this is especially true for the root chakra. Here you may completely surrender into gravity and stillness, letting down into the earth and feeling the support of solidity beneath you.

1. Lie down on your mat, centering your body from head to toe.

2. Extend your tailbone down toward your feet.

3. Arrange your arms and legs symmetrically alongside your body, palms facing upward.

4. Center your head over your torso, lengthening the back of the neck.

5. Roll your shoulder blades underneath you so your shoulders move down toward your feet.

Guidelines

- Allow yourself to surrender deeply while remaining awake and alert.

- Follow the lines of solidity in your body. Feel your body's edges and weight.

- Feel how the earth plane holds you perfectly.

- Be grateful for your body as the vehicle that carries you through life and through your practice.

- Allow your body to rest and receive nourishment from the earth.

Benefits

- Gives the body deep rest

- Allows the body to integrate your practice

- Promotes surrender and receptivity

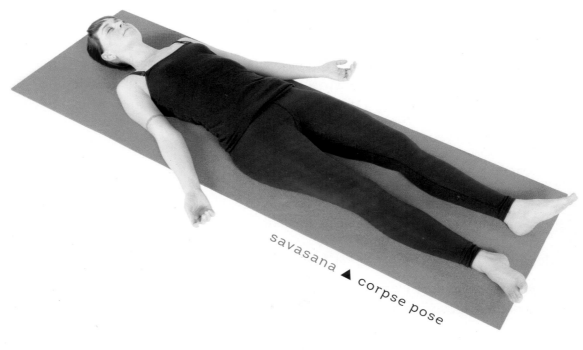

savasana ▲ corpse pose

First Chakra Posture Flow

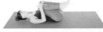

Apanasana: Knees to Chest Pose

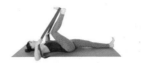

Opening the Leg Channels

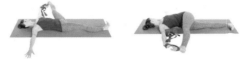

Supta Padangusthasana: Reclining Hand to Big Toe Pose

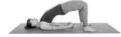

Setu Bandha Sarvangasana: Bridge Pose

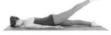

Salabhasana: Locust and Half Locust Pose

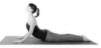

Bhujangasana: Cobra Pose

Adho Mukha Svanasana: Downward Facing Dog Pose

Uttanasana: Standing Forward Fold

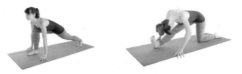

High Lunge and Reverse Lunge

Standing Bioenergetic Grounding

Utkatasana: Awkward Chair Pose

Utkata Konasana: Goddess Squat

Vrksasana: Tree Pose

Utthita Hasta Padangusthasana: Extended Hand to Toe Pose

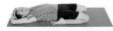

Supta Virasana: Reclining Hero Pose

Siddhasana: Baby Cradle Pose

Janu Sirsasana: Head to Knee Forward Bend

Paschimottanasana: Seated Forward Bend

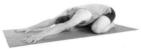

Balasana: Child's Pose

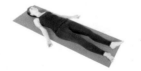

Savasana: Corpse Pose

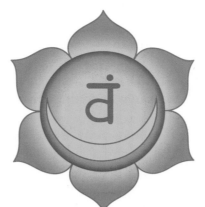

Svadhisthana
ONE'S OWN PLACE

Element	Water
Principle	Polarity
Purposes	Movement, flow, expansion, pleasure
Properties	Flowing, feeling, changeable, yielding, pleasurable
Body parts	Hips, sacrum, abdomen, sexual organs, inner thighs, knees, and joints
Practices	Opening and widening the hips, tuning in to sensation and feeling as a guide, movement in general, working with polarities
Actions	Inward rotation of thighs, balancing polarities, especially expansion/contraction, rooting down/lifting up, and opening to flow, fun, and play
Poses	Hip openers, forward bends, splits
Masculine	Extending, seeking, penetrating, cleansing, holding
Feminine	Feeling, receiving, attracting, nurturing, passionate
Deficient	Rigid, stiff, dry, numb
Excessive	Poor containment, watery, sloppy, indulgent
Balanced	Full yet contained, graceful movement

Align...

*It is not how far you move into a pose
but how deeply you feel the pose that
you are in.* ~ ANODEA JUDITH

Once you enter the temple of the body and establish your ground in chakra one, the next step is to align your body along the central axis that runs through your core, called the sushumna. In yoga, alignment means finding the optimal arrangement between various parts of your body to maximize the flow of prana and grace. Your sushumna is the most direct connection between the polarities of heaven and earth, and the central organizing channel for aligning various parts of your being: your emotions and will, your head and your heart, your mind and your body, your values and your actions.

Chakra yoga seeks to define alignment from the inside, by feeling the flow of prana through the body and finding the best way to enhance that flow through the core and the chakras. You could call it alignment for the subtle body. It's where the sacred architecture of the soul aligns with the architecture of the body. While a good yoga teacher will point out instructions for body alignment in various poses, ultimately alignment is something you feel when the ease of a pose clicks into place, opening you to the grace of a pose.

Alignment is how you set up the movement of energy between where you are and where you want to go. When you travel in a car, for example, your journey may have many twists and turns, yet you could look at a map and draw a line from one point to the other. When you drive, you align with the roads and highways that will take you to your destination. Let's look at how this plays out in moving from chakra one to chakra two.

The first chakra represents a single point. This is your ground—the place your body occupies. It is the singularity of your selfhood, as you have only one body,

2

which can occupy only one place at a time. A point gives you a location, a place on the earth. When you move from chakra one to chakra two, you go from singleness to duality, from one point to two. Two points define a line.

Alignment orients your body to a line or sometimes to several lines. When you are standing upright in a basic standing pose like Tadasana, your orientation is to the central vertical line through your core. You arrange your physical body and subtle energy symmetrically along that line, balancing left and right, front and back. By drawing a line on your mat, either literally or in your imagination, you can align your core to the center line of your mat as you bow forward or step back into a lunge. When doing a more complex pose, such as a triangle, there are several lines to consider: one through each leg, another line from base to crown, and yet another line moving across the heart and through the arms.

While simple in theory, core alignment is not always easy. Blocks in the chakras take us out of our core, fixating the energy in elaborate defenses. These blocks then manifest in the body as muscular tension, stiffness, shortened connective tissue, excess weight, pain, or chronic energetic contractions. In outer life, chakra blockages manifest as defensive or distracting behaviors that divert the energy in unhealthy ways and may leave us anxious or exhausted.

Working with Polarities

Just as a line has two points and denotes movement, the number two implies polarity. It is here where you move from the singularity of the body to the dualities of self and other, mind and body, up and down, expansion and contraction, inside and outside, and many other properties you'll see listed in the table below.

Polarities can move toward each other, such as pressing your right palm into your left palm, or they can move apart, such as stretching your arms open and moving your left and right fingertips away from each other. Likewise, a line can join two things together or it can define a separation, such as drawing a line in the sand.

In yoga, we consciously work with polarities to direct the flow of prana. You stretch your fingertips up overhead while rooting down into your heels, which creates a line of energy that flows between the higher and lower extremes of your body. You hug into your core while extending your arms outward, and this

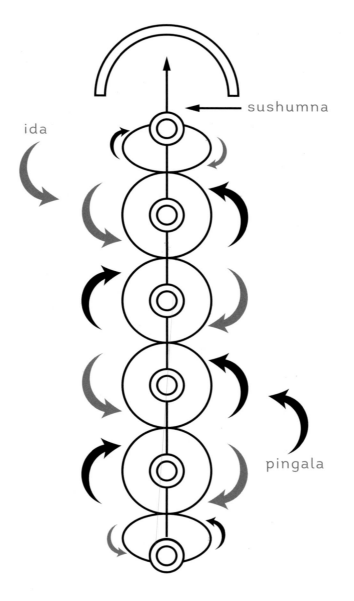

figure ▲
chakras spin as a result
of the polaric currents
ida and pingala

simultaneous contraction and expansion allows both expressions to be more dynamic. Keeping your center while utilizing polarities is one of the main tasks of the second chakra. This action takes you deeper into a sense of your core even as it expands your limits. The stronger your sense of core, the easier it is to expand. We saw in the first chapter how opening your hand chakras occurs through a combination of expansion and contraction. The table below shows a few of the polarities that yoga embraces to help energy move through your body. To expand your yoga, find both sides of a polarity within a pose. Find the effort and the surrender, the containment and the freedom. If you are creating a sequence for a class or simply for your own practice, try to embrace a balance of polarities.

Rooting down/Rising up	Containment/Freedom
Left/Right, Front/Back	Expansion/Contraction
Will/Surrender	Inside/Outside
Mind/Body	Holding/Releasing
Knowing/Feeling	Activity/Rest, Movement/Stillness
Leading/Following	Creation/Dissolution
Expression/Reception	Fullness/Emptiness
Action/Resistance	Masculine/Feminine

You could even say that it is polarity that contributes to the spinning of the chakras, as the upward and downward currents cross between the chakras through the ida and pingala nadis, spinning the chakras in opposite directions like gears, as shown in the figure. By working with both the upward and the downward currents, you actually run more energy through the chakras. As a chakra expands, its movement contributes to the movement of the chakra above or below it.

Tantra: The Yoga of Polarities

The chakra system arose during the Tantric period of yoga philosophy, approximately AD 500–1000. This was a time of weaving together many of the philosophies of India. While the West mistakenly sees Tantra as primarily sexual, it is really about the unity of archetypal polarities within the self and embraces a much larger context. Tantra embraces a weaving of the archetypal polarities of existence: mind and body, heaven and earth, spirit and matter, God and Goddess, masculine and feminine. Through the integration, or weaving, of these polarities, the fabric of life is restored into balance.

In the chakra system, as in Tantra, the most basic polarity is between *prakriti* and *purusha*, or matter and consciousness. The integration of these polarities is a path to wholeness and one of the goals of yoga. Once you are grounded, the thirst for higher consciousness awakens the upward journey and takes you to the next step.

In reflection of the true Tantric origins of the chakra system, chakra yoga benefits from utilizing the opposite forces inherent in any polarity to help balance the chakras. Some of this occurs through the way you practice your postures. Other aspects are the alignment you create between your mind and your heart, your self and others, your attitude and intention. When alignment occurs, power is generated, which will bring you from chakra two to chakra three.

Feeling and Sensation

The second chakra's Sanskrit name, *Svadhisthana*, means one's own place. You access your own place through inner sensation. Because it is internal, you cannot see it any more than you can see a thought; you can only feel it. To occupy your own place here at the second chakra is to fully feel your core rising out of your roots on its journey to the infinitely blooming lotus at the crown.

Your desires, needs, longings, and urges are said to arise from this chakra. You experience them as sensations that are pleasurable or uncomfortable, things you want to move toward or things you want to move away from. The limbic system that processes your experience seeks to increase pleasure and reduce pain. The limbic system is the mammalian brain, responsible for emotional bonding and well-being. This is a much older part of the brain than the cerebral cortex, yet it is more advanced than the earlier reptilian brain, which is focused on survival. When all is well, this mammalian part of the brain hums with an underlying feeling of connection and well-being. When there is pain, it alerts you that something is wrong and needs your attention, fixating consciousness until the pain is addressed. When pain is chronic, however, consciousness begins to shut down the sensation, and this creates blockages. Numbing the pain allows us to function, but it comes at the cost of reducing awareness.

We tend to move toward pleasure and away from pain. Likewise, our prana expands when the body and soul are in an enlivened, pleasurable state, and it contracts when we are in pain. So if you want to expand your prana, create pleasurable movement and flow throughout the body. When practicing yoga, pushing yourself into pain in order to progress further is detrimental in the long run, as it encourages a pranic contraction that can lead to injuries.

However, there is a kind of sensation bordering on pain that occurs right at your edge. It is the sweetness of stretching into intense sensation, similar to the way a good massage digs into your sore muscles. The key to finding this delicate boundary between beneficial stretching and harmful stretching occurs entirely through the realm of feeling and sensation. You can only find it from within as you move into and out of poses, sensing your edge. This internal monitoring is an essential guide to your practice.

Feeling brings consciousness into the body and simultaneously brings the body toward consciousness. It is the ultimate connector between awareness and the body. We feel where we are in space. We feel our orientation to gravity, the rise and fall of the breath, the tingling of limbs or loins. The feeling function is of crucial importance in developing your practice and coming to understand the gifts of yoga. A society that teaches us to deny our feelings and sensations leads people to hurt themselves in a yoga class; by failing to pay attention to the cues their body sends them about their limitations, people push past their limits into injury.

Sensation is also the gateway between inner and outer worlds. We see something, we hear it, smell it, touch it, or taste it, and this brings knowledge of what's outside of us into our inner consciousness—it gives us "in-form-ation" about ourselves and the world around us. This knowledge, in turn, allows us to move through space and to navigate the physical world. We reach out to the world through our senses. In reaction to pleasure or pain, we extend or recoil. Thus feeling and sensation guide our movement from inside to out and from outside to in.

Physiologically, the feelings of the second chakra move toward the satisfaction of hunger and sexuality. Emotionally, the second chakra's drive is toward connection and fulfillment. Spiritually, the urge is toward higher consciousness, liberation, and connection with the Divine.

Emotion

Sensations and feelings contribute to emotions, another aspect of the second chakra. Emotion—from the Latin *e,* meaning out, and *movere,* to move—is the moving of prana through the tissues of the body. Emotions are the result of feelings stored up in the body. For example, you may have a feeling of irritation at something, but if that feeling is repeatedly stored in your tissues, it can become the emotion of anger. I like to think of sensations as the words, feelings as the sentences, and emotions as the story that emerges.

When you repress emotion, you restrict the body's natural movements. You become rigid, creating the opposite of the second chakra's watery flow, inhibiting flexibility. Therefore, developing flexibility in your body may require willingness to feel old emotions that are stored in your body.

When you start to move more deeply into your poses, you may stumble upon pockets of emotion that spontaneously emerge without connection to current events. I remember doing a twisted triangle about six months after a car accident in which I had broken a rib. The rib had long healed and I had done that pose many times since, but when the teacher gave me an added adjustment, taking me a little deeper into the twist, suddenly the months of holding myself rigid against the pain in my ribs sprang forth in sobs. When I ask my students how many have burst into tears on a mat for no apparent reason, invariably most of them raise their hands—even men! If you can allow such emotions to flow and release, embracing their truth, your body will regain its fluidity and flexibility.

Ultimately you move from earth to water, or from solid to liquid, by melting. When you can melt into a pose internally while firmly holding the external shape, you have the combination of matter and movement that is the first and second chakra combined. It is from this combination that we create power in the third chakra.

Second Chakra Practice and Postures

Second Chakra Subtle Energy

In the second chakra you tune in to the subtle sensations within the whole body, especially within the sacral area. Learning to sense ever subtler energies is part of the refinement of moving up the chakras. The second chakra invites consciousness through sensation.

Sitting and Sensing

1. Find a comfortable seated position. Make sure you can easily keep your spine upright. If you are sitting cross-legged on the floor and your knees are higher than your hips, then sit upon a folded blanket or cushion. If you are on a chair, be sure to uncross your legs and allow each foot to touch the floor so that your hips are level.

2. Begin by extending your roots downward and your crown upward. Find the center line that runs between your crown and base: your sushumna nadi, the central axis of your inner temple. Imagine this center line extending from your vertical center all the way up to the heavens and all the way to the center of the earth.

3. As you deepen your breathing, feel as if you could draw the breath up your core on each inhalation and all the way down on each exhalation. Extend the height of your crown as you inhale, and extend the depth of your roots as you exhale. Keep the depth of your roots even as you inhale. Keep the lift you've gained even as you exhale.

4. Now that you've established your core, gently increase the curve of your sacrum, as if someone were pressing softly on your sacral vertebrae from behind. Keep your shoulders relaxed and your crown extended upward.

5. Keeping that nice curve in the sacrum, firm up the muscles of your abdomen, drawing the front and back of the second chakra toward each other.

2

6. At the same time, slightly rotate the inner thighs downward and imagine your thigh bones moving subtly apart from each other, widening your hips. In other words, the front and back of the second chakra move toward each other, while the left and right hips move apart.

7. Now move your navel forward and back slowly. Notice what happens to the thigh bones as you change the angle of your pelvis, flexing and extending your sacral vertebrae. Can you feel your thigh bones move slightly apart as you increase the curve of your sacrum and move slightly toward each other as you flatten your sacrum to the back? Can you feel the subtle movements of lifting and descending in the ribcage? What about your core—can you feel it expanding and contracting? What happens to the rest of your spine? Can you allow the movement of your pelvis to undulate all the way up in the spine, emanating from the sacrum?

8. Feel the differences between the polarities of forward and back, and find a resting place in the middle where you feel the core of your second chakra settling into your midline. Feel your own place inside the inner temple. Imagine this as the stem of your lotus, flowing serpentlike through a beautiful and sacred pool of water.

Pelvic Pulses

Because the sacrum gets stiff through too much sitting, repressed emotions, or simply guarding against injuries, it helps to begin your second chakra practice by rocking the sacrum loose and opening to the pleasurable surrender that is the second chakra's key attribute.

1. Lie on your back, bend your knees, and place your feet hip-width apart, heels within a foot of your buttocks.

2. Gently push into your feet, rhythmically rocking the pelvis forward and back effortlessly, moving from position A to position B.

3. Allow your whole body to surrender to the pulsing as if you were made of gelatin.

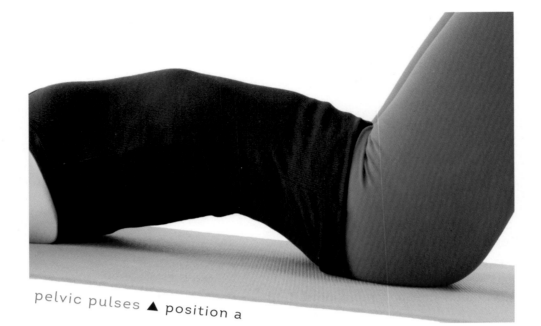

pelvic pulses ▲ position a

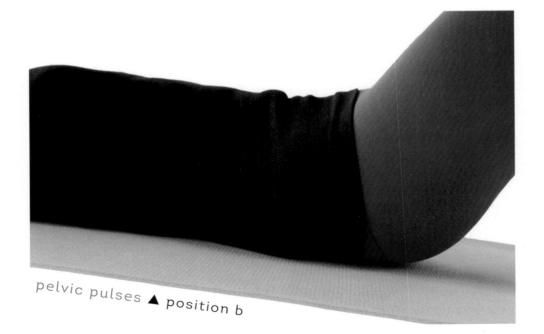

pelvic pulses ▲ position b

Guidelines

- Allow your belly to fully relax so that the movement happens from the legs only, without contracting your belly muscles.

- Open to the fluidity of the second chakra by allowing your whole body to move in a wavelike manner, undulating throughout the whole spine, with the chin bobbing up and down with each pulse.

- Find an easy rhythm that allows you to surrender without effort. Make it pleasurable.

Benefits

- Eases low back pain

- Promotes flow of cerebrospinal fluid

- Relaxing and soothing for emotional pain

- Sometimes releases held emotions

- Good for both second chakra excess and deficiency

Pelvic Breath

Now that you have loosened the pelvis, you can begin more concentrated movements for the second chakra.

1. Begin on your back with feet parallel, hip-distance apart, heels placed within a foot of your buttocks. Imagine that your shoulders, hips, knees, and feet form two parallel lines defining each side of the body.

2. With a long, slow breath, inhale and increase the curve of the sacrum as you press the tip of your tailbone down toward the floor (position A, page 127).

3. As you do so, imagine drawing the breath all the way up the front of your body.

4. With a long, slow exhalation, press the back of your
   spine into the mat, beginning with the upper back and
   moving downward, flattening the sacrum into the floor,
   and tilt your pelvis upward (position B, page 127).

5. As you complete the exhalation, press your feet into the floor
   and push energy from the earth up into your pubic bone.
   Keep the back of your sacrum pressed into the floor.

6. As you inhale repeat steps 2 and 3, and as you exhale repeat
   steps 4 and 5. Allow your breath to be full and deep. Continue
   for 3–5 minutes, stopping if you feel dizzy or uncomfortable.

Guidelines

- Allow the breath and movements to be completely correlated.
  Let the breath move the body and change the direction of your
  movement only at the top of the inhalation or the bottom of the
  exhalation. Imagine you can breathe directly through your pelvis.

- At the peak of your inhalation, the small of your back curves
  off the floor just enough to slide a hand underneath it.

- At the peak of the exhalation, press into your feet and tip the pubic
  bone upward, pushing the small of your back into the floor.

- Keep everything above the waist on the floor
  at all times. Do not lift your hips.

- Let your breath be full, deep, and slow.

Benefits

- Distributes prana up and down the torso

- Increases fluidity in the sacrum

- Relaxes lower back

2

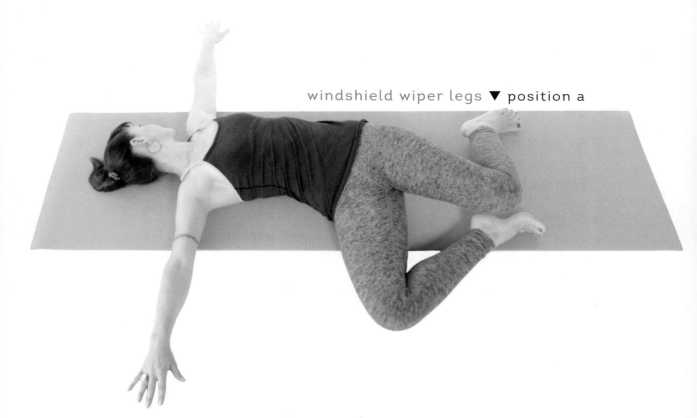

Windshield Wiper Legs

1. With your knees still bent, move your feet
   as wide apart as your yoga mat.

2. Bring your arms out to the side like a T, palms facing downward.

3. Inhale as you roll across the back of your sacrum, taking both knees
   toward the floor on the right while your head rolls toward the
   opposite side (position A). Pause and feel the stretch as you exhale.

4. Inhale and move your knees to the left, rolling your head to the
   right (position B). Pause and feel the stretch on this side.

5. Once you have moved to each side slowly, begin to pick up
   the pace. Move your knees to the right and then to the left
   more rapidly, allowing the sacral area to release and let go.

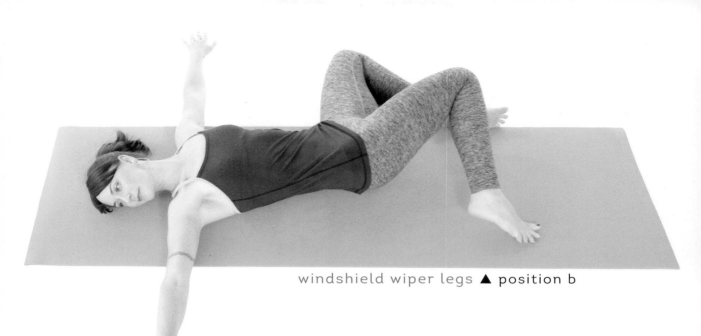

windshield wiper legs ▲ position b

Guidelines

- Be sure to feel the sensations of the floor massaging your hips and sacrum as you roll from side to side.

- Experiment with different rhythms, moving fast or slow. When moving quickly, try to be fluid and effortless. When moving slowly, pause to feel and breathe into any parts that feel blocked or tight.

Benefits

- Eases low back pain

- Massages hips and sacrum

- Lubricates hip joints

2

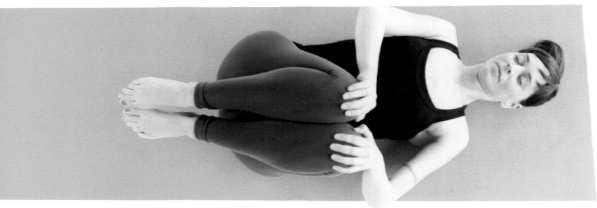

knee circles ▲

Knee Circles

1. Draw both knees into your chest, flattening
   your low back into the floor.

2. Place your hands on your knees and slowly circle your knees in a
   clockwise motion, pausing whenever you feel tightness to breathe
   into the stretch, exhaling as the knees move in toward the chest.

3. Make complete circles, feeling where your back body touches
   and lifts from the floor as you breathe and move.

4. After three slow rounds moving clockwise, change
   direction and circle counterclockwise.

5. Complete by bringing your knees back into your chest
   again, shoulders and hips toward the floor.

6. Realign your core.

2

Guidelines

- Keep your knees together, allowing both legs to move as a single unit.

- Keep your shoulders pulled down to the mat and your head centered, in line with your spine.

- Relax your feet, toes, and ankles.

- Imagine your contact with the floor is creating a circle around the back of your second chakra.

Benefits

- Lubricates hip joints

- Relaxes lower back

- Good for menstrual cramps

- Good for digestion

Avoid or Use Caution

- Lower back injury

- Hip injury or hip replacements

- Advanced pregnancy

2

Part 1: Supta Baddha Konasana

1. Lie on your back with your knees bent and your feet placed close to your buttocks.

2. Bring the soles of your feet together, and allow your knees to extend outward. If this is uncomfortable, place a pillow, a block, or a bolster beneath the side of each knee so that you can relax without being in pain.

3. Imagine opening your second chakra as you continue to breathe slowly and fully in and out, feeling your sacrum undulate with each breath. Slowly allow your inner thighs to release.

Part 2: Flapping the Butterfly Wings

1. Begin from the open position in part 1. As you exhale, press your sacrum into the mat and slowly move your knees together, turning the soles of your feet to the floor.

2. As you inhale, slowly move your knees apart, returning to the full Supta Baddha Konasana, with the soles of your feet touching each other.

3. Continue back and forth, aligning your movements with your breath. Begin slowly and then experiment with moving more quickly, still aligning the movements with your breath.

Guidelines

- If you experience trembling in your thighs, allow that to happen. In the journey between open and closed, notice exactly where the trembling occurs most and spend more time making micro-movements in that area to allow the trembling to increase.

- This exercise brings a lot of prana, or charge, into the pelvic area. If this is uncomfortable for you or if you feel overcharged in this area, stop the exercise or do some rapid movements

supta baddha konasana ▲
reclined bound angle
or butterfly pose

such as the Pelvic Pulses or the Windshield Wiper Legs to
distribute that charge throughout your whole body.

Benefits

- Promotes reproductive health

- Lubricates hip joints

- Good for second chakra deficiency, as it increases prana in the pelvis

Avoid or Use Caution

- Hip injuries or hip replacements

- Low back pain—stop with any discomfort

- Unhealed sexual trauma

2

Ananda Balasana: Happy Baby Pose

Let yourself be a playful baby just discovering your body and loving the feel of movement.

1. Begin on your back with your knees drawn in toward your chest as in Apanasana, Knees to Chest Pose (page 62).

2. Reach your arms through the inside of your shins and grab onto the outside of your feet with your hands. Lift the bottoms of your feet upward while drawing your knees in toward your shoulders.

3. Gently pull your feet toward your shoulders.

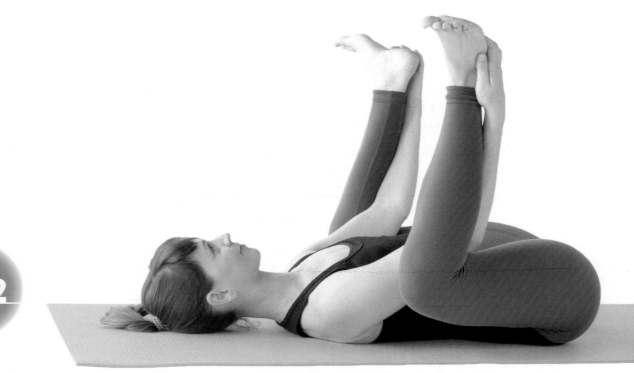

ananda balasana ▲ happy baby pose

2

Guidelines

- For people who are tight in their inner thighs, this pose may feel like a crying baby rather than a happy one. If you feel discomfort or if you can't reach your feet, place a strap over both feet and push up into it.

- Allow yourself to be playful like a baby as you rock side to side, allowing your body to find its own expression.

- Keep the four corners of your torso pulled down toward the floor.

- You can gently push your legs wider by pressing your elbows against your inner shins.

Benefits

- Promotes digestion

- Eases menstrual pain

- Lubricates hip joints

- Good prenatal pose

Avoid or Use Caution

- Hip injuries or hip replacements

- Knee injuries

Sucirandhrasana: Eye of the Needle Pose

This exercise gives you a nice massage in the hips and is a good preparation for Pigeon Pose (page 166).

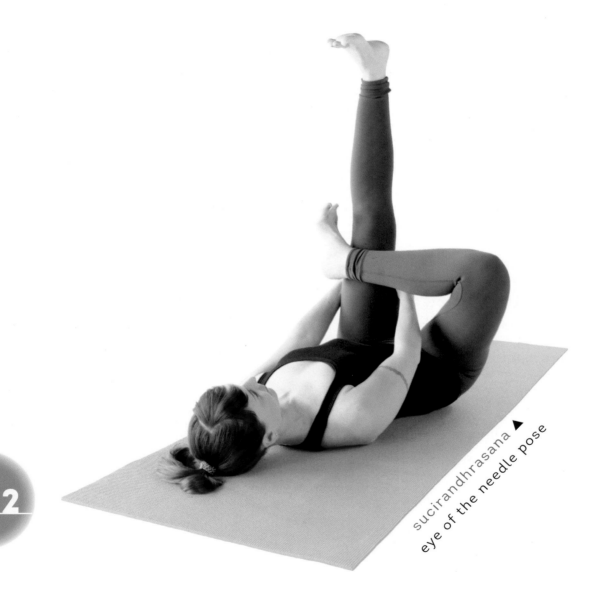

sucirandhrasana ▶
eye of the needle pose

2

1. Lying on your back, lift your left leg straight up over your left hip, flexing your foot.

2. Cross your right foot over your left leg just above the knee on the lower thigh, as shown. Keep your right foot flexed and active.

3. Reach with two hands around the back of your upright leg and gently pull it in toward your chest.

4. Breathe deeply and feel into your right hip.

5. Hold long enough to feel some release, then switch legs and repeat on the other side.

Guidelines

- You can make the pose easier by bending the left knee or using a strap over the foot.

- Pull the four corners of the torso down to the mat.

- Press your tailbone toward the back body.

- Keep both feet flexed and legs active. Extend into the upper heel.

Benefits

- Relaxing and grounding

- Releases first and second chakras

- Lubricates hip joints

- Stretches hamstrings

Avoid or Use Caution

- Hip injuries or hip replacements

- Knee injuries

Jathara Parivartanasana: Knee-Down Twist

1. Lie on your back and bring your arms to a T position, wrists level with each shoulder, palms facing downward.

2. Bend the left knee and place the left foot gently on the right thigh just above the knee. Inhale and lengthen the vertical line from crown to heel.

3. Exhale and use the right hand to guide the left knee toward the floor on the right side of your body, twisting the lower spine as you roll onto the outer right hip.

4. Turn your head to the left, the opposite side as the bent knee.

5. Lower your left hip toward the foot of your mat, lengthening the left side body.

6. Breathe and hold for several breaths, inhaling to lengthen and exhaling to move deeper into the twist.

7. Release with an inhalation, then switch legs and repeat on the other side.

Guidelines

- Attempt to keep both shoulders on the floor.

- Press the tip of your tailbone toward the back and increase the curve of the sacrum.

- Press your opposite palm into the floor to increase the twist.

- Keep your lower leg straight with the foot flexed. Press the outside of the extended foot into the mat to bring more firmness to your straight leg.

Benefits

- Releases held second chakra tension in the hips

- Improves digestion

2

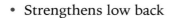

jathara parivartanasana ▼
knee-down twist

- Strengthens low back

- Lengthens the spine

- Relieves stress and deepens relaxation

- Cooling and soothing

Avoid or Use Caution

- Heavy menstruation

- Advanced pregnancy

2

Open Leg Twists

This movement was introduced to me by Selene Vega, co-author of our book *The Sevenfold Journey*. It is good for strengthening the abdominal muscles, stretching the inner thighs, massaging the lower back, and simply having fun. It takes concentration to keep your legs open as long as possible while you move side to side.

1. Lie on your back, opening your legs out to the sides with your knees straight (position A). If this is uncomfortable, bring your legs a little closer or bend the knees slightly.

2. Flex your feet and push into your heels.

3. Place your arms to the side, forming a T, with palms facing downward.

4. Allow your right leg to move toward the floor on the right side while keeping your legs as open as possible (position B).

5. When the right leg touches the floor, slowly bring the left leg over to join it, bringing your legs together on the right side (position C).

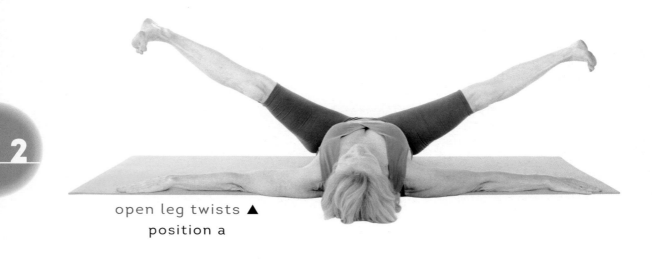

open leg twists ▲
position a

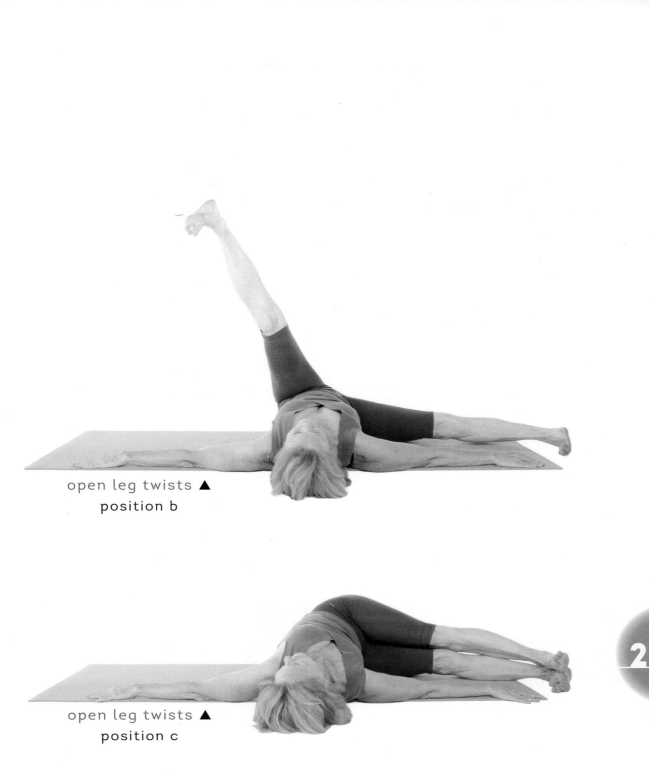

open leg twists ▲
position b

open leg twists ▲
position c

6. Pause here and line up the edges of your feet. (The top foot tends to slide back a little.)

7. Extend the tailbone toward the back body and gently arch the small of your back. Allow that movement to travel up the spine and out to your left fingertips as you turn your gaze to the left. Breathe.

8. Then, keeping both legs straight, begin to lift the left leg, moving it apart from the right leg (position B again).

9. When you reach the maximum openness of your legs, slowly move the left leg toward the floor, keeping the legs as open as possible (position D).

10. When the left leg touches the floor, the right slowly moves to join it on the left side (position E).

11. Slowly go back and forth between these positions, pausing as you go through the open position in the middle.

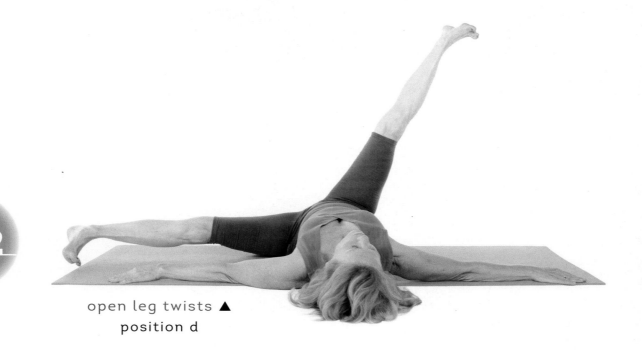

open leg twists ▲
position d

Guidelines

- Turn your head in the opposite direction from your feet as you move from side to side.

- Feel the floor massaging the back of your sacrum and your hips as you move.

- Keep your legs open as long as possible as you move from side to side.

- Keep your legs straight and your feet flexed.

- When your legs are together on one side, seek to line up the soles of your feet so that the top foot is directly above the lower foot. From this position, direct the tip of your tailbone toward the back body, increase the curve of your sacrum, and send the energy up the spine and out your outstretched hand.

Benefits

- Massages abdominal organs

- Increases core strength

- Stretches hamstrings

- Lubricates hip joints

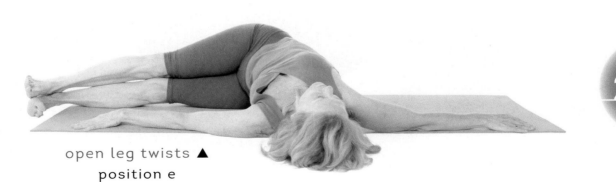

open leg twists ▲
position e

Avoid or Use Caution

- Hip injuries

- Lower back injuries

- Hernia

- Heavy menstruation

Having warmed up with the previous exercises, you can now take your second chakra stretches a little deeper. Elevate your hips onto a blanket or bolster if your inner groin muscles are too tight to keep your spine upright.

• • • • • • • • • • • • • • •

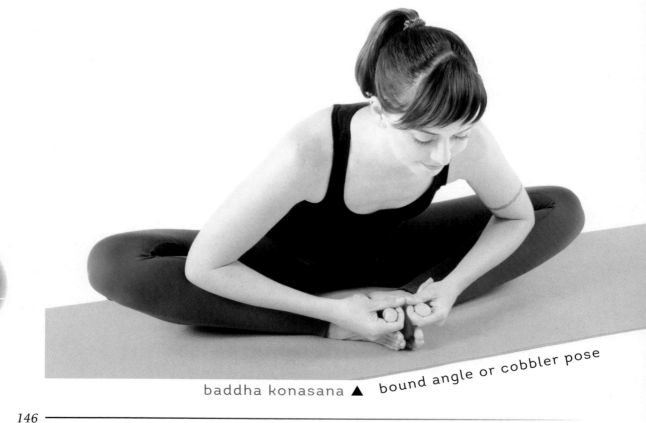

baddha konasana ▲ bound angle or cobbler pose

Baddha Konasana: Bound Angle or Cobbler Pose

1. Begin in Dandasana, Staff Pose.

2. Bend your knees and pull your feet in toward your groin as close as you can comfortably manage, bringing the soles of your feet together.

3. Wrap the first two fingers of each hand around your big toes.

4. Lengthen the front of your torso, lifting the sternum and extending upward to the crown while extending your tailbone toward the back and increasing the sacral curve. Draw the tops of the shoulders back and extend the tips of the shoulder blades downward.

5. Deepen the stretch by slowly moving the torso forward, keeping your spine lengthened and the crown lifted as you do so.

6. Come out of the pose by drawing into your core, tucking your tailbone, and gently lifting to an upright spine.

Guidelines

- If you cannot pull your torso upright as you bring your feet together, it is important to raise your hips by sitting on a folded blanket, block, or bolster.

- Keep the torso lifted and the pelvis tilted, and rotate the front of the hip bones toward the floor.

- Avoid rounding the spine in order to get your head lower down. Be satisfied with less forward movement and keeping the spine extended.

- Pause when you reach your edge, being careful not to push yourself into pain. Breathe into any tightness and allow your consciousness to explore where you might be holding. Gently relax with each breath rather than pushing yourself forward.

2

Benefits

- Opens and lubricates the hip joints

- Increases flexibility in general

- Massages abdominal organs

- Promotes digestion

- Good for second chakra deficiency or constriction

Avoid or Use Caution

- Pregnancy (second or third trimester)

- Hip injury or replacement

- Knee injury

Upavistha Konasana: Open-Leg Forward Fold

Now you are ready for deeper stretches to the hips and inner thighs. Don't worry if you don't look like Sarah, our beautiful model; most people are much less flexible. Stretching the connective tissue in these joints takes a long, long time, and must be done slowly and carefully.

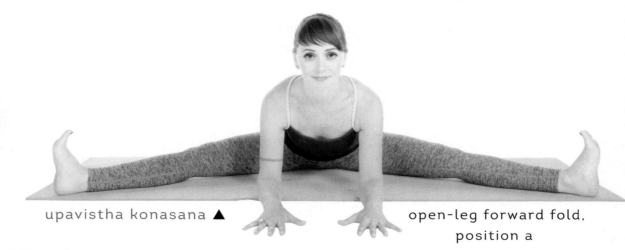

upavistha konasana ▲

open-leg forward fold,
position a

1. From Baddha Konasana, Cobbler Pose, allow your legs to straighten and open to each side to the degree of your flexibility. (Use a bolster or folded blanket if necessary.) With your spine upright, press your hands into the floor to lengthen and lift.

2. Slightly rotate your inner thighs downward, creating more space in the hip sockets. Firm up your legs by sending energy down the core of each leg out to your heels, flexing your feet and hugging the muscles of your thighs in toward the bones. Keeping your muscles active in this way will help to prevent injury and allow you to move more deeply into the pose.

3. Extend your tailbone toward the back body and tilt your pelvis to accentuate the natural curve in your sacrum. Extend the spine upward to the crown and downward into your root, hugging into your core.

4. Lift the sternum and rotate the heads of the arm bones toward the back body. Inhale.

5. Keeping your spine extended, reach your hands to the floor in front of you (position A). Draw earth energy up your arms as your hands press into the floor, drawing the heels of your hands toward your pelvis. Exhale as you slowly bend at the hips, pressing the tailbone toward the back body and being careful not to round your shoulders (position B).

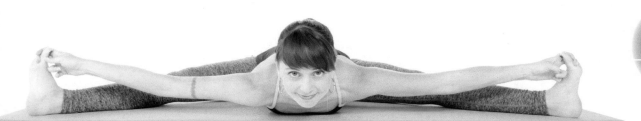

upavistha konasana ▲ open-leg forward fold,
position b

6. Find your edge and allow your breath to gently soften the tissues that are holding you back. Do not push yourself forward into pain, as the muscles will contract. Allow your consciousness to explore where you are holding. With each exhalation you can relax just a little more deeply, without pushing.

7. To come out of the pose, inhale and lift your head, allowing the rest of the torso to follow as you walk your hands back. Exhale and establish your upright position and core once again.

Guidelines

• Be sure to lift your hips onto a folded blanket or cushion if your hamstrings are too tight to sit easily with a straight spine.

• If you are a more novice practitioner, don't worry if your knees are slightly bent—you can work the back of your knees down to the floor over time. It is more important that you lengthen your spine.

• Be satisfied with less movement but maintaining an extended spine.

• Take time to settle into the pose until you feel an absence of pain or a subtle moving of your edge. This may take several minutes. Avoid pushing. If you are uncomfortable, back it off a little and let your breath do the work.

Benefits

• Deep stretch to the inner thighs and groin area

• Strengthens the lower back

• Stimulates digestion

• Massages lower organs

• Good for deficient second chakra, as it combats contraction

Avoid or Use Caution

- Hip injuries or replacements

- Hamstring injuries

- Low back injury

- Advanced pregnancy

Agnistambhasana: Fire Log or Double Pigeon Pose

1. Begin in a simple cross-legged pose with your spine erect.

2. Place your left shin directly over your right shin, aligning your shins like fire logs placed on top of each other. Sit on a folded blanket or cushion if your hips are too tight to extend your spine upright. (If it is too difficult to stack your shins directly on top of each other, you can begin with a simpler cross-legged pose.)

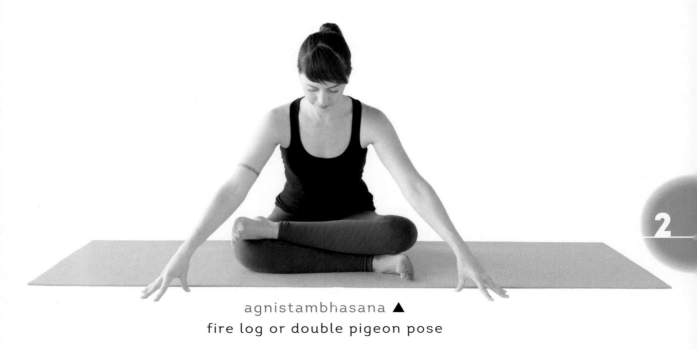

agnistambhasana ▲
fire log or double pigeon pose

3. Keeping your spine extended, reach your hands to the floor in front of you, pressing your hands into the ground. Inhale as you extend from your pelvis up into your heart and crown, pressing your tailbone toward the back body. Exhale as you slowly bend at the hips, keeping your chest lifted and sliding the shoulder blades down your back.

4. Find your edge and allow your breath to gently soften the tissues that are holding you back. Do not push yourself forward into pain. Allow your consciousness to explore just where you are holding, and slowly release that tension with your breath.

5. To come out of the pose, inhale, then lengthen and lift your head, allowing the rest of the torso to follow as you walk your hands back. Exhale and establish your upright position and core once again.

6. Switch legs and repeat on the other side, noting any differences.

Guidelines

- Place the shins on top of each other. Activate your muscles by flexing the feet.

- Extend your tailbone and shoulders toward the back body. Extend the spine simultaneously upward and downward, hugging into your core. As in the previous forward folds, keep your spine extended as you bow forward.

- Stop at your edge and breathe.

Benefits

- Promotes hip flexibility

- Combats second chakra contraction

- Lengthens the spine

- Strengthens the lower back

- Stimulates lower chakras in general

- Massages digestive and reproductive organs

Avoid or Use Caution
- Hip injuries or replacements

- Knee injuries

- Menstruation

*Now that you have given your second chakra area
a good stretch, your standing postures will feel
a little different. As you come to a stand, your
hips should feel more open and spacious.*

• • • • • • • • • • • •

Uttanasana: Standing Forward Fold

This pose was also introduced in the first chakra. For second chakra focus, press the inner edges of the feet into the mat, rotate your inner thighs toward the back, and imagine widening the back of the sacrum. Let your upper body be fluid and relaxed as it flows forward. Experiment with swaying back and forth, lifting and lowering, to feel the serpentine motion of your spine.

1. Begin in Tadasana with feet hip-distance apart, parallel
   to each other. Ground the four corners of your feet.

2. Extend your roots down and lift your crown up, aligning between
   heaven and earth through your core. Press your thighbones
   toward your hamstrings, extend your tailbone down, and lift the
   torso up out the hips, creating space in the front groin areas.

3. Open your arms out to the sides and keep the spine
   lengthened as you fold forward into the pose.

2

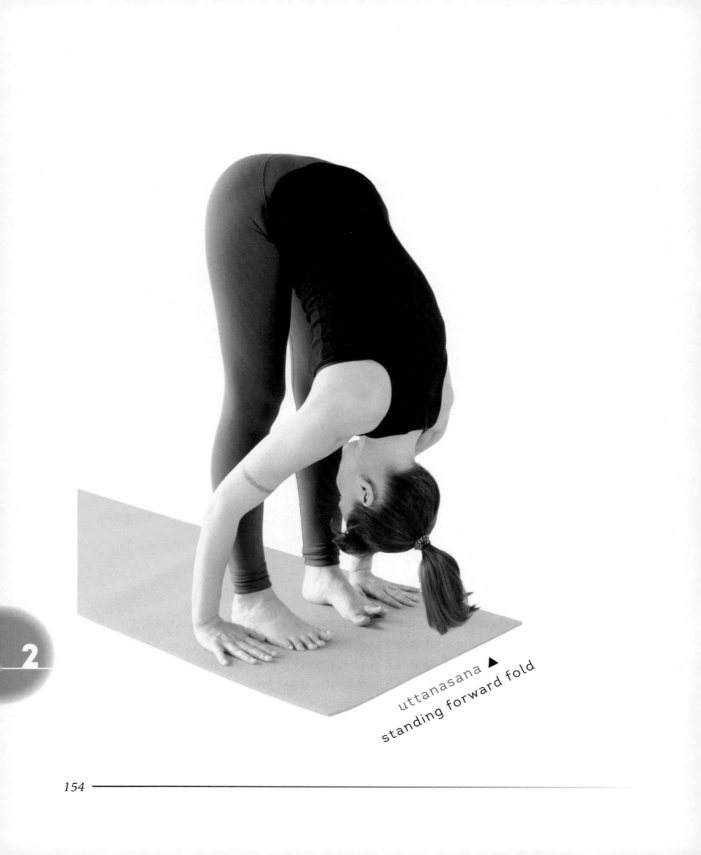

uttanasana ▶
standing forward fold

2

4. Ideally your legs are straight but your knees are not hyperextended or locked. If your knees need to bend a little, you can gently push them back over time, being careful not to push farther than the natural limits of your body.

5. Rise up out of the pose on an inhalation, softening the knees.

Guidelines

- Rotate the inner thighs toward the back, widening the pelvic floor and the back of the sacrum while lifting the sitting bones.

- Allow your legs to be strong like posts while letting your torso soften and let go. This letting go takes time and breath, so linger in this pose while you allow your torso to gradually release. Imagine space opening up between your vertebrae.

Variations

- Refer to chakra one, pages 82–83.

Benefits

- Stretches the hamstrings and calves

- Opens the hips

- Improves digestion

- Eases menstruation

- Releases back tension

- Calms the nervous system

- Cools excess heat

2

Avoid or Use Caution

- Advanced pregnancy

- Low blood pressure (can get dizzy coming back up)

- Low back injury

- Hamstring injuries

Adho Mukha Svanasana: Downward Facing Dog Pose

This pose was introduced in the first chakra. For a second chakra focus, widen the pelvic floor and the back of the sacrum with a slight inward rotation of the thighs. Experience the energy generated by having both hands and feet pushing into the mat, with a focal point in the pelvis. Draw the pubic bone back and up and firm up your belly. Alternately bend and straighten each leg, wiggling your hips.

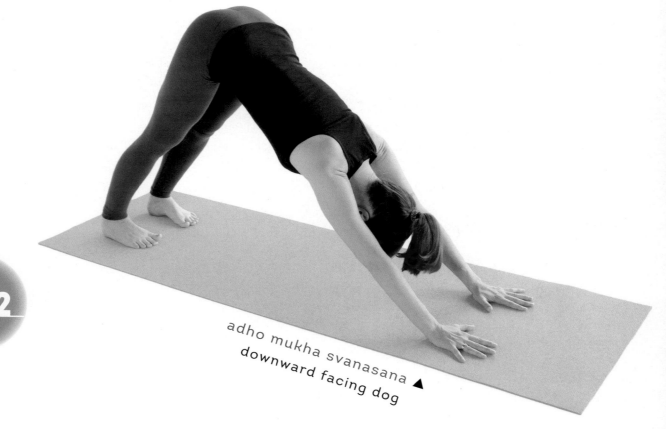

adho mukha svanasana ▲
downward facing dog

1. Begin in Table Pose. Place your palms firmly on the mat, fingers spread wide, first fingers parallel to each other, wrist creases parallel to the front of the mat.

2. Engage by tucking your toes into the mat and pushing your feet and hands into the floor. Firm up your shoulder blades, drawing them downward. Feel this engagement with the ground before you lift your hips.

3. From that engagement, lift your hips until your body forms a triangle, with the floor as the base.

4. You may wish to alternately bend and straighten your knees a few times as you "walk your dog" and wiggle your way into the pose.

5. With feet hip-width apart, press your heels down toward the mat. Don't worry if your heels don't touch; it may take years of practice to get your heels all the way down.

Guidelines

- Energize the pose by pressing both hands and feet more firmly into the floor, as if you were trying to lengthen your mat from top to bottom, distributing your weight evenly among the four corners of this pose: your two hands and two feet. Notice how this rooting action energizes the body.

- **Legs:** Hug your muscles in toward the bones, lifting your kneecaps. Press the front of your thighs toward the back, with a slight rotation of the inner thighs toward the back, creating more space in the pelvic floor and widening the back of the sacrum.

- **Arms:** The fleshy part of the hand between the thumb and first finger contains a point in Chinese medicine used for grounding. Pressing this part firmly into the ground will give you a slight inner rotation of your forearms. Simultaneously outwardly rotate your upper arms, opening the shoulders and chest. Draw the muscles of your arm up from the earth and into your shoulders.

2

- Soften the heart as you extend from the heart to your wrists and from the heart to your pelvis.

- Be wary of hyperflexion in the shoulders. Ideally, there should be a straight line from your hips to your wrists.

- Experiment with bending and straightening your knees, rising up on your toes and lowering your heels, and bending and straightening your arms to experience different dynamics in the pose.

Benefits

- Creates core strength and increases steadfastness

- Opens the arms and shoulders, stretches the hamstrings, and loosens the hips

- Improves digestion

- Energizes the body

Avoid or Use Caution

- Late-term pregnancy

- Carpal tunnel syndrome

- High blood pressure

- Headaches

Anjaneyasana: Deep Lunge

1. From Downward Facing Dog Pose, inhale as you step your left foot forward, placing it between your hands, in line with the left hip.

2. Lower your back knee down to the floor and place your hands on your front knee as you deepen the stretch by allowing your front knee to move forward. Point your tailbone downward and draw the front and back of the second chakra toward the midline.

3. On an inhalation lift your arms up overhead and arch
   back, palms facing each other (position A).

4. To come out of the pose, lower your hands back down to the floor and
   step back to Downward Facing Dog or step forward to Uttanasana.

5. Repeat on the other side.

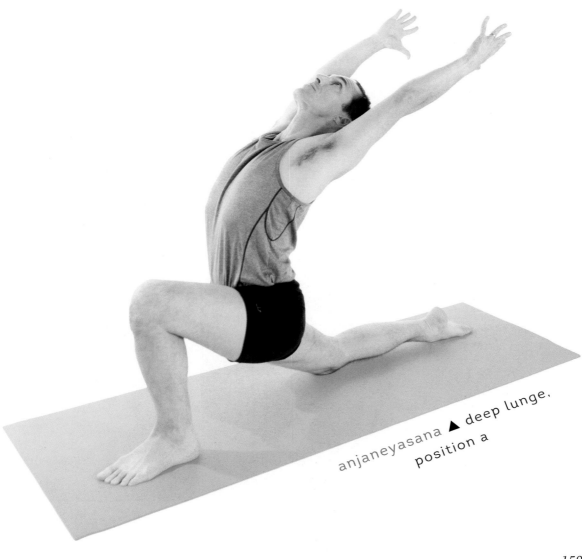

anjaneyasana ▲ deep lunge, position a

Guidelines

- Press both the front foot and back knee into the mat and energetically draw them toward each other.

- Allow your shoulders and chest to be relaxed and your head lifted, with eyes gazing straight ahead. Point the tips of your shoulder blades down your back.

- Inwardly rotate the thigh of the back leg and draw the back hip slightly forward.

- Keep both hips and shoulders square to the front, avoiding side rotation.

- For a deeper stretch, bend your back leg in toward your buttocks (position B).

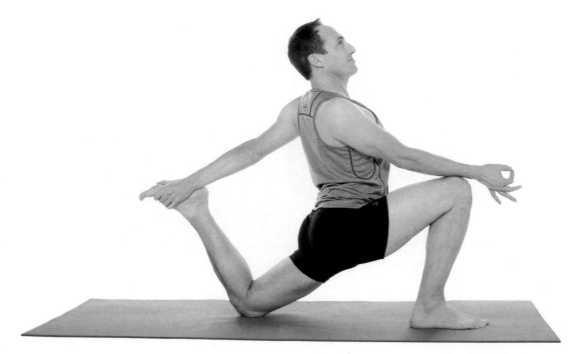

anjaneyasana ▲ deep lunge,
position b

Benefits

- Opens second chakra by stretching hip flexors and quadriceps

- Promotes balance and steadfastness

- Energizing

- May relieve sciatica

- Excellent for athletes and runners

- Stimulates the heart chakra

Avoid or Use Caution

- Heart problems

- Hernia

- Hip injury

Uttan Pristhasana: Lizard or Humble Warrior Pose

1. From Uttanasana, step your right foot back to a lunge, with your hands on either side of your front foot. Your left knee should be directly above your left ankle.

2. Lower your right knee down to the mat. (You can raise it again later if you want to deepen the pose.)

3. Bring your left arm inside your left leg and place your left hand next to your right hand on the inside of your left foot. If this is enough stretch for you, stop here.

4. To deepen the pose, lower onto your forearms, hugging your front knee in close to the shoulder.

5. To come out of the pose, straighten your arms, take your left hand back to the outside of your left knee, and step back to Downward Facing Dog or step forward to Uttanasana, Standing Forward Fold.

6. Repeat on the other side.

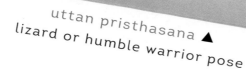

uttan pristhasana ▲
lizard or humble warrior pose

Guidelines

- Tone up your abdomen, hugging into the core. Lengthen the spine and extend from the pelvis up to the heart.

- Draw the hip of the back leg slightly forward and the hip of the bent knee slightly toward the back to keep the hips square to the front of the mat.

- To increase the stretch, tuck your back toes into the mat, lift your back knee off the floor, and pull your back heel farther toward the rear of the mat.

Benefits

- Opens the second chakra by opening the groins and stretching the hip flexors

- Tones abdominal organs and strengthens the legs

Avoid or Use Caution

- If you have low blood pressure, keep the head higher than the heart

- Knee or hip injuries

- Pregnancy

2

Open-Leg Child's Pose to Hanging Cobra

This is not a common yoga flow, but it's a great hip opener and one I have found to embrace both the masculine and feminine aspects of the second chakra—important qualities at this level!

Part A: Open-Leg Child's Pose

1. Sit upright on your heels, spine erect.

2. Separate your knees about as wide as your mat, keeping your big toes next to each other. (**Note:** you may wish to put a blanket under your knees if you are on a hard floor.)

3. Extend your roots down and your crown up, aligning with your core.

4. Keeping your spine lengthened, bow forward between your knees, extending your arms toward the front of your mat.

5. Allow your sacrum to relax as your hips sink down between your thighs.

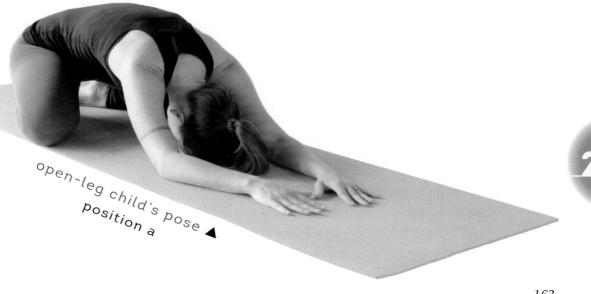

open-leg child's pose ▲
position a

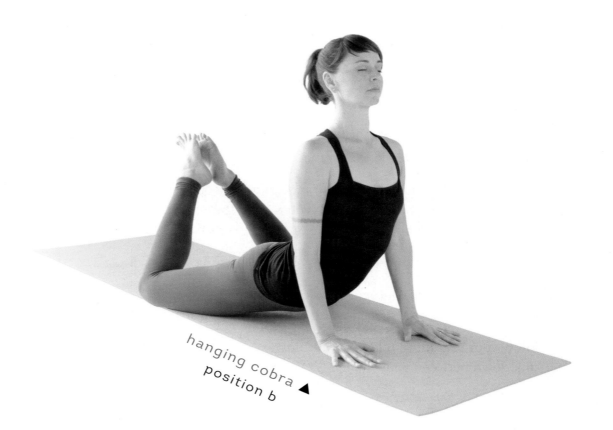

hanging cobra
position b ▲

Part B: Hanging Cobra

1. Lift your hips and come onto your hands and knees while keeping your knees as wide as the sticky mat.

2. With weight on your wrists, allow your pelvis to come forward, hanging in the air.

3. Roll your shoulders back, outwardly rotate your upper arms, lift your chest and head, and look up.

4. Pressing your hands into the floor, twist side to side to accent the stretch on the right and left groin separately, then return to the central position.

2

Part C: Vinyasa

1. Go back and forth slowly between part A and part B, taking time to really feel your stretch in each position, including the transition between them. Inhale as you move forward and exhale as you move back.

Guidelines

- Feel the feminine, receptive aspect of the second chakra in the open-leg child's pose. Feel the masculine extension in the hanging cobra.

- For those who are highly flexible, your pelvis might go all the way to the floor. Raise your upper body higher by placing each hand on a block.

- Take time while hanging to fully release the lower back. Press your chest forward as in a regular cobra, rolling your upper arms outward.

Benefits

- Stretches the front of the groins and opens the hips

- Lubricates the hip joints

- Moves from active to passive in the second chakra

Avoid or Use Caution

- Low back injury or soreness

- Pressing the pelvis forward with the legs wide can scrunch the lower back if held too long. The best benefit of the pose comes from twisting side to side.

Eka Pada Kapotasana: Pigeon Pose

1. Begin in Downward Facing Dog.

2. Pressing firmly into your hands, lift your right leg up into the air behind you, knee straight, pointing your toes. Extend from the heels of your hands all the way to your right toes as you inhale deeply.

3. Exhale and swing your right leg through between your hands, bending the knee and placing the outer edge of the right calf on the mat, moving your right foot as far forward as you can comfortably manage without discomfort.

4. Extending your left leg straight behind you, inwardly rotate the top of your back thigh so that the front of the entire leg, knee, ankle, and foot press downward onto the mat.

5. Extend your tailbone toward the back end of your mat. Press your hands down, lift your crown, move the head of the armbones toward the back, and take a deep breath (position A).

6. Exhale and lower your upper torso down to the floor, keeping your spine lengthened and your core in line with the center of your mat. You may use your hands to make a pillow for your forehead or extend your arms straight in front of you, resting on your forehead (position B).

7. Remain here for several minutes to get the full benefit of the pose. Practice letting go with each breath.

8. To come out of the pose, inhale, lift your head, and walk your hands back to either side of your front leg. Press your hands into the mat and lift your hips up into Downward Facing Dog.

9. Repeat on the other side.

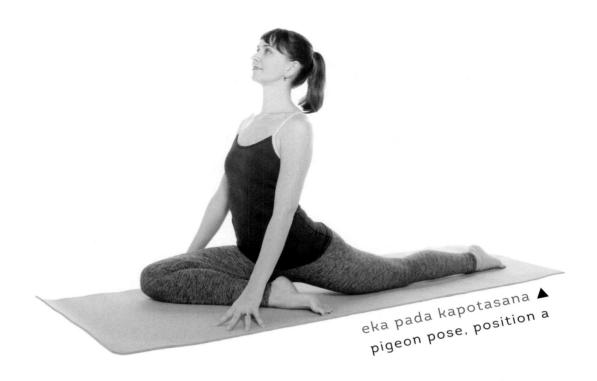

eka pada kapotasana ▲
pigeon pose, position a

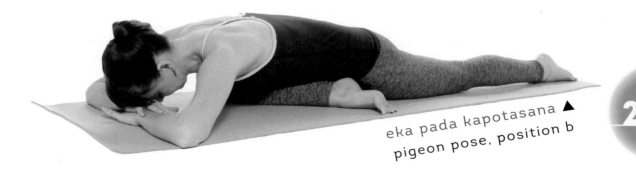

eka pada kapotasana ▲
pigeon pose, position b

2

Guidelines

- It is important for the body to be warmed up before entering this pose. Good warm-up poses for Pigeon Pose are the seated poses listed above, such as the ankle to knee hip stretch, or Firelog Pose, as well as lunges and forward folds.

- Gently work the outside of your front foot forward toward the top of your mat until you find your edge of flexibility. The advanced form of the pose is with the shin parallel to the top edge of the mat, but few people can do this without years of practice.

- Keep your front foot flexed and active. You can use your hands to move your front foot forward to find your edge.

- If your hips are not square to the mat, extend the back hip slightly forward and pull the front hip slightly back. Press the front of the hip points down into the mat.

- Square your shoulders by facing directly forward, aligning your spine with the midline of your mat.

- Point your tailbone to the rear of your mat and extend your crown toward the front of your mat.

- For beginners, it may be helpful to place a folded blanket under the hip on the side with the bent knee.

- To increase the stretch, tuck your back toes into the mat, lift your back knee to a straight leg, and pull your heel toward the rear of the mat.

- Stay in this pose a little longer than some others. It takes a while for the hips to let go. Use your breath to relax in the pose.

Variations

There are many variations in this pose:

1. Bend your back knee and lift your foot toward your buttocks. Catch your foot in the hand on the same side and press on the top of the foot to deepen the stretch (position C).

2. Catch your back foot in the elbow crease of your arm on the same side. Reach back with the opposite arm and interlace your fingers. Be sure to square your shoulders to the front, as reaching back tends to twist the body toward the back leg (position D).

3. The full pose reaches back with both hands and holds the foot to the back of the head. This is not shown, as the model couldn't do this pose; it is very difficult.

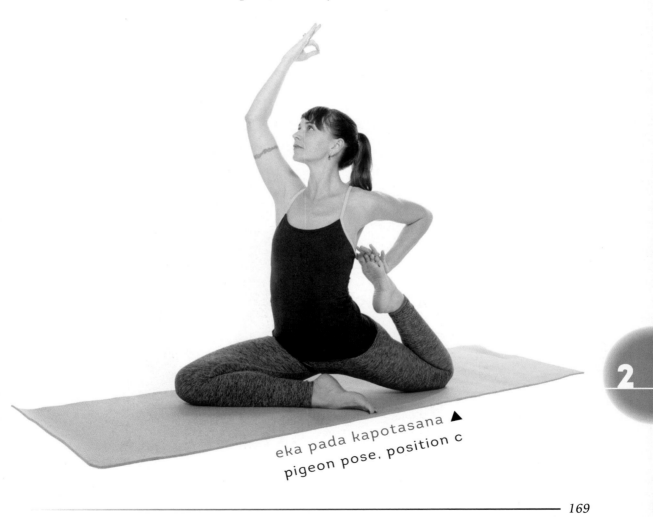

eka pada kapotasana ▲
pigeon pose, position c

Benefits

- Opens the second chakra and releases stagnation from the hip joints

- Energizes the whole body

- Promotes spinal flexibility and is good preparation for backbends

- Stretches thighs, groins, back, and psoas

- Opens chest and shoulders

Avoid or Use Caution

- Hip or knee injuries or hip replacements

- Advanced pregnancy

- Shoulder injury, if reaching for the back foot

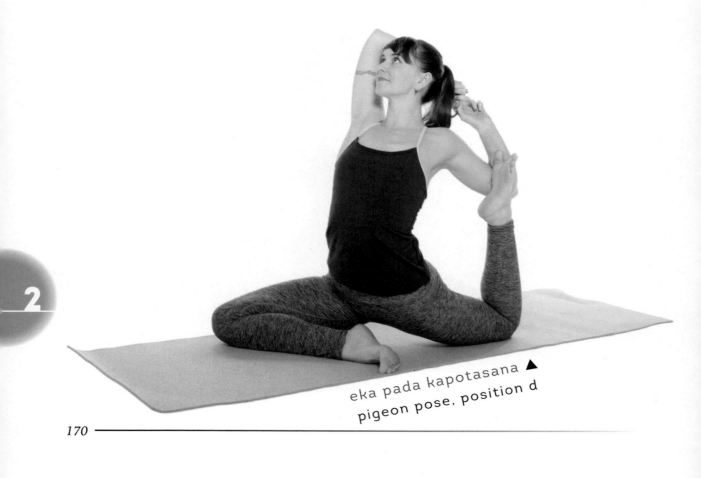

eka pada kapotasana ▲
pigeon pose, position d

Supta Baddha Konasana: Savasana with Open Legs

The second chakra focus in Savasana reflects the element of water. Direct your consciousness toward fully feeling the experience of your body. Allow yourself to surrender to the internal rivers of prana within you. Notice where you are flowing freely, and allow that feeling of fluidity to flow toward any places of tension or stagnation. Notice the profound state of pleasure that can occur when the body relaxes into its own flow after a good practice. Let that pleasure register deeply in your consciousness and become a baseline to your day.

For a second chakra Savasana option, consider lying in Supta Baddha Konasana. If this is uncomfortable, support each knee with a bolster. Make sure there is no strain on your inner thighs and you can completely relax.

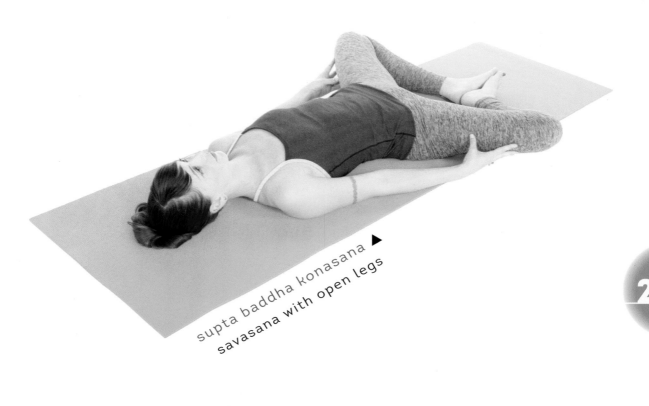

supta baddha konasana ▶
savasana with open legs

Second Chakra Posture Flow

Pelvic Pulses

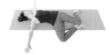

Windshield Wiper Legs

Knee Circles

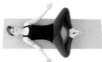

Supta Baddha Konasana: Butterfly Pose

Ananda Balasana: Happy Baby Pose

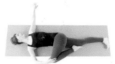

Sucirandhrasana: Eye of the Needle Pose

Jathara Parivartanasana: Knee-Down Twist

Open Leg Twists

Baddha Konasana: Bound Angle or Cobbler Pose

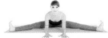

Upavistha Konasana: Open-Leg Forward Fold

Agnistambhasana: Fire Log Pose

Uttanasana: Standing Forward Fold

Adho Mukha Svanasana: Downward Facing Dog

Anjaneyasana: Deep Lunge

Uttan Pristhasana: Lizard Pose

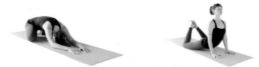

Open-Leg Child's Pose to Hanging Cobra

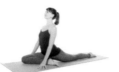

Eka Pada Kapotasana: Pigeon Pose

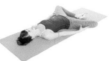

Supta Baddha Konasana: Savasana with Open Legs

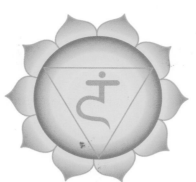

Manipura
LUSTROUS GEM

Element	Fire
Principle	Combustion
Purposes	Energy, strength, will, mastery
Properties	Heat, strength, power, deliberateness, energy
Body parts	Ribs, adrenal glands, solar plexus, digestive organs
Practices	Strengthening the will through discipline, using polarities to create power, using movement to generate energy, strengthening the core, balancing will and surrender
Actions	Lengthening side bodies, combining matter and movement to generate energy, guiding pranic flow toward desired results, overcoming inertia, practice, practice, practice
Poses	Balance, warriors, torso toners, twists, plank
Masculine	Initiating, willing, forcing, making
Feminine	Warmth, dexterity, skill, radiance
Deficient	Weak, passive, tired
Excessive	Controlling, dominating, constantly active
Balanced	Mastery

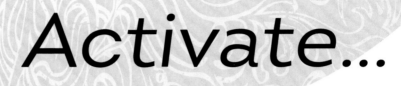

Activate...

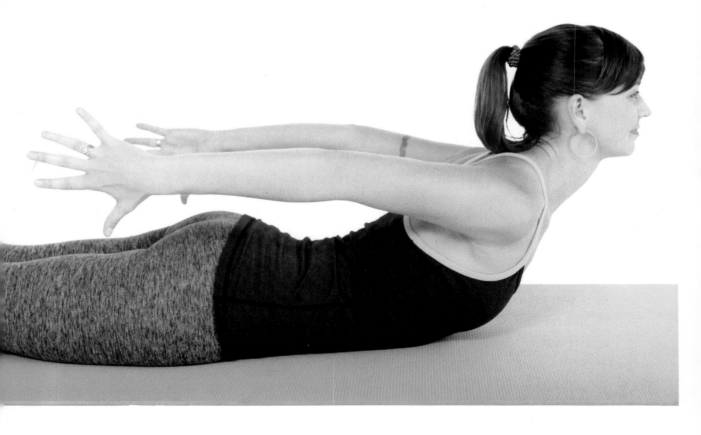

To be a warrior is to learn to be
genuine in every moment of your life.
~ *CHOGYUM TRUNGPA*

After entering your body in chakra one and aligning your core between heaven and earth in chakra two, the next step is to activate your energy body and direct that energy in a way that is masterful. Now, at the third chakra, we add a third point to the two points of the line we discussed in chakra two. With a third point we define an area. Finding more room in your inner temple, Kundalini begins to dance, building up energy.

The first chakra represents getting inside your vehicle and learning how it operates. The second chakra is about getting your vehicle moving. You could push the car down a hill to do that, and as long as nothing is in the way and the road flows downhill, it will keep moving. But to take a successful journey you need a way to steer the vehicle, as well as provide an engine to keep it energized so it can climb hills or accelerate when necessary. This is the task of what is often called the power chakra, located in the solar plexus.

Let's look at it another way: the first chakra gives you your foundation, a ground to root into in order to reach the stars. Without the solidity of matter, you have no edges or boundaries for containment, no way to build up energy, nothing to push against in order to rise.

In the second chakra you get matter moving—you move your body, your joints, your breath, your emotions, and your prana. The faster you move, the more heat you create. This heat is caused by friction: matter moving against matter. So matter and movement combine to generate the element of the third chakra, which is fire.

In Vedic mythology, Agni is the god of fire. His name is the first word in the most ancient of texts, the Rig Veda. He is the primordial fire that sparks all other fires, from which we get the word *ignite*. As the receiver of sacrifices, he is ever young, his energy constantly renewed by the flame of life. His vehicle is the animal related to the third chakra, the ram. Invoke Agni when you begin your third chakra practice to ignite your fire.

Having a strong internal fire gives you the spark to do anything in your life. In yoga internal fire is called *tapas*, the fire generated through practice, discipline, austerities, concentration, focused activity, and personal will. Once generated, tapas becomes a spiritual fire that burns through blockages. As a yogic principle, tapas is often joined with *svadhyaya*, self-inquiry and study, and *isvara-pranidhana*, devotion to the Divine.

Cultivating Fire in the Body

Earlier you learned how to open your hand chakras by rapidly opening and closing your palms. Now rub your open palms firmly together for thirty seconds or so. Notice how this creates heat. It takes just the right combination of resistance and freedom for heat to be generated. If there was too little movement as you rubbed your hands or if you didn't press your palms together firmly enough, you wouldn't generate much heat. Too much movement and the energy is scattered. Too much containment and the energy doesn't even get started. This combination of matter and movement is the combined qualities of chakra one and chakra two. Together they create the fire of chakra three.

Move your body rapidly and you get warm. Things start to loosen up, which is why a good yoga class always starts with a warm-up practice. Your joints lubricate, your cells metabolize, and you may even sweat. Energy is generated and released, and the rest of your practice involves channeling that energy into different parts of the body. This is the third chakra in action.

The subtle body in which the chakras reside is often called the energy body because it consists of a subtle energy or life force. The chakras handle that life force, acting much like the capacitors and resistors of electronic equipment. The chakras either increase the energy (capacitate) or slow it down (resist). The chakras are not the source of the energy, but they are the organizers and managers

3

of it. The energy lies within you, but, like a furnace, it needs to be ignited and channeled appropriately.

Activating your energy body means that you are igniting the prana in your body and distributing it wherever you want it to go—guided by your will. This awakens the will as a director within you, channeling your energy to rise up the spine or to move downward, moving energy into your core or expanding it out into your limbs. Energy is the fuel for action and the fire of the third chakra. Without energy the will has no power behind it. Intentions go unfulfilled, and the strength of the will is diminished.

To generate energy in your practice is to find just the right combination of resistance and freedom, containment and release, holding on and letting go. This is the art of yoga. Its goal is mastery: mastery of yourself and your life. All it takes is consciousness, effort, and many, many years of practice.

Your motive in working should be to set
others, by example, on the path of duty.

• • • • • • • • • • • • • •

THE BHAGAVAD GITA

Power and Mastery

Humans are the only animals to control fire. We alone are capable of complex acts of will. We alone can rise above our instincts, choose to evolve, and make changes in our world. As humanity has evolved through time, we are now at a place where individuals have more power than at any time in history. With this power we can save or destroy our world.

What do we do with this power? While the answers to this question are many and varied, the yoga practitioner develops their power for the purpose of mastery. If activation of the energy body is the task of the third chakra, mastery is its ultimate goal. This occurs through a precise combination—honed and cultivated over time—of will and surrender, purpose and practice.

Mastery is the ability to transform intention into reality, live deliberately, and create your life on purpose. But even more important, mastery is fulfilling your intentions with ease. If a portrait painter captures the likeness of a child's face and does so in a few quick strokes, you would say he or she is a master painter. A virtuoso singer or piano player can let go fully into the music because the mechanics of singing or playing no longer require effort or concentration. A true master creates effortlessly. A master at yoga moves into a pose with grace and elegance, making it look easy. Diligent practice, dedicated to a purpose, is needed to bring this about.

In the practice of yoga, mastery occurs when years of effort and discipline reach a point of ease. In the Yoga Sutras Patanjali states: "Perfection in an asana is achieved when the effort to perform it becomes effortless and the infinite being within is reached."[7] In yoga terminology this is a combination of *abhyasa*, or effort, and *vairagya*, detachment. We practice with focused determination yet release any attachment to a goal.

Practice requires intense effort and discipline. It takes a strong will to carry you through the months and years of effort to reach the place where something becomes effortless. Over time it gets easier; there is more appreciation for the subtleties of what you are doing. There is more grace and enjoyment in the process, hence more reward. You get the feeling of yoga in your bones, then long for that feeling when you miss your practice for a few days.

Will is the engine of the third chakra. Will overcomes the inertia of what is, so you can move toward what you want it to be. As the third chakra is a higher level than the second, will trumps the desire of the second chakra when desire wants to move in another direction. We may desire to stay in bed in the morning, but the will gets us up and moving instead, and soon we no longer feel sleepy. But you have to train the will to become stronger than the desires of the second chakra. Will utilizes the energy created by matter and movement coming up from the bottom two chakras.

But will also requires intention, which originates in consciousness and descends down to the third chakra to meet the energy rising up. You set an intention to meditate or to hold a pose for a certain amount of time or to simply get to class on time, but it takes energy to fulfill that intention. When your will can successfully harness your energy into your intention, you have true power.

---

7 Yoga Sutra 1.47 as translated by B. K. S. Iyengar in *Light on the Yoga Sutras* (London: Thorsons, imprint of HarperCollins, 1996), 159.

Cultivate your energy so that it is available to you. Set an intention, and allow your energy to flow into it. Develop your will by aligning with your purpose, picking goals, and achieving them. Build your strength by using your muscles—both the muscles of your body and the muscles of your will. Become the director of your life and you will be its creator as well.

The Three Gunas

In the second chakra you utilize polarities as a way to find internal alignment. In the third chakra you move from harnessing polarities to exploring the basic trinity of matter, energy, and consciousness. In yoga terminology these fundamental aspects of reality relate to the three *gunas*, or qualities, which are *tamas*, *rajas*, and *sattvas*.

Like three strands of a braid, matter, energy, and consciousness are always present in various combinations. In meditation, for example, the sattvic guna is most present, as consciousness is heightened while the body and its actions are calmed. In active vinyasa practice or any vigorous exercise, the rajasic guna is more present, as you are moving and expending energy, but you may not be thinking very much. And when looking at the physical aspect of the body's resistance, or even its bones and flesh, you are dealing with the tamasic guna. Eating and sleep are very tamasic, yet all three gunas are present in any experience and in every pose. There is always an aspect of consciousness present, there is always a flow of energy, and there is always the container of the physical body subject to gravity.

In addition, the chakras themselves relate to these three gunas, as the lower two chakras are more tamasic, the middle three chakras more rajasic, and the upper two chakras more sattvic. To be well balanced, you want to honor each of these aspects in your practice—from your opening meditation to your peak poses to your Savasana at the end.

Classically, the three gunas are not seen as equal in importance, with the tamas guna often viewed as an obstacle to spiritual growth. Personally, I do not agree; I feel that the grounding and containment of the body and the physical world is equally important, even essential to supporting the other two gunas. However, if the tamas guna is dominating, then indeed we feel sluggish and dull and lack the energy needed to ignite the will.

The following chart looks at how these three gunas play out in relation to yoga:

TAMAS	RAJAS	SATTVAS
Matter	Energy	Consciousness
Inertia at rest	Inertia in movement	Balancing intermediary
Chakras 1 and 2	**Chakras 3, 4, and 5**	**Chakras 6 and 7**
Personal chakras	Interpersonal chakras	Transpersonal chakras
Body	**Energy**	**Consciousness**
Ayurvedic Constitution		
Kapha	Pitta	Vata
Yoga Focuses		
Postures, body alignment	Movement, vinyasa	Meditation, stillness
Diet, nutrition, exercise	Breath, pranayama	Philosophy, understanding
Rest, stillness	Emotion, action, karma yoga	Awareness, study
Purposes		
Foundation	Energy	Intelligence
Stability	Movement	Consciousness
Containment	Power	Guidance
Consistency	Will	Intention
Steadfastness	Vitality	Knowledge
	Prana	Wisdom
	Charge	Awareness
Student Experiences		
Form, function, tension, pain, resistance, freedom, tightness, grounding, alignment, substance	Charge, emotion, trembling, expansion, heat, movement, tingling	Awareness, insight, awakening, knowledge, insight, memory, changes in belief or story

Sensing the Subtle Energy

Effort generates energy because it requires energy. When the effort ceases, the energy generated can then flow into the tissues. When charge is flowing freely through the body, it feels like gentle warmth pervading your flesh. It is this subtle energy that you want to distribute into various parts of the body through the calm direction of the will.

1. Stand upright, placing your palms against a wall at about the height of your solar plexus, or third chakra. This makes your forearms parallel to the floor, with your elbows by your sides.

2. Find your vertical alignment and core as if it were the trunk of a tree and your arms were branches extending out from the trunk. Root down through your legs and find your ground. Lift up into your crown.

3. Press firmly into the wall until you feel a mild trembling in your arms. Remember to breathe deeply as you do so. Be careful not to lean forward, but keep your core upright. Push out from your core, but don't push the core itself forward.

4. Hold for as long as you comfortably can, then very slowly relax your arms while keeping your hands in place on the wall.

5. Feel the difference between energy generated from effort and energy flowing from the relaxation of effort. Play with that difference by pushing again for a few seconds, then releasing again. Imagine how you might do this in a pose.

6. For an interesting variation, try this with another person. Stand upright, facing a partner, pressing your palms into each other at the height of your third chakras. Look eye to eye as you do so and be fully in your power, facing another who is fully in their own power.

7. Ignite the energy by pushing from your core into each other's hands. Release the energy slowly without pulling your hands away—just release the effort. Notice the difference. Can you feel energy flowing both within you and between you?

Third Chakra Practice and Postures

Uddiyana bandha contracts the third chakra area of the belly and draws prana up into the heart. It also massages many of the digestive organs, thereby improving digestion. While it is good for third chakra excess, make sure you practice this on an empty stomach.

1. Begin in Tadasana. Bend your knees slightly and gently round your back, placing your hands on the front of your thighs, above your knees.

2. Inhale deeply, expanding your ribs, then exhale fully, contracting your abdominal muscles to push out as much air as possible from both your chest and your belly.

3. Hold the breath empty, preventing any air from coming back in, while expanding your chest as if you were inhaling. The result is a kind of vacuum that draws your navel toward your spine.

4. Once here, you can either hold the contraction or pump the belly in and out, still without allowing any air to come in to the lungs, an action called *Agni Sara*.

5. When your body signals the need for air, inhale deeply and return to standing.

6. Repeat three times.

Guidelines

- Use the action of expanding the chest while holding your breath to move the belly inward.

- Though it may seem counterintuitive, relaxing the belly muscles allows for a deeper contraction.

- Release the bandha before inhaling again. Inhale slowly and steadily.

- Do not perform this bandha on a full or even partially full stomach.

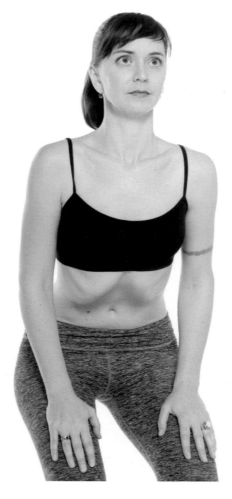

uddiyana bandha ◀
upward abdominal lock

Benefits

- Improves digestion

- Good for constipation

- Tones abdominal muscles

- Purifying

- Good for third chakra excess or deficiency

Avoid or Use Caution

- Pregnancy

- Menstruation

- High blood pressure

- Glaucoma

- Headaches

- Stomach or intestinal ulcers

Kapalabhati: Breath of Fire

The name *Kapalabhati* means shining skull. This is a rapid diaphragmatic breath that actively snaps the belly inward and passively releases it outward in rapid succession. It tones the muscles over the solar plexus, which is both energizing for a third chakra deficiency and a good discharge for third chakra excess. It also mirrors the effort-and-release dynamics of the third chakra. Feel free to use this breath when holding any upright poses to increase the activation of the third chakra.

1. Sit with an erect spine and take a few full, natural breaths through the nose with your mouth closed. Place your hand over your third chakra to feel its movement as you focus on breathing into your belly.

2. When you are ready to begin, inhale and then contract the muscles of your belly toward your spine with a rapid snap of the diaphragm. Notice that the air expires from the nostrils in a short burst. This is an active exhalation.

3. Next, simply relax your belly muscles and notice how the air comes in through the nostrils without effort. This is a passive inhalation.

4. When the natural inhalation process is full, snap your belly in again.

5. Repeat rapidly like a bellows, gaining speed as you find your rhythm.

6. Return to a natural full breath. Notice the effects.

Guidelines

- Begin with cycles of 20–30 snaps of the diaphragm, followed by at least four full natural breaths. Gradually increase to 100 or more.

- Gradually increase your speed to two rounds per second.

- Once you are adept at doing this practice while sitting, you can then use it during postures in which your belly is upright.

- It's often good to have tissues nearby to clear the nostrils.

- After experiencing this breath with both nostrils, you may wish to try closing off one nostril at a time. Finish the practice by breathing in and out of both nostrils.

Benefits

- Expels toxins

- Tones the abdomen and belly

- Purifies and energizes

- Stimulates third chakra while reducing excess

Avoid or Use Caution

- High blood pressure

- Heart disease

- Strong menstruation

- Pregnancy

- Do not practice this breath after eating

Standing Side Stretch

It is good to begin third chakra practice by cultivating your inner flame. In this posture imagine your flame rises up your core, with your joined hands forming the tip of the flame. Keep your core steady as your flame flickers from side to side.

1. Stand in Tadasana, Standing Mountain Pose, pressing down into your feet, lifting your crown, and activating your core.

2. Lift your arms up overhead, interlacing your fingers to a steeple position, with the first fingers pointing upward. Hug your arms in close to your ears and keep your elbows as straight as possible.

3. Lift your chest, draw the shoulders back, and firm your belly. Take a few deep breaths here as your stretch upward, drawing your belly in with each exhale. You may also choose to do Kapalabhati while you are vertical.

4. Inhale fully, then exhale and bend your body to the right, keeping your straight arms close to your ears. Keep your left shoulder back and your sternum lifted while hugging into your core.

5. Hold for several full breaths.

6. Inhale and come back to center, then exhale and stretch to the left, being careful now to keep your right shoulder back and your chest lifted.

7. Inhale and return to center.

8. Next, lift your ribs up out of your hips and arch slightly backward, pointing your fingertips toward the back wall. Imagine you are making room for your third chakra to shine outward by lifting the cage (your rib cage) that contains your power.

9. Inhale and return to center. Keep the lift in the torso and the length in your side bodies while lowering your arms to your sides.

3

Guidelines

- Keep the arms close to the ears and the hands clasped tightly.

- Pull your top shoulder back and avoid collapsing the chest, even if it means you don't bend quite as far to the side.

- Imagine you are doing this pose between two panes of glass. Keep your torso squared to the front and only move sidewise.

- Hug into your core from your waist down to your feet while releasing and expanding your upper body.

Benefits

- Strengthens the core

- Stretches intercostal muscles and expands rib cage

- Opens the shoulders and chest

Avoid or Use Caution

- Shoulder injuries

- High blood pressure

- Headaches

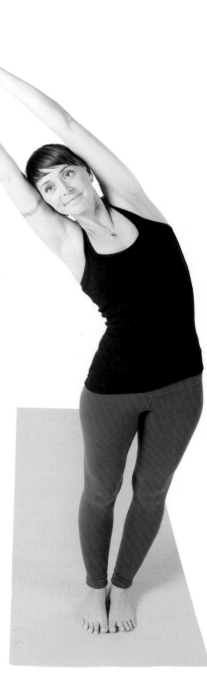

standing side stretch ▲

Virabhadrasana: Warrior Poses

Virabhadra was an ancient warrior from Hindu mythology. *Vira* means hero and *bhadra* means auspicious. When Shiva tore his hair out over the death of his wife, Sati, Virabhadra sprang from Shiva's locks. Think of this as your spiritual warrior, triumphantly arising from the strength of your third chakra. There are many variations of this pose, all of which are good for the third chakra. Practice Virabhadrasana with firm determination, awakening the warrior within you.

Warrior I

1. Begin in Tadasana, Standing Mountain Pose, with arms raised, standing at the front of your mat. Energize your torso by lifting your ribs upward, stretching into your fingertips, with elbows straight and arms firm. Spread your fingers wide and feel them as the flame of your third chakra fire.

2. Exhale and bow forward into Uttanasana, Standing Forward Fold. Bring your belly toward your thighs, firm up your legs, widen your hips, and extend your ribs down toward the floor. Place your hands on the floor beside your feet.

3. On the next inhalation step your left foot back about four feet, keeping your right foot between your hands, knee directly over the ankle. Spin your back heel down to the floor while firming up your back leg by hugging the muscles to the bones.

4. Inwardly rotate the thigh of your back leg while pulling the front leg's hip slightly toward the back. Feel the stability this creates in your root chakra.

5. Once you feel that stability, lift your torso upward. Press through the core of your front leg to bring earth energy into it.

6. When stable, lift your arms up overhead, pressing energy through the core of each arm into the fingertips as if your arms were rays of the sun emanating from your third chakra. With this energy, straighten your arms fully.

3

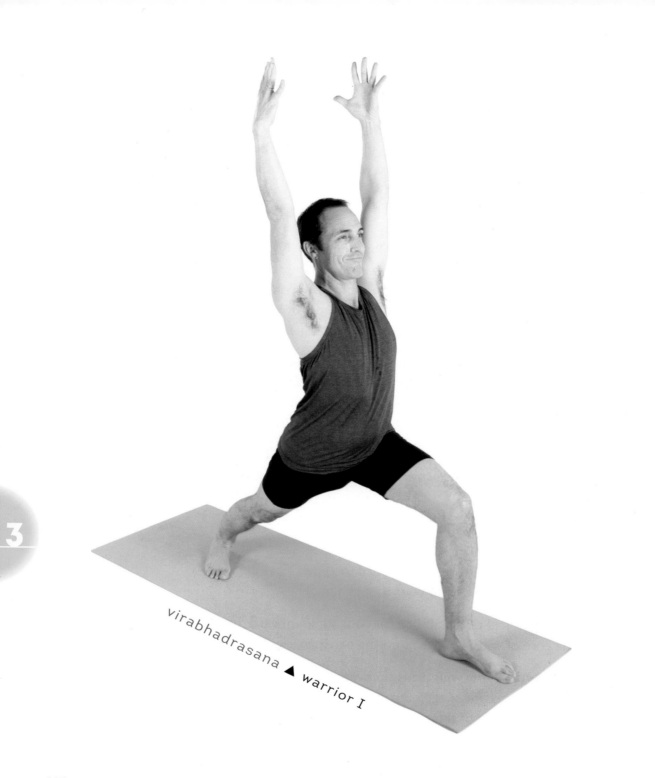

virabhadrasana ▲ warrior I

7. Hold for several breaths, lifting and expanding the ribs. You may choose to perform Kapalabhati, Breath of Fire.

8. Come out of the pose by returning to Tadasana or Uttanasana or moving to Downward Facing Dog.

9. Repeat on the other side.

Guidelines

- If you feel wobbly, place both hands on your front knee until you feel steady.

- Press both feet firmly into the mat and draw them slightly toward each other.

- Create stability by inwardly rotating the thigh of the back leg and outwardly rotating the front leg.

- Ideally, the bottom of the front thigh should be parallel to the floor.

- The inside of your back foot should be in line with your front heel.

- Lift your ribs up out of your hips, but keep your hips steady and grounded.

- Fire up your arms as if they were rays of the sun, your fingers as flames. Draw the muscles of the arms down into the shoulders, firming up the shoulder blades.

- Internally place the first chakra directly below your second chakra. This allows more freedom in the upper body for your ribs to move upward, making room for a slight backbend.

- Gradually increase the time you hold this pose to build up strength and steadfastness.

Benefits

- Strengthens the legs and hips

- Opens the shoulders

- Broadens the chest

- Generates energy and focus

- Relieves sciatica

- Strengthens the will

- Builds focus

Avoid or Use Caution

- High blood pressure

- Heart problems

- Shoulder problems

- Neck injury—keep the eyes level with the horizon

Warrior II

1. Take a wide stance along the length of your mat, feet parallel or toes slightly inward. Extend through the core of each leg as you firmly press all four corners of each foot into the floor.

2. Raise your arms to shoulder height on each side and extend out through the fingertips.

3. Looking out over your right arm, turn your right foot 90 degrees outward so that the toes point toward the front of the mat.

4. Bend your right knee, placing it directly above the right ankle. More advanced practitioners can seek to have the base of their right thigh parallel to the floor.

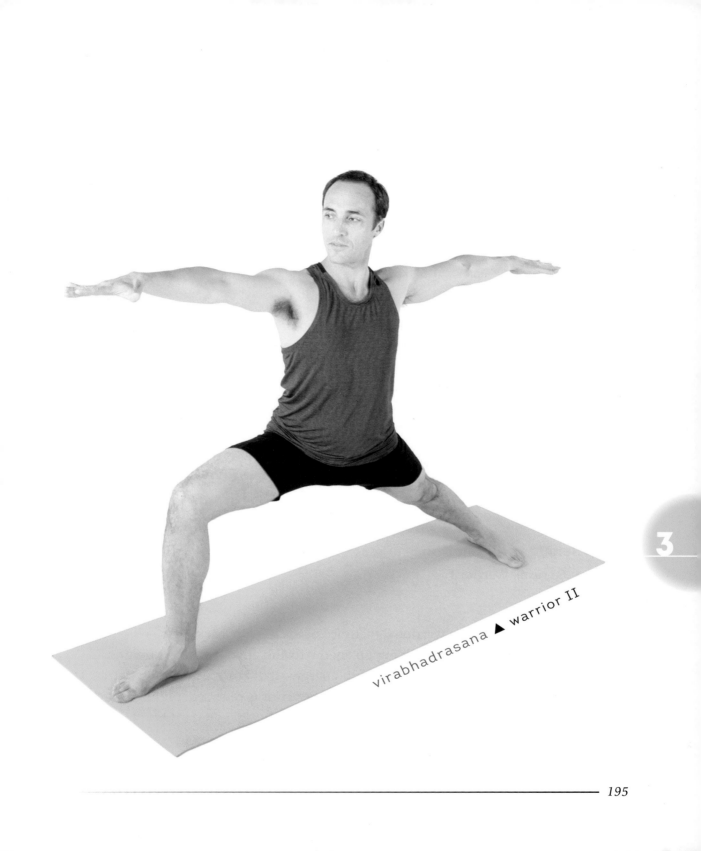

virabhadrasana ▲ warrior II

5. To come out of the pose, straighten your right leg and turn your feet parallel once again.

6. Repeat on the other side.

Guidelines

- When you first extend your arms, try turning your palms upward to rotate your upper arms toward the back. Firm up your shoulder blades, pointing the tips down your back, then turn your palms back downward, keeping the same openness in the chest and shoulders.

- Allow your arms to be like arrows shooting out from your core. Keep your gaze steady and still.

- To avoid the fatigue that tends to happen in the bent leg, push that leg more firmly into the floor, pushing energetically through the core of the leg, as learned in chakra one.

- Draw energy from the earth, through your legs, and into your core.

- Lift the third chakra and let it radiate power.

- Find the determination to be a warrior in your life and let this be expressed in your pose.

- You may choose to use Kapalabhati to further energize the third chakra.

Benefits and Cautions

- Same as Warrior I

Viparita Virabhadrasana: Reverse Warrior Pose

To maintain strength, a warrior sometimes needs to draw back. This is like pulling back the arrow on a bow, building up energy to aim at your target intention. This is an essential principle of third chakra energy—that at times we must retreat in order to keep on advancing. In this pose the warrior is reversed, pulling into himself and reaching up to the Divine.

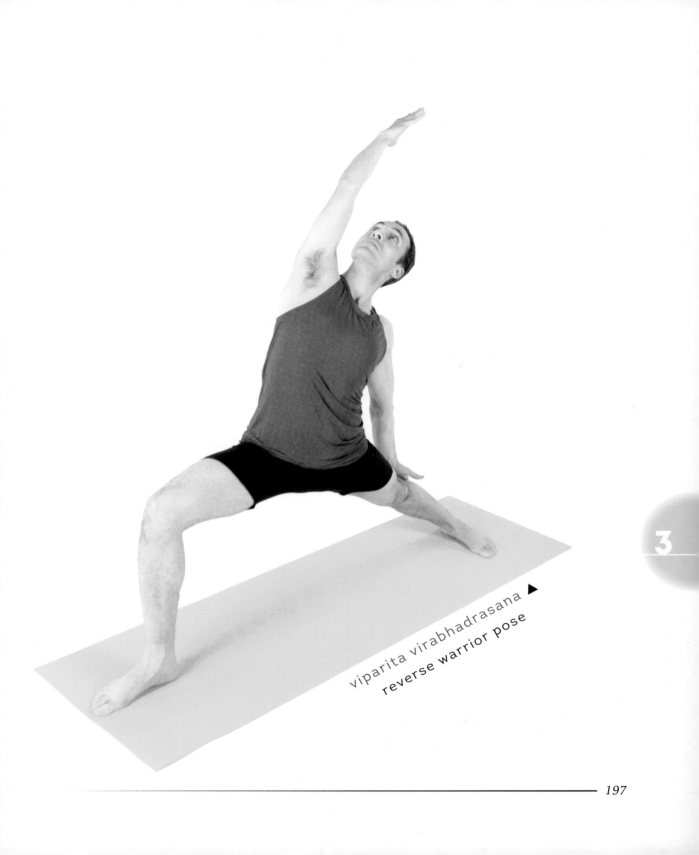

viparita virabhadrasana ▶
reverse warrior pose

1. With your right foot forward and right knee bent as in Warrior II, turn your right palm upward and lean forward slightly into the hand extended over your bent knee.

2. Keeping both arms fully extended and energized, slide your left arm down your back leg and lift your right arm upward.

3. Press the right shoulder backward as you lengthen the right side body and open the chest. Look up past your top arm.

4. Inhale to come out of the pose, returning to Warrior II. Then repeat, starting with Warrior II on the other side.

Guidelines

• Energize the line from the core of your back leg and up through your torso, upper arm, and fingertips. Extend from the pelvis through the heart and into the neck, stretching the ribs.

• Keep your front knee bent over your ankle. Press your front leg into the earth with determination to hold your ground.

• Extend your arm firmly as if you were reaching for power from above.

Warrior III

1. Begin in Tadasana, Standing Mountain Pose.

2. Take a step back with your right foot, placing it about two feet behind your left foot.

3. Bring your weight onto your left leg and find your core stability. Place your hands on your hips, making sure your hips are square toward the front of your mat.

4. Extend out through your back leg as you hinge your whole torso forward, lifting your right leg parallel to the floor.

5. Root into your standing leg and, with hands on hips, find your stability. Attempt to keep the front of both hips parallel to the floor.

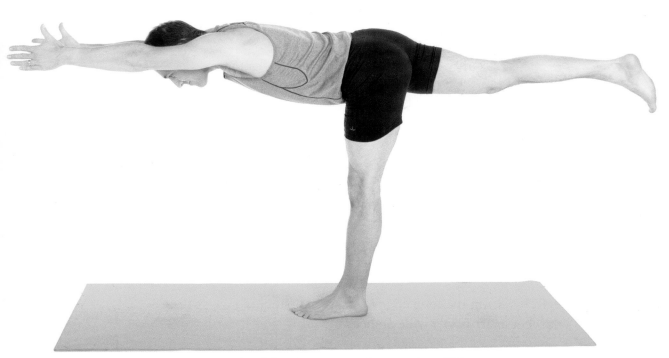

virabhadrasana ▲ warrior III

6. When stable, extend both arms forward, palms facing each other.

7. Radiate outward from the third chakra. Push down into your standing leg and out toward the toes of your lifted leg and up the core of the torso into each hand. Feel the crown of your head in line with your root chakra, and hug into your core.

8. Hold for as long as you feel stable. To come out of the pose, inhale and lift your arms overhead as you hinge back upright, bringing both feet together in Tadasana, with your arms by your sides.

9. Repeat on the other side.

Guidelines

- Move slowly and deliberately, seeking steadiness and balance at each stage. If you fall out of the pose, you can always come back in.

- Pull your shoulder blades toward each other, firming up the back as you reach forward. Firm up your belly into your ribs and soften your heart (upper back) toward the floor.

- Turn your back toes down toward the floor to help level the lifted leg's hip.

- Extend from the back toes to the front fingertips in one energized line.

Trikonasana: Triangle Pose

This basic pose is one you can do again and again, finding deeper levels of alignment over the years. It begins to coordinate the complexity of the third chakra by directing energy lines through the legs, torso, and arms, all moving in different directions. Imagine that these lines all radiate outward from your third chakra like rays of the sun.

1. Begin by facing the long edge of your mat, stepping your feet apart into a wide stance.

2. Turn your right foot out 90 degrees and square your left foot with the rear of your mat.

3. Establish your roots through each leg. Hug the muscles to the bones and draw the earth energy up into your third chakra.

4. Lift your arms up to shoulder height, elbows straight.

5. Outwardly rotate the upper arms to roll your shoulders back, firming up your shoulder blades.

6. Extend out through the right arm as far as you can, keeping a strong line in your core between your root and your crown.

7. When you cannot extend any farther, tip the right arm downward, reaching for the floor directly below the right shoulder, either behind or in front of your ankle; alternately, place your hand on a block. Raise the left arm so that a straight line runs from right to left fingertips. Spread your fingers wide and energize both arms.

8. Look up toward your upper fingertips, keeping the neck in line with the spine.

9. Inhale to come out of the pose, firming your legs and belly for support.

10. Repeat on the other side.

Guidelines

• Bend from the hip joint, not the waist. Imagine you are doing yoga in an airplane aisle and you have very little room in front or behind you.

• Align the arch of the back foot with the front heel along the midline of your mat.

• If you cannot easily reach the floor with your lowered hand, use a block or let your hand fall to your knee, shin, or ankle.

trikonasana ▲ triangle pose

- If your neck is uncomfortable looking up,
  you can look forward or down.

- If you have full extension, you can place your
  hand behind the ankle on the floor.

- Lift your outer hip, rotating the lower ribs forward.

- Let the arms sparkle with energy. Spread your fingers wide and draw
  the head of the upper armbone back, expanding the ribs and chest.

- Ideally your legs are separated enough to form an equilateral
  triangle between your feet and the length of each leg. Too short
  a stance makes bending sideways more difficult. Your ankles
  should be as far apart as your wrists when your arms are raised.

- Imagine lines of energy running from your third chakra out to
  each of your extremities. Radiate equally in each direction.

- Move to Ardha Chandrasana, below, or repeat on the other side.

Benefits
- Improves digestion

- Relieves sciatica

- Strengthens the legs and midsection

- Opens the chest

- Creates strength and steadfastness

- Strengthens the will

Avoid or Use Caution
- Low blood pressure

- Heart disorders

- Hip injuries or replacements

I think of this pose more like a radiating star than a moon. Balancing requires core strength, consolidating the third chakra, while extending into your legs and out through the arms encourages the energy to radiate outward like a star.

1. From Triangle Pose, bend your left knee and reach your left hand to the floor (or a block) about a few inches out from the right foot and slightly behind (position A).

2. Place your right hand on your right hip and lift your right leg (position B).

3. Push down through your standing leg and turn the upper hip toward the sky, extending out to the heel of your lifted leg, with your foot flexed.

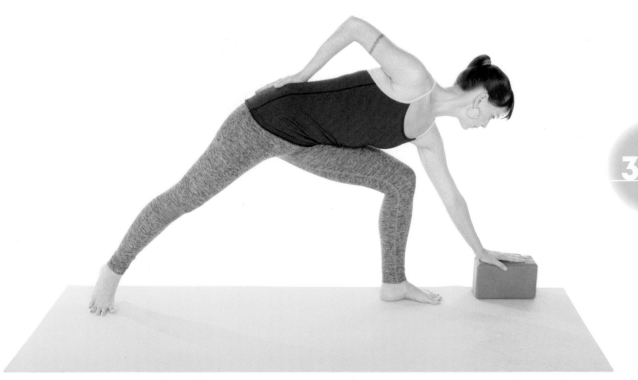

ardha chandrasana ▲ standing half moon pose, position a

4. When stable, raise your right arm directly above your left arm so a straight line extends from hand to hand (position C).

5. Extend into the heel of your lifted left leg and align the core of your lifted leg with your crown, making another straight line.

6. Turn your chest upward toward the sky. If possible, look up toward your upper fingertips.

7. For a full expression of the pose, grab the big toe of your upper leg with your first two fingers and lift high.

8. To come out of the pose, bend your front knee and bring your upper leg back down into triangle, then come up to standing.

9. Repeat on the other side.

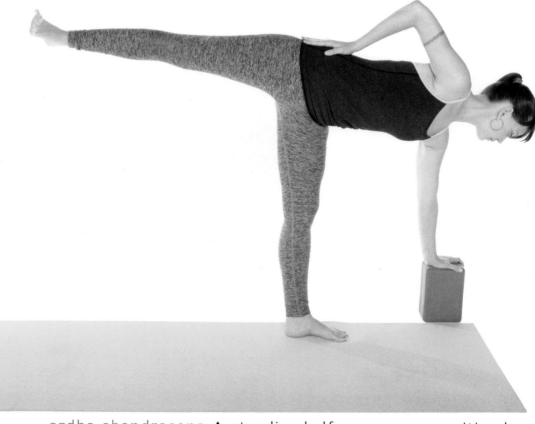

ardha chandrasana ▲ standing half moon pose, position b

Guidelines

- Beginners should use a block beneath their lower hand to make balancing easier.

- Use a wall to support your backside to help with balance while you get used to opening your hips in the pose. Press your upper hip and thighbone back into the wall.

- Remember Padangusthasana from chakra one and let each leg be a root branching out from your first chakra. Let the root support of Muladhara bring you freedom in the pose.

ardha chandrasana ▲ standing half moon pose, position c

- Don't force your neck to look upward if it is uncomfortable or if it makes you lose your balance. Allow yourself to look straight ahead. Just don't allow the head to drop, bringing your head out of alignment.

- For extra challenge, try Ardha Chandra Chapasana, Sugar Cane Pose. Grab the outside of your upper foot with your upper hand, bend your knee, and open the front of the body in a bow by pressing the upper foot firmly into the hand.

Benefits

- Energizing

- Combats fatigue

- Develops strength and balance

- Improves focus and willpower

- Strengthens the legs

- Opens the chest and hips

- Good for constipation

- Strengthens digestion

Avoid or Use Caution

- Low blood pressure

- Headaches

- Neck problems

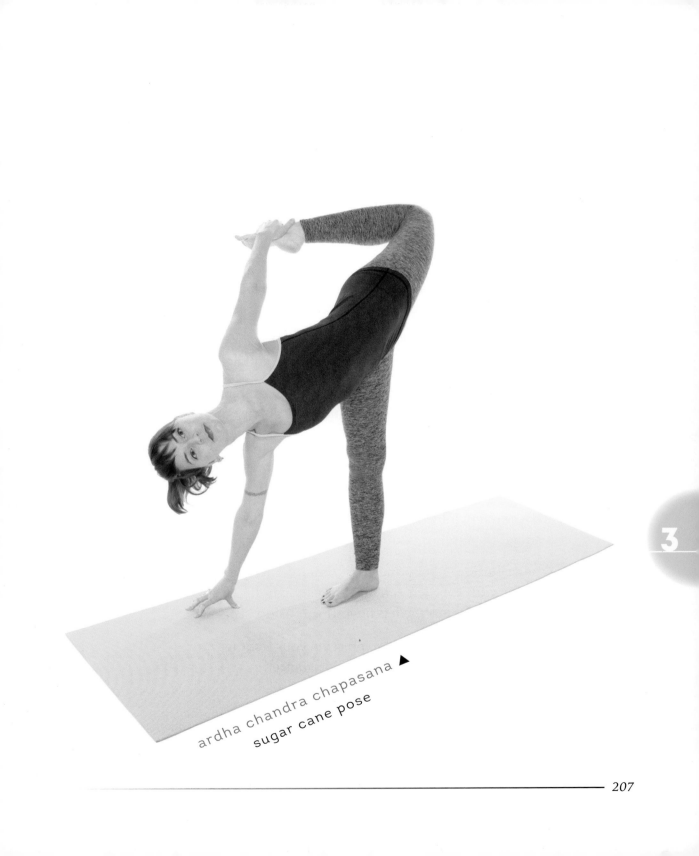

ardha chandra chapasana ▶
sugar cane pose

This is a foundational standing posture with a long, lateral stretch from heel to fingertips that stretches the intercostal muscles between the ribs. Work this pose from your third chakra, radiating both down to the legs and out to your fingertips. This pose strengthens and stretches the legs, groins, and hamstrings while opening the chest and shoulders.

1. Facing the long edge of your mat, step into a wide stance.

2. Raise your arms to shoulder height, palms down. Roll your shoulders back with a slight external rotation of the upper arms.

3. From your third chakra, extend energy down each leg, out through each arm, and up into your crown.

4. Turn your right foot out 90 degrees and your back foot parallel to the back of the mat. Align the front heel with the middle of the back foot.

5. Bend your right knee, bringing the base of your thigh parallel to the floor and your left hand on your left hip.

6. Bring your right hand to the floor in front or behind your right calf or on a block. (The front is a bit easier, while placing the hand behind the knee is a bit more difficult but correct for the pose's full form.)

7. While extending fully down into the right arm, bring your left arm straight up, in line with your right arm (position A).

8. Rotating your lower belly and chest upward, bring your left arm in line with your left ear, making a straight line from the arch of the left foot to the left fingertips (position B).

9. Inhale to come out of the pose, pressing your front leg into the floor. Return upright to a wide stance.

10. Repeat on the other side.

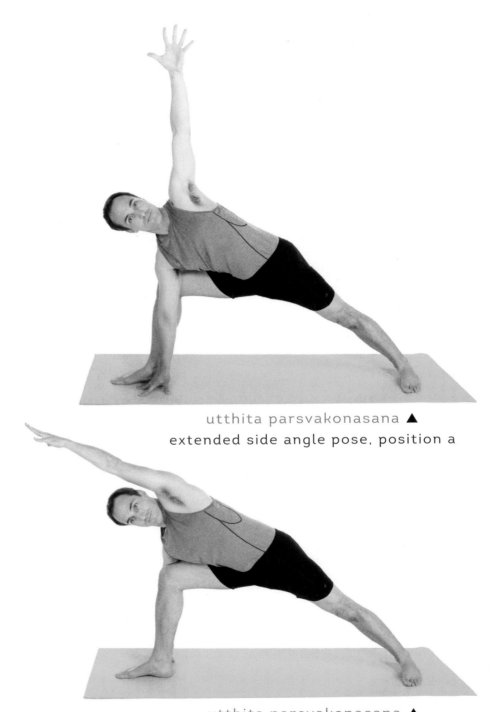

utthita parsvakonasana ▲
extended side angle pose, position a

utthita parsvakonasana ▲
extended side angle pose, position b

Guidelines

- To make the pose easier, bend your right elbow and place above the knee on the right thigh.

- To stretch the side bodies even more, extend your upper arm alongside your ear (position B).

- Press your lower ribs forward, your upper ribs back. Try to create length along both sides of the torso.

- Firm your shoulder blades against the back ribs.

- Pull the upper shoulder toward the back. Press your right arm against your knee to twist a little more.

- From your third chakra, fire up the power line from your straight leg to your extended fingertips.

Benefits

- Builds energy and strength throughout the body

- Opens the shoulders and chest

- Stimulates third chakra and strengthens the will

- Improves digestion

- Relieves constipation

- Increases lung capacity

Avoid or Use Caution

- Knee injuries

- High or low blood pressure

- Hernia

- Insomnia

Adho Mukha Svanasana: Downward Facing Dog Pose

When I was a beginner holding this pose, I remember a teacher saying Downward Facing Dog was a resting pose. Under my breath I quietly muttered, "You gotta be kidding!" But as the years have gone by I have come to love this pose as a stabilizing moment of rest during a vinyasa practice or between other vigorous poses. In the third chakra, use this pose to build strength, alignment, and determination. It strengthens the arms and legs and helps the body firmly define its edges and boundaries. For a more pointed third chakra focus, think of bringing your solar plexus toward your thighs.

1. Begin in Table Pose. Place your palms firmly on the mat, fingers spread wide, first fingers parallel to each other, wrist creases parallel to the front of the mat.

2. Engage your legs by tucking your toes into the mat and pushing your feet and hands into the floor. Firm up your shoulder blades, drawing them downward. Feel this engagement with the ground before you lift your hips.

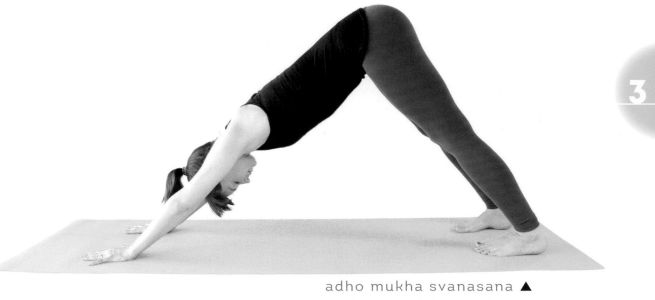

adho mukha svanasana ▲
downward facing dog

3. From that engagement, lift your hips until your body forms a triangle, with the floor as the base.

4. You may wish to alternately bend and straighten your knees a few times as you "walk your dog" and wiggle your way into the pose.

5. With feet hip-width apart, press your heels down toward the mat. Don't worry if your heels don't touch; it may take years of practice to get your heels all the way down.

Guidelines

- Energize the pose by pressing both hands and feet more firmly into the floor, as if you were trying to lengthen your mat from top to bottom, distributing your weight evenly among the four corners of this pose: your two hands and two feet. Notice how this rooting action energizes the body.

- **Legs:** Hug your muscles in toward the bones, lifting your kneecaps. Press the front of your thighs toward the back, with a slight rotation of the inner thighs toward the back, creating more space in the pelvic floor and widening the back of the sacrum.

- **Arms:** The fleshy part of the hand between the thumb and first finger contains a point in Chinese medicine used for grounding. Pressing this part firmly into the ground will give you a slight inner rotation of your forearms. Simultaneously outwardly rotate your upper arms, opening the shoulders and chest. Soften the heart as you extend from the heart to your wrists and from the heart to your pelvis.

- Be wary of hyperflexion in the shoulders. Ideally, there should be a straight line from your hips to your wrists.

- Experiment with bending and straightening your knees, rising up on your toes and lowering your heels, and bending and straightening your arms to experience different dynamics in the pose.

Benefits

- Grounds the whole body

- Creates core strength

- Increases steadfastness

- Opens the arms and shoulders, stretches the hamstrings, and loosens the hips

- Improves digestion

- Energizes the body

Avoid or Use Caution

- Late-term pregnancy

- Carpal tunnel syndrome

- High blood pressure

- Headaches

Phalakasana: Plank Pose

When you step on a plank stretched over a chasm, you trust it will have sufficient strength and integrity to hold you. In the same way, Plank Pose invites you to make your body solid and strong. This pose can be used to generate energy throughout the whole body. It requires that you hold yourself firmly, hugging into the core. It will strengthen your arms, your back, and your belly muscles, toning the entire third chakra area. It is often incorporated into Sun Salutations, but practiced on its own and held for a minute or more can give you a sense of how to use your strength and will to create energy. Variations can be used to increase core strength or increase your inner fire, the element of the third chakra.

The pose can be entered from Table Pose, from Downward Facing Dog, or by walking or jumping your feet back from Standing Forward Fold. Here we will start from Downward Facing Dog.

3

1. Begin in Downward Facing Dog, pushing firmly into your hands and feet to energize your limbs.

2. On an inhalation, lower your hips and draw your torso forward until your shoulders are over your wrists, making as straight a line as possible through your core, from the center of your crown to your tailbone and down to the space between your feet.

3. As in Down Dog, rotate your upper arms slightly outward and your forearms inward, pressing down through the thumb side of each hand.

4. Hug all your muscles to the bones.

5. Come out of the pose by bending the elbows and lowering down to the ground, keeping your body rigid until it touches the mat. If that is too difficult, lower the knees first, then slowly lower the belly and shoulders to the mat. You can also push back up into Downward Facing Dog Pose.

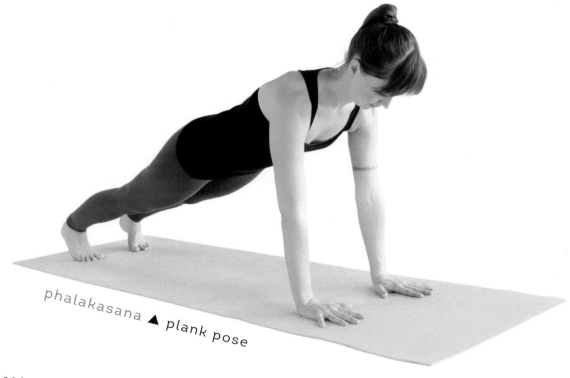

phalakasana ▲ plank pose

Guidelines

- Beginners may wish to lower their knees to make the pose easier.

- Firm your shoulder blades against your back and draw inward to your third chakra, holding your belly firm. Hug your muscles to the bones from head to toe.

- Don't let the back or belly sag toward the earth. Keep the belly firmly tucked in, with the kidney area on the back of the third chakra lifted into the back body.

- Draw the heels of your hands toward your feet to increase third chakra activation.

- Hold the pose until you feel the edge of your strength. If you count your breaths while you're holding, you can then know if you increase your ability to hold the pose over time. When Plank Pose is part of a vinyasa flow, as in Sun Salutations, it is held only briefly.

- Notice what happens when you begin to tire. If you feel a need to collapse, try to stay a few more seconds and see what it's like to summon your will and experience the energy generated through your arms and the rest of your body.

- Instead of thinking of holding yourself up, which can be tiring, think of pushing the floor away. You will have more strength in the pose.

Benefits

- Increases strength and endurance throughout the body

- Activates the core and tones the belly; good for third chakra deficiency

- Energizing when held; releasing when stopped

Avoid or Use Caution

- Carpal tunnel syndrome

- Wrist and shoulder injuries

Variations

1. **Leg Lifts:** To increase the challenge of Plank Pose and develop more core strength, practice lifting one leg at a time, keeping both knees straight. Try not to lose the central line of your body, but hug in even more to your core. Notice the increased effort and the energy this generates. Find your edge and use some determination to expand your edge.

2. **Forearm Plank:** It is slightly more challenging to do Plank Pose from your forearms instead of your wrists, but if you have pain in your wrists this can also be good variation for you.

   • Place your elbows beneath your shoulders with your forearms parallel to each other, fingers spread wide.

   • Lift your hips until your body is straight and firm, and hold until you reach your edge.

   • For extra challenge, lift each leg for a count of ten to twenty.

3. **Pulsing Plank:** To really fire up the third chakra and experience generating instant heat, try Pulsing Plank; note that this pose is not recommended for pregnancy or carpal tunnel syndrome.

   • Holding Plank Pose, first inhale fully, then exhale while pushing the hips rapidly upward, as if going toward Downward Dog but not all the way into that pose.

   • Return to Plank on the next inhalation and repeat, pulsing rapidly with the breath, approximately ten times (once for each petal of this chakra).

   • After ten pulses, hold Plank again for a few moments and then release to the ground. Feel the rush of heat generated by the fire of the third chakra.

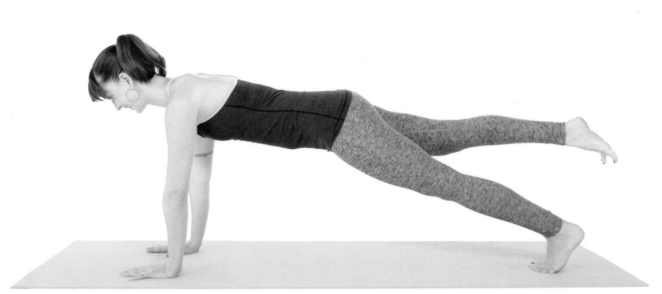

phalakasana ▲
leg lift variation

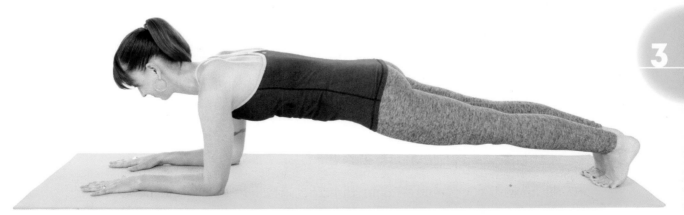

phalakasana ▲
forearm variation

This pose is good for developing core strength, toning the abdominal muscles, and focusing the will. Unless you have pain, challenge yourself to hold it a little longer each time you practice.

1. Begin in a seated position, with knees bent at right angles to the thighs and feet placed hip-width apart on floor.

2. Place your hands so that you can wrap your fingers around your thighs, near the knees.

3. Lean your torso back at right angles to your thighs without collapsing your chest or belly.

4. Extend from your tailbone to your crown. Hug into your core and draw the muscles into the bones. Firm your belly, lift your ribs, and anchor your shoulder blades onto your back.

5. Fix your gaze on a focal point in front of you and lift your feet up off the ground, balancing on your sitting bones. Begin with position A and, if stable and strong enough, continue to position B.

6. Continue to lift your feet as long as you are able to keep your spine straight and chest lifted, extending from base to crown.

7. The full pose extends the legs straight at a 45-degree angle to the floor, with arms parallel to the floor and the chest lifted (position B).

8. Hold for several breaths as long as you are steady. If you fall out of the pose, repeat the above steps and come back into the pose again.

9. To come out of the pose gracefully, slowly bend your knees and place your feet on the floor.

10. Sit up with your spine straight and cross your legs in a simple pose.

11. Take a few breaths and feel the effect on your third chakra.

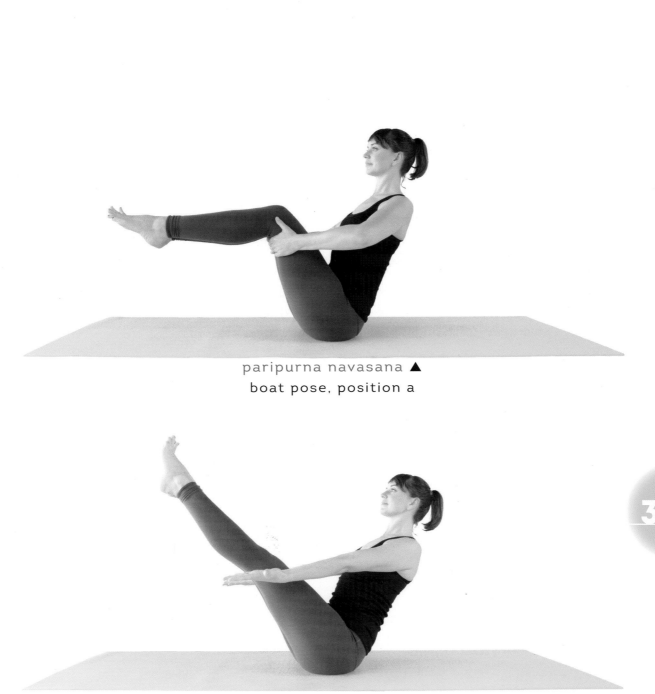

paripurna navasana ▲
boat pose, position a

paripurna navasana ▲
boat pose, position b

3

Guidelines

- Bending the knees makes the pose easier. Beginners may wish to hold on to the backs of their thighs while developing strength. You could also use a strap behind the thighs.

- Press your root into the ground and extend through the pelvis up to the crown. Be careful not to round your back, but keep the natural curve of the sacrum.

- Hug your legs together, drawing into the core.

- Tone your feet by half flexing your ankles while flexing and spreading your toes wide.

- Keep your chest lifted. Draw the arms muscularly into the shoulders, rotating the head of the armbones back, pressing your shoulder blades down your back.

Benefits

- Builds strength and energy throughout the body

- Accentuates the core

- Tones the belly over the third chakra

- Increases will

- Improves balance

- Increases circulation

- Improves digestion

- Excellent for third chakra deficiency

Avoid or Use Caution

- Pregnancy

- Low back issues

- Low blood pressure

- Menstruation

- Cardiac issues

- Insomnia

Desk or Table Top Pose

This is a good pose to do to counteract the effects of sitting at a desk, though its name comes from its resemblance to a flat, tablelike surface. This pose strengthens one's sense of backbone, right behind the third chakra, and generates heat. Pulsing upward from this position activates even more heat.

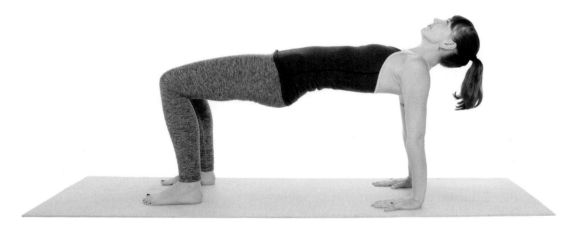

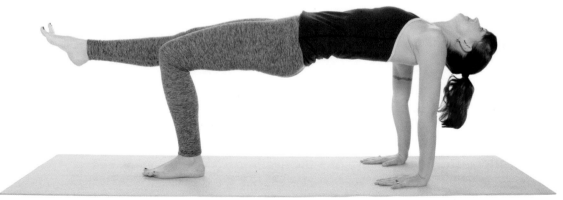

desk or table top pose ▲
position a, top, and position b, bottom

1. Begin in Dandasana, Staff Pose.

2. Bend your knees and place the soles of your feet hip-width apart on the mat.

3. Place your hands on the mat next to your hips, fingertips facing forward.

4. Lengthen your spine by rooting into your tailbone and lifting your crown. Tone up your belly. There is a strong tendency to collapse the chest in this pose, so keep your chest lifted and your upper arms rotated outward, shoulder blades down the back.

5. Inhale into your core and press down into your feet, especially pushing the inside edges of the feet into the floor.

6. Lift your hips upward, attempting to make a straight line from your knees and through your hips to your shoulders (position A).

7. Hold for several breaths, then lower back down to Staff Pose.

Guidelines

- Keep the chest lifted and lengthen the tailbone toward the knees.

- Press outward with your third chakra.

- If you have pain in your wrists, you can place them on a rolled-up mat or turn them slightly outward.

Variations

- For more challenge, hold this pose while lifting one leg out straight (position B), then switch legs.

- To generate more energy, rapidly pulse the hips upward on an exhalation and lowering as you inhale, similar to Pulsing Plank. Feel the heat!

Purvottanasana: Inclined Plane Pose
(literal translation: Intense Stretch of the East)

If Desk Pose was difficult, stick with that until you can hold your hips level with your knees. When that becomes more comfortable, Purvottanasana will take you to the next step.

1. Begin in Dandasana, Staff Pose.

2. Bring your feet together, pointing your toes.

3. Place your hands slightly behind your hips, fingertips pointing forward.

4. Extend into the crown and root into your base.

5. As you inhale, lift your hips until your body forms a straight line from heels to crown. Hug into the core. Rotate your upper arms outward to keep your chest lifted and your shoulders expanded.

6. Take several deep breaths or practice Kapalabhati (page 187).

7. To come out of the pose, lower your hips back to the floor on an exhalation and return to Dandasana. It is nice to follow this with a forward bend such as Paschimottanasana (page 108).

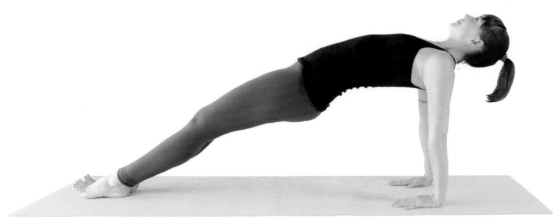

purvottanasana ▲
inclined plane pose

Guidelines

- If you have pain in your wrists, turn your hands slightly outward or place them on a rolled-up mat.

- Draw the feet and legs together to make them stronger.

- Hug the shoulders into the core of the back.

- Lengthen your tailbone toward your feet.

- Lift on an exhalation.

- Pulse as above to activate more third chakra heat, exhaling as you pulse upward, inhaling as you return to the line of your plane.

- For an advanced and more difficult version used to develop strength in the back, lower onto your forearms, placing your elbows beneath your shoulders, and lift from there.

Benefits

- Produces heat and increases energy

- Develops focus and willpower

- Strengthens the arms, wrists, and back

- Tones abdomen and belly

- Accentuates the core

- Releases shoulder tension

- Relieves constipation

- Increases circulation

Avoid or Use Caution

- Carpal tunnel syndrome or wrist injuries

- Shoulder issues

- High blood pressure

- Advanced pregnancy

Vasisthasana: Side Plank

Vasistha, whose name means most excellent, was a great sage. This pose requires both strength and balance, and it helps develop a powerful core. If you feel trembling in the pose, allow this to happen—push through the trembling to find the core of your arms, torso, and legs.

1. Begin in Plank Pose but with your feet close together.

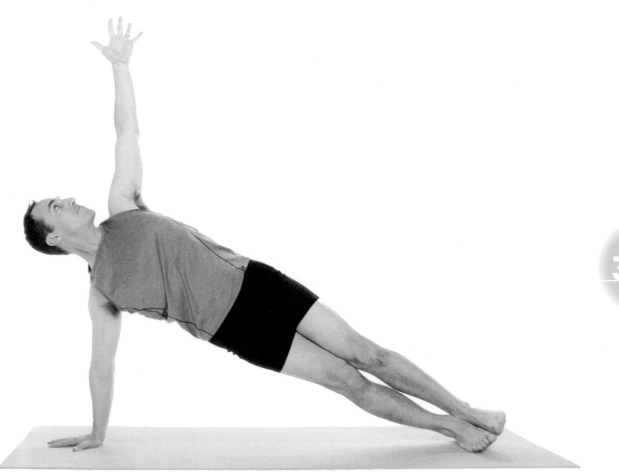

vasisthasana ▲ side plank, position a

2. Simultaneously roll onto your right hand and outer right foot, with the left foot directly on top of your right foot.

3. Push directly into the ground with your right arm as you firm up the core, and place your left hand on your hip. The right hand should not be directly under your shoulder but slightly toward the front edge of your mat, as shown. Find your stability here by hugging the muscles of the arm into the bones and rooting the heel of the hand into the floor.

4. Firm your shoulder blades into your back and draw your legs together, rooting through your heels. Align your whole body along the midline. Lengthen your tailbone down toward your feet.

5. If you are stable here, lift your left arm upward, making a straight line across your shoulders, pressing from right hand to left hand (position A).

6. To come out of the pose, swing the upper arm back down, roll forward, and return to Plank or to Child Pose. Downward Facing Dog is also a good resting pose between sides.

7. Repeat on the other side.

Guidelines

• Find the line of energy that runs from hand to hand across your shoulders and chest. Push the lower hand firmly into the ground to root, and rise up to the upper hand.

• Press your supporting shoulder blade directly behind your heart.

• Keep your neck in line with your torso and your upper shoulders back.

• Flex your feet and hug your legs together.

• Find and hold your midline.

Variations

- To make this pose easier, bend your top knee and place it on the floor in front of your straight leg for balance (position B).

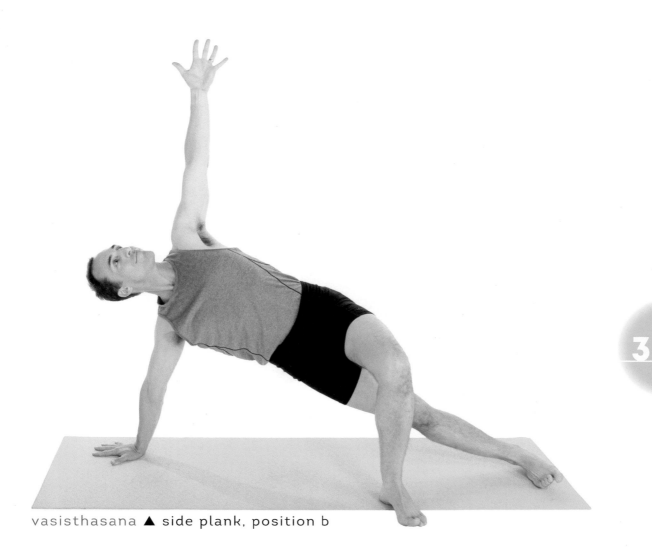

vasisthasana ▲ side plank, position b

- Lift the top leg so that it is parallel to the floor. If you are stable here, bend your knee, grab your big toe with your first two fingers, and lift your leg high for the full pose (position C).

- Another option (that is not pictured) is to take the top leg foot against the shin or thigh as in Vrksasana, Tree Pose.

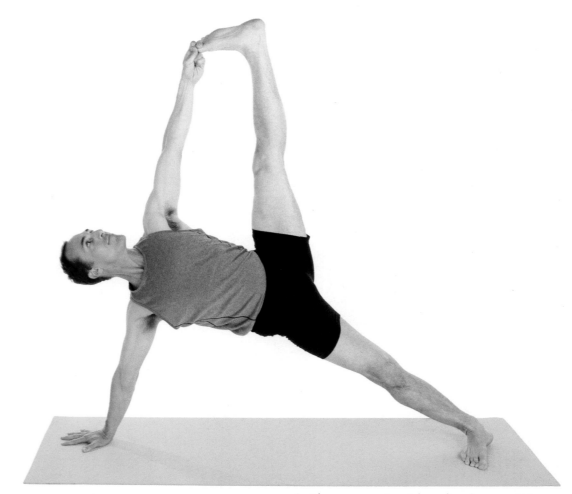

vasisthasana ▲ side plank, position c

Benefits

- Develops balance

- Builds strength in upper body, legs, and torso in general

- Accentuates the core

- Builds stability in the wrists for further arm balances

- Energizing

- Develops will and focus

Avoid or Use Caution

- Carpal tunnel or wrist issues

- Shoulder injuries

Parighasana 1: Gate Pose

Think of opening the gate to your power as you stretch your ribs in this pose. Reach for the power in your upper hand and receive it in your lower hand. When you return to center, bring your palms over your third chakra.

1. Begin in a kneeling position, with your knees hip-distance apart. Lift your chest and crown, bringing your shoulders back and lengthening your spine.

2. Stretch your right leg out to the right side, knee straight, rotating your leg so that the knee points upward and the toes are pointed outward. If desired, you can roll a blanket underneath your extended toes, though it is also permissible to flex your foot. Engage the muscles of the leg by lifting the kneecap.

3. Extend the arms out to each side at shoulder height. Stretch across the heart by pressing the arms wide. Inhale.

3

4. With an exhalation, bend the trunk to the right side, aligning with the plane of your straight leg and sliding your right hand down your right leg. Rest your hand on your ankle, shin, or knee, as your flexibility allows.

5. Stretch the left arm up and over the ear, keeping the shoulders square with the hips and being careful not to collapse the chest. Keep the spine lengthened as you bend sideways, rotating the chest slightly upward.

6. Inhale to come out of the pose, rising up and returning to the original kneeling position.

7. Repeat on the other side.

Guidelines

- Turn your pelvis slightly toward the side of the bent knee.

- Point the kneecap toward the ceiling on the extended leg.

- Press into the extended leg's heel to avoid hyperextension.

- Lift the lower ribs toward the upper shoulder.

- Fold the mat under your knee if kneeling is uncomfortable.

Benefits

- Lengthens the side bodies and stretches intercostal muscles located between the ribs

- Tones the abdominals and midsection

- Opens the shoulders

- Increases breath capacity

- Energizing and warming

- Develops will and focus

- Improves digestion

Avoid or Use Caution
- Knee injuries

- High blood pressure

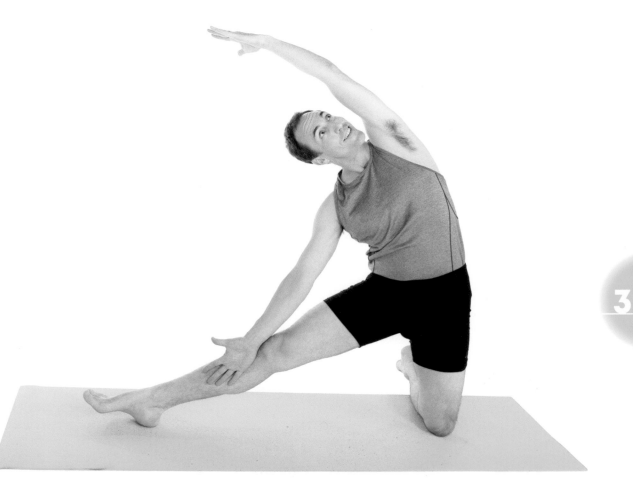

parighasana 1 ▲ gate pose

Salabhasana: Locust Pose

We first visited this pose in the first chakra, lifting only the legs. We then learned baby cobra, using only the muscles of the back to lift the chest and shoulders. Now these two poses are combined. This requires a focused third chakra determination and is very energizing. Holding the pose is good for a deficient third chakra, while coming out of the pose releases the stagnant energy of an excessive third chakra.

1. Lie on your belly, centering your chin on the mat and aligning your core.

2. Externally rotate your arms alongside your body, palms facing upward.

3. Activate your legs by drawing them toward each other and pushing down to the toes.

4. On an inhalation, lift your legs up behind you and simultaneously lift your shoulders and head.

5. Reach your hands back toward your feet, using the muscles of your back and belly.

6. Exhale to come out of the pose, turn your head to the side, and relax.

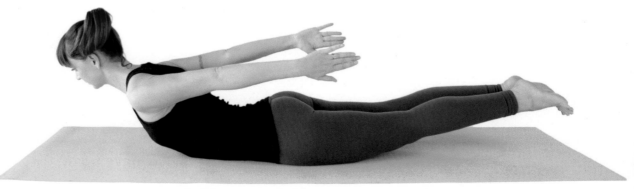

salabhasana ▲ locust pose

Guidelines

- Warm up first with Cobra, Baby Cobra, or other back-bending poses.

- Let the breath lift and lower your ribs. Draw your shoulder blades onto your back.

- Actively press the legs together and lengthen through the inner thighs. Keep your knees straight.

- Root your tailbone downward.

- Activate your arms by extending into the fingertips and hugging the muscles to the bones.

Benefits

- Strengthens the spine

- Energizes and activates third chakra

- Tones abdominal organs

- Improves digestion

- Opens the chest and shoulders

- Develops strength in the legs and tones hamstrings

- Stimulates circulation

- Channels stress into strength and focus

Avoid or Use Caution

- Pregnancy

- Headaches

- Stomachaches

- High blood pressure

3

Dhanurasana: Bow Pulling Pose

Think of stringing the arrow of your intention upon the bow of your will as you lift into this pose. Imagine shooting that arrow straight out of your third chakra at whatever task your will needs to address. Dhanurasana will help you build energy, stimulate your digestion, and open the spine for backbends. This pose stimulates third and fourth chakras equally but is more third chakra related as it requires effort and determination. Use your breath to rock the body forward and back.

1. Lie on your belly, hands alongside your body, palms facing upward. Take a few breaths here, feeling the third chakra press against the mat with each inhale.

2. Bend your knees, bringing your feet toward your buttocks. Energize your feet by spreading your toes. Reach back and wrap your hands around the outside of your ankles, fingers pointing inward.

3. Press a line of energy from your third chakra to your knees, energizing the front of the thighs so that they begin to lift off the floor.

4. Send another line of energy from the third chakra up to the crown as you lift the chest, shoulders, neck, and head.

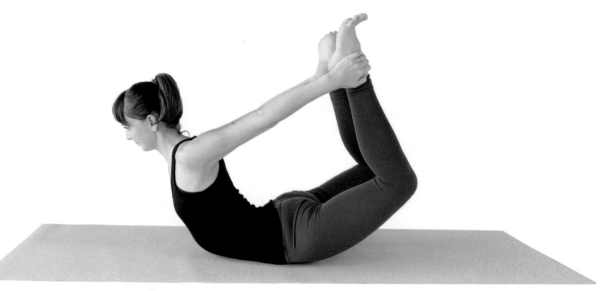

dhanurasana ▲ bow pulling pose

5. Hold for a few breaths, rocking back and forth.

6. Exhale and come down slowly, releasing your ankles, turning your head to the side, and bringing your arms alongside the body. Take a few moments here to relax and let the energy generated distribute through your body.

Guidelines

- Avoid straining your back muscles by letting the arms and legs do the work. Push your feet into your hands. Work toward engaging your belly while allowing your back muscles to soften.

- Keep your shoulders low, away from your ears. Press your shoulder blades down the back and allow the fire of the third chakra to melt the heart.

- Breathe deeply and experience how your breath can rock you forward and back.

- Can't reach your feet? Use a strap around your ankles, with an end in each hand (see variation).

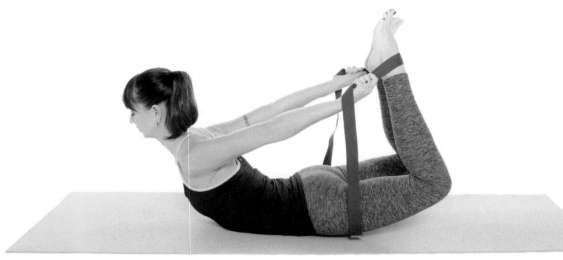

dhanurasana ▲ variation with strap

- The knees tend to splay apart in this pose. Draw the thighs toward each other to keep the knees hip-distance apart.

- Want to deepen the pose? Draw your thighs, knees, and feet toward each other. Lift your feet higher.

Benefits

- Opens the shoulders and the entire front of the body

- Good preparation for back-bending

- Energizes third chakra

- Increases breath capacity

- Improves digestion

Avoid or Use Caution

- Pregnancy

- Low back issues

- Shoulder injury

- Migraines

- Insomnia

Ardha Matsyendrasana: Half Lord of the Fishes or Seated Twist Pose

The third chakra rules metabolism, and this pose is excellent for massaging the digestive organs. Twists are generally cooling postures that are good for winding down from a hot third chakra practice. This pose gives a "squeeze and soak" phenomenon to the liver, spleen, and digestive organs. This means that the twisting squeezes out blood and toxins, and the release of the pose allows new blood to come in. For this reason it is purifying and stimulating for third chakra–related organs.

1. Begin in a simple cross-legged seated position.

2. Place your left foot on the floor, just to the outside of your right thigh. Your left knee will naturally point upward. (Straightening your right leg can make the pose a bit easier.)

3. There is a tendency for the left hip to lift up off the floor, so try to push both sitting bones evenly into the floor. Find your center line and square your torso, taking the four corners toward the back and extending upward from root to crown.

4. Place your left hand on the floor behind your spine. Reach upward with your right hand and lengthen your spine while rooting down into your sitting bones.

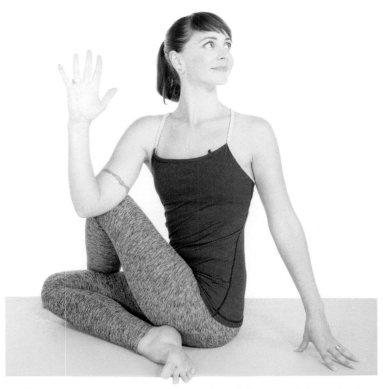

ardha matsyendrasana ▲ half lord of the fishes
or seated twist pose, position a

5. Bend your right elbow and place it on the outside of your left knee (position A). If this is too difficult, you can wrap your right arm around the outside of your knee (position B).

6. Establish your vertical axis so that it remains upright while you twist.

7. Inhale and lift. Exhale and twist to the left, keeping your crown above your base and looking over your left shoulder. Use your right arm as a lever to twist into your edge. With each inhalation, send energy up to your crown and down into your root. With each exhalation, twist a bit more.

8. Come out of the pose on an exhalation and return to a simple cross-legged pose.

9. Repeat on the other side.

ardha matsyendrasana ▲
seated twist variation, position b

Guidelines

- Twist on your axis (your vertical core), but keep your axis straight up and down as you twist.

- Lead with the ribs on the side you are moving from. If you are twisting to the left, lead with the right ribs. If you are twisting to the right side, lead with the left ribs.

- Keep both sitting bones solidly on the floor as much as possible.

Benefits

- Purifies and regenerates digestive organs, liver, and kidneys

- Stretches shoulders

- Opens chest

- Cools and releases third chakra

- Old texts say it destroys disease and awakens Kundalini

Avoid or Use Caution

- Spinal injuries

- Advanced pregnancy

- After eating

Savasana: Corpse Pose

After a good third chakra practice, Savasana is most needed and welcome. Now effort turns to complete surrender and action becomes stillness. This allows the energy generated through your practice to enter the cells of the body.

As you lie in Savasana, settling into stillness, imagine dissolving your physical body into your energy body. Imagine that your energy body—glowing and pulsing with prana—is the only thing on the mat. Notice where that prana is most present and notice where it might be missing. Imagine the available prana is flowing into those places most in need of it. Allow your prana to flow until it is evenly distributed throughout your whole body.

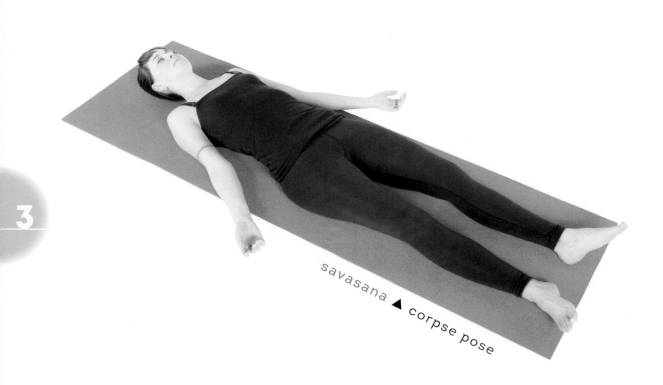

savasana ▲ corpse pose

Third Chakra Posture Flow

Kapalabhati: Breath of Fire (no picture)

Uddiyana Bandha: Upward Abdominal Lock

Standing Side Stretch

Adho Mukha Svanasana: Downward Facing Dog

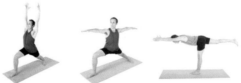

Virabhadrasana: Warrior Poses I, II, and III

Viparita Virabhadrasana: Reverse Warrior Pose

Trikonasana: Triangle Pose

3

Ardha Chandrasana: Standing Half Moon Pose

Utthita Parsvakonasana: Extended Side Angle Pose

Phalakasana: Plank & Pulsing Plank Pose

Paripurna Navasana: Boat Pose

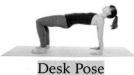

Desk Pose

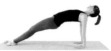

Purvottanasana: Inclined Plane Pose

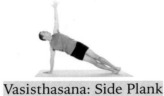

Vasisthasana: Side Plank

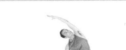

Parighasana 1: Gate Pose

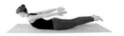

Salabhasana: Locust Pose

Dhanurasana: Bow Pulling Pose

Ardha Matsyendrasana: Seated Twist

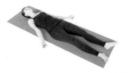

Savasana: Corpse Pose

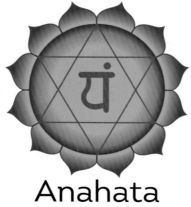

Anahata

UNSTRUCK, UNHURT

Element	Air
Principle	Equilibrium
Purposes	Love, dissolution of ego and separateness, expansion
Properties	Softness, openness, expansion, integration, radiance
Body parts	Chest, lungs, diaphragm, shoulder blades, ribs, heart, respiratory system
Practices	Opening the chest, expanding the breath, surrendering the ego, generosity, forgiveness, empathy, radiating from the core
Actions	Lifting the sternum, shoulders back, pranayama, bandhas
Poses	Chest openers, shoulder openers, breath openers, backbends
Masculine	Protecting, guiding, supporting
Feminine	Giving, nurturing, connecting, joining, radiant
Deficient	Fear of intimacy, judgmental, isolating
Excessive	Codependent, desperate for love and attention
Balanced	Radiant, joyful, generous

chakra four

Soften...

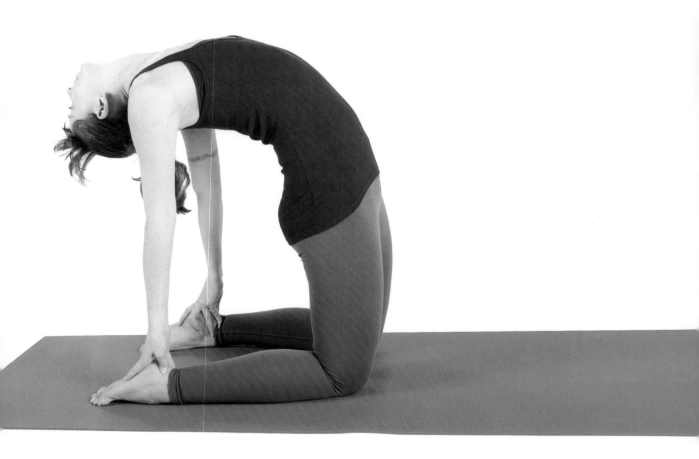

Your task is not to seek for love, but merely to seek and find all the barriers within yourself that you have built against it. ~ RUMI

Take a moment to celebrate your breath. Each breath is free, and there is an infinite supply—you will never run out. Each inhalation is an opportunity for a new moment; each exhalation is a chance to release the old. Each breath expands your interior, softens your resistance, and allows you to open wider. From your very first inhalation to your last exhalation, the breath defines the length of your life. It is a constant example of the perpetual exchange between inner and outer worlds.

Welcome to the heart of the journey! Now that you have entered, aligned, and activated your lower three chakras, the key to opening the fourth chakra is to soften, which will then allow you to open and expand. In the hard, masculine world of today there is too little emphasis on softness, and this is as true in yoga classes as anywhere else. Third chakra yoga uses effort and strength to push to new levels. Fourth chakra yoga moves from doing to being, from effort to surrender, from muscular strength to yielding tenderness.

Softening opens the gateway to the heart. That could mean softening your body or your breath, but it also points to softening your judgments or your stance toward another person or situation. Next time you find yourself holding a hard line with someone, try softening your stance and see what happens. Softening allows things to join, to match their edges together. It invites openness, connection, and reception. Once you find your alignment in a pose, notice if you are rigid or if you have the ability to soften your face, your eyes, your shoulders—and, most of all, your heart.

You are now halfway through the chakra journey as you expand into the mid-point of the chakra system. With three chakras above and three chakras below, the Anahata chakra (accent on the second syllable) takes you to the exact center of your core. Within this sacred chamber lies the jewel of the heart chakra: the inner beloved, whose teachings are always about love. Opening the heart brings expansion and joy through a profound sense of universal love and connection to all that is. As the heart of the chakra system, this chakra is the integrator of all that you are, taking you yet another step closer to the essential meaning of yoga as union.

Love is a natural state of being, not only within your inner temple but through all of creation—myriad interconnecting relationships, the exchange of energy and information, singing together, vibrating, sparkling. Even though love is the universal force of connection and healing, we simultaneously fear it and long for it, and this creates blockage in the heart. Opening the heart chakra breaks through the bondage of that conflict into ecstatic joy, radiant love, tender compassion, and a deep intimacy with your own (and another's) interior.

Moving from a point to a line to an area (chakras one, two, and three), you now enter the dimension of spaciousness in chakra four. When you create space inside yourself—as well as spaciousness in your life—you have room to truly enter your heart. Spaciousness can mean free time, peace and quiet, relaxation in the body, or physical space that is expansive, such as being outside.

As Rumi has suggested in the quote above, our key to finding love is to remove the barriers we've built against opening to love. The reasons for these defenses are many: past hurts and betrayals, childhood wounds, and the exquisite sensitivity—and therefore potential pain—of a center that holds the very essence of our core and the unifying force of life.

Opening the heart chakra involves taking down those defenses to experience the love that is the natural state of our being. Unfortunately, defenses get hardwired into the body and become permanent body armor. This rigidifies the upper back, chest, and shoulders. It constricts the breath and can even shorten the connective tissue in the front of the body, drawing the shoulders forward and collapsing the chest. Then it becomes more difficult to breathe and to align your posture, and the heart feels depleted.

4

*Opening the heart chakra involves taking
down those defenses to experience the love
that is the natural state of our being.*

. . . .

ANODEA JUDITH

When the heart chakra is blocked, people often experience a kind of pressure against their chest, as if someone were pushing down against it. The tissue around that area may be sore or tender to the touch, especially over the sternum. The shoulders may round forward in protection or the heart area may collapse from lack of energy, indicating a fourth chakra deficiency. Alternatively, the chest may be frozen in a puffed-up fashion like a military chest, and it becomes difficult to exhale fully, which makes it harder to relax or yield.

Yoga for the heart chakra seeks to remedy this armoring of the heart by opening the chest and upper back and by working with the breath. The result is more spaciousness in the inner temple, more freedom and relaxation through the chest and shoulders, more softeness, and more room for the natural state of love and joy. In this way, the subtle energy that is activated in the third chakra expands in the fourth chakra, escaping its boundaries to gradually dissolve the barriers between inner and outer.

With a solid base to support you, softening the body—combined with the intense effort of the third chakra—opens the windows of your temple to a sweet surrender, allowing the cool breeze of Shakti to blow through your chakras. Like the air that is the associated element of the heart's lotus, this breeze both cleanses and softens. You open to the breath and, in turn, the breath's softening enables you to expand even more.

How Do You Get There?

As you rise up the chakras, your inner actions become more complex. Here at the heart chakra you have several tasks:

- Raise the lower chakra energy up to the heart

- Get out of your head and bring the upper chakra energy down to the heart

- Utilize the breath so that you can surrender and expand from the heart

- Stay centered within yourself as you open to the radiant ecstasy of love

Let's look at each of these in turn.

Raising energy up to the heart. This occurs through proper integration of the lower three chakras: by generating sufficient energy through matter and movement, then directing that energy into different parts of the body by holding and releasing as appropriate. The body is the container that keeps you centered, the second chakra generates the movement, and the will guides the energy gently upward. Fire naturally moves upward and causes things to expand, so the more you develop your inner fire, the more you can cook up the steamy passion of your lower chakras to rise into the heart.

Descending down to the heart. It is said that you take many journeys in life, but perhaps the most difficult are those eighteen inches between your head and your heart. If the body is too contracted, then there is not enough room on the inside of the temple to descend down into it, leaving no choice but to live in your head. By expanding and softening the body, you open a place in the deep interior of your being that can receive the divine spirit that you are.

Working with the breath. Think about the element of air. It is soft. It has no hard edges or boundaries—yet as wind it can have great power. In the same way, your breath has great power to bring spaciousness into your body and to help your muscles soften and release. We guard against the vulnerability of love through tensing and hardening the body. The heart, however, requires softness, melting your edges. The breath is the central tool for softening. The heart is more about allowing than pushing—more about being rather than doing.

Staying centered in yourself. While doing all of the above, you have to stay centered in your core in order to expand and soften. With a strong core that is activated and aligned, you are safer to expand and have less need for boundaries and protection. A strong core allows you to surrender. Loving yourself, you can love another without losing yourself. You will have less need to be filled from other people, and that leaves more room for genuine love. Always orient from your inner axis, connecting to spirit above and the earth below.

As the great integrator of above/below, inside/outside, self/other, masculine/feminine, and mind/body, the heart is the center of the self. In addition, every yoga pose has a center of focus. Try to feel for the heart of each pose as you practice and breathe into your heart. Be loving with yourself and encourage softening rather than achievement. Use your breath as a guiding mantra in every pose.

*Mind-body integration is more than a
personal health strategy. It is a movement of
consciousness that can change the world.*

· · · · · · · · · · · · · ·

MATTHEW SANFORD

Sensing Subtle Energy

1. Sit quietly and align your core.

2. Press your roots downward, pushing your sitting bones into the mat or cushion.

3. Slightly increase the curve of your sacrum while simultaneously firming up your abdominal muscles.

4. Lift your ribs up out of your hips and extend upward with your crown.

5. Relax your shoulders and shift the tops of the armbones toward the back.

6. Imagine someone gently putting a hand on the back of your heart chakra, giving you support, while gently pressing your heart slightly forward and up.

7. Imagine that you are enveloped in a field of universal love that is wrapping itself around you with complete compassion and understanding. Each breath you take fills you with an embrace of unconditional love.

8. Tune in to your breath, becoming the witness of the breath's natural flow in and out.

9. As you inhale, imagine softening your whole chest area so that you can receive more of this wondrous breath of love, feeling your whole body expand like a balloon. Notice where there might be resistance to receiving the breath of love.

10. As you exhale, keep the chest high and allow the breath to be expired by pressing the muscles of the belly inward. Let your lower body do the muscular contraction while the upper body stays soft and open.

11. Keep the spine firm and erect, yet soften everything around it. Soften your skin, your eyes, your jaw, your shoulders.

12. Imagine that your lower chakras form your roots and stem while the heart chakra is a flower that blossoms upward, opening to the front, sides, and back in a full circle around you. Imagine your favorite flowers with many petals in a soft pink with green leaves.

13. Imagine each breath is a caress that knows you deeply, intimately, and loves you unconditionally. Imagine that caress is gently calling you to open, inviting you to greater presence.

14. Continue inhaling and exhaling slowly and deeply until you feel a spaciousness inside your heart chakra and your whole body feels soft and peaceful.

15. Bring your hands together over your heart and lift the corners of your mouth gently toward your ears.

4

Breathe, and all will be revealed. Love,
and all will be healed. This is yoga.

. . . .

SEANE CORN

Pranayama: The Vital Breath

The breath is the central key that unlocks the body and opens the realm of the heart. Each breath you take puts you in constant exchange with the world around you. Each breath is, therefore, a relationship—receiving and expressing from inside to out. While breath is a fundamental part of any yoga practice, relevant to every chakra, the heart chakra's element of air makes the breath especially conducive to softening, opening, and expanding.

Breath brings spaciousness into the body. All you have to do is inhale to feel that principle in action. Every breath you take expands your chest and belly, making more space on the inside. When you learn to direct your breath into tight places in your body, especially while stretching, you create a slow, gentle release. The result is a combination of joyous expansion and tender softening.

Breath has long been equated with spirit, from which we get the words *inspire* and *expire*. When we are full of breath, we are full of inspiration. Recently I sat at the bedside of a friend who was dying. Barely conscious, she took small inhales and long exhales, holding the breath empty for half a minute or more before her next inhalation. I could see why we say that something that has come to its end has "expired." To remain alive, to say nothing of being energized and inspired in your life, the breath is essential. But the amount of breath you can take in depends on the openness of your heart.

In yoga terminology, breath practices are called pranayama. Prana represents the basic energy of life—the first unit—and *yama* means to reign in, such as connecting a chariot to its horses. This control gives tremendous power in yoga; pranayama is the control, or mastery, of the breath. Pranayama practices are highly potent and bring about direct changes in consciousness. No yoga practice is complete without the inclusion of pranayama.

The intent of this section is not to write a whole treatise on pranayama, as there are excellent books on the subject, but to share ways to integrate the breath with the chakras.

The Chakras and the Five Vayus

Through their exploration of yoga and breath, the ancient yogis discovered that prana occurred through various *vayus,* or winds. These reflect the flow of prana through the body, especially as directed by breath.

Apana vayu relates to the lower two chakras and pervades the lower abdomen. The flow of apana vayu is down and out, and it is the only vayu that descends. It nourishes the organs of reproduction and elimination, including elimination of toxins. Simply visualize the breath moving downward as you exhale, releasing your pelvic floor. The imbalance of apana vayu leads to retention and blockages in the process of elimination.

Samana vayu is your third chakra breath, related to digestive fire. Its flow moves inward from the periphery of the body to the navel and the core in general. It governs digestion in terms of assimilation of all substances: food, air, experiences, emotions, and thoughts. Feel your breath rising and falling in the front, sides, and back of the torso. Imbalance of this vayu leads to digestive problems.

Prana vayu moves into the fourth chakra through the heart, chest, and lungs. It is an inward-moving vayu, which is energizing and uplifting. When it is blocked, it may affect the heart and energy levels.

Udana vayu is related to the throat chakra. It flows in a circular pattern around the neck and head. It governs speech, self-expression, growth, and higher consciousness. Ujjayi breath (in chakra five) is a good practice for contacting this vayu. When it is blocked, it may affect self-expression.

Vyana vayu relates to the whole body and governs circulation on all levels. It moves from the core to the extremities. Deficiency can lead to poor circulation and numbness in the limbs.

Yoga postures and pranayama work with the various vayus to distribute prana throughout the whole system. Some postures, such as Apanasana (Knees to Chest Pose, or Wind-Relieving Pose) stimulate a specific vayu. Bandhas hold back the vayus to concentrate prana in certain areas.

4

Inhale, and God approaches you. Hold the inhalation, and God remains with you. Exhale, and you approach God. Hold the exhalation, and surrender to God.

• • • • • • • • • • • • •

KRISHNAMACHARYA

Coordinating the Breath: Inhalation and Exhalation

The main thing to remember is that breath is energy. Taking in more breath is charging; it increases your sensitivity, vitality, and aliveness. Letting your breath out is discharging; it facilitates letting go, relaxation, and helps dissolve pain and tension. Lengthen your inhalations or exhalations according to where you want to go. If you want more energy, focus on bringing in more oxygen. If you want to release, let go, relax, or soften, allow longer exhalations.

Inhaling is related to *brahmana*, which means to expand. It tonifies, nourishes, heats, and builds energy. Increase the inhalation for active, energetic poses or when you need strength and power.

Exhaling is related to *langhana*, which means to fast. It is used for relaxation, contraction, purification, cooling, and conservation of energy.

In general, rising up to a stand, raising your arms overhead, opening the front of the body, or back-bending are best assisted with an inhalation, as it allows you to expand. Forward folds, twists, and anything that makes the body pull into itself are best done on an exhalation, as it enables letting go. Bioenergetic grounding (page 59) is an exception. Here, you exhale as you push into the ground and inhale as you bend your knees, drawing up from the earth.

In addition, breathing into the belly stimulates the parasympathetic nervous system, which is calming and regulating. Breathing into the chest stimulates the sympathetic nervous system and is more energizing. Too much chest breathing can put us into a panic, however, as it stimulates the fight or flight response. Too much belly breathing can leave us overly loose and relaxed.

Ideally, we want to distribute prana evenly throughout all our chakras and be able to relax when desired and become energized whenever we need an extra boost.

Kapalabhati: Breath of Fire

This breath cleanses and energizes while strengthening the belly. Find a detailed description in the third chakra on page 187.

Ujjayi

Ujjayi breathing is made with a slight constriction of the throat, so it is also stimulating to the fifth chakra. Its technique is discussed in that chapter on page 325.

Nadi Shodhana: Alternate Nostril Breathing

Because this breath brings balance to the nervous system, it is excellent for the heart chakra or any upper chakra states of consciousness. It is both cleansing and calming, balancing the two hemispheres of the brain, and it is also recommended for insomnia.

1. Sit quietly in a comfortable upright meditation posture. Elevate your hips on a cushion if it is difficult to hold the natural curve of your spine.

2. Take a few deep, complete breaths.

3. With your right hand, fold down your first two fingers, making what is called the Vishnu mudra. This leaves your thumb and ring finger available for closing your nostrils as you switch sides.

4. At the top of an inhalation, close off your right nostril by pressing on the side of it with your right thumb (position A).

5. Exhale through the left nostril.

6. Inhale through the left nostril.

7. When the breath is full, use your ring finger to close off the left nostril (position B).

8. Exhale through the right nostril.

9. Inhale through the right nostril.

4

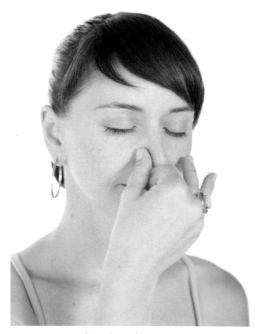

nadi shodhana ▲
alternate nostril breathing,
position a

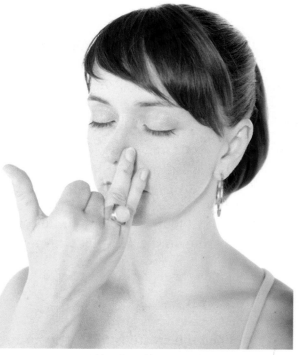

nadi shodhana ▲
alternate nostril breathing,
position b

10. This constitutes one full round. Repeat steps 4 through 9 for 10–20 full cycles, then return to a moment of meditation with relaxed natural breath.

Guidelines

- Keep your head centered over your midline. Do not tilt your head or move your head from side to side.

- Begin by counting slowly as you breathe, allowing the inhalation and the exhalation to be equal. Gradually increase the length of each breath as you expand your capacity.

- More advanced practitioners may extend the length of the exhalation up to twice as long as the inhalation.

- For extra credit, see if you can mentally trace the ida and pingala nadis crisscrossing between the chakras as you breathe in and out.

Benefits

- Calms and clears the mind

- Lowers the heart rate

- Is said to synchronize the two hemispheres of the brain

- Stimulates the ida and pingala nadis (the figure-eight currents around the chakras)

- Good for insomnia

- Purifying

- Quiets the heart and is good for anxiety

Avoid or Use Caution

- If you are stuffed up from a cold

- Do not practice forcefully

4

Kramas

The word *krama* means step, and krama pranayamas break the breath up into steps. Krama breathing utilizes either a short series of inhalations followed by a long exhalation or a long inhalation followed by short, contained exhalations or short breaths in both directions. Kramas are a good way to focus the attention on each chakra and are a good meditation technique for beginning meditators.

Anuloma krama focuses on the in-breath and is good for drawing energy up the chakras. In this breath you take a short inhale, pause without exhaling, then another inhale, pause, and continue until the breath is full, then follow with one long exhalation. To use this breath as a chakra meditation, take seven short inhalations, focusing on each chakra from bottom to top, holding the breath for a few moments at the top, then imagine clearing the chakras as you release. This stimulates the liberating current that moves upward.

Viloma krama focuses on the out-breath and is one long inhalation and seven short exhalations. Take a long, full breath in, then exhale and hold seven times, focusing on each chakra from top to bottom. When the breath is empty, pause again briefly, then take one full inhalation. This is good for grounding and bringing energy down the chakras.

Pratiloma krama retains the breath in steps on both the inhalation and the exhalation. This is good for focusing on the core and balancing the upward and downward currents.

Kundalini Chakra Breathing

This is a set of movements coordinated with rapid breathing, designed for stimulating the rise of energy up the chakras. It can be done as a quick pick-me-up or as preparation for yoga or meditation. It's a good exercise to do in the morning to get your energy going for the day. It's long been a favorite among my workshop students.

Note: Each movement begins in a seated cross-legged pose with an erect spine. Each breath is an inhalation through the nose and an exhalation through the mouth.

4

Chakra One

1. Bring your hands to your shoulders, elbows out to the side at shoulder height (position A).

2. Inhale through the nose and lift both arms overhead, lifting your knees at the same time (position B).

3. Exhale through the mouth and pull both your arms and your knees downward rapidly (position A).

4. Repeat 10–20 times, increasing in speed, then return to a normal breath.

5. Close your eyes and feel the charge of pranayama at your base chakra.

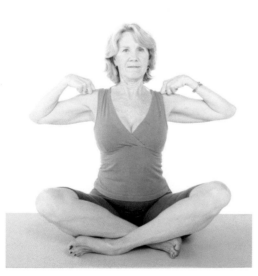

chakra one ▲
position a

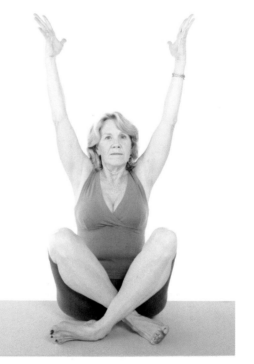

chakra one ▲
position b

Chakra Two

1. Place your hands on the front of your knees, palms down.

2. Inhale while pressing the back of your sacrum forward, bringing the navel toward the front. Pull gently on your knees to enhance the curve of the spine and the lift in the chest (position A).

3. Exhale and round your back, taking your navel toward the spine (position B).

4. Repeat 10–20 times, then return to a normal breath and straight spine.

5. Take a moment to feel the effects in your second chakra area.

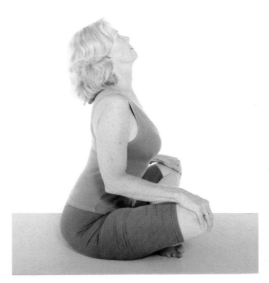

chakra two ▲
position a

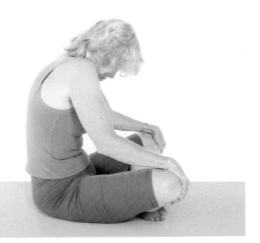

chakra two ▲
position b

This time you're going to move the middle of your torso around in a circle, as if you were trying to touch the sides of your midsection to the sides of a wine barrel. Start slowly, then pick up speed as you get the hang of it.

1. Inhale, bringing your belly forward as in chakra two, then exhale as you bring your right side body around to the right and toward the back.

2. When the exhale is complete, inhale and bring your left side body forward around the left side.

3. Continue, slowly picking up speed, trying to keep your shoulders stationary over your hips.

4. As there are ten petals to this chakra, complete ten circles clockwise, then repeat with ten circles counterclockwise.

4

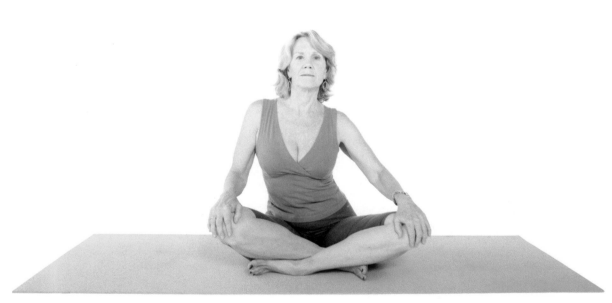

chakra three ▲

Chakra Four

1. Place your hands on your shoulders once again, elbows out to the side at shoulder height.

2. Inhale and twist your torso and elbows to the right.

3. Exhale and twist all the way to the left.

4. Repeat at least twelve times (once for each petal of this chakra), inhaling to the right and exhaling to the left.

5. Then repeat twelve times, inhaling to the left and exhaling to the right.

4

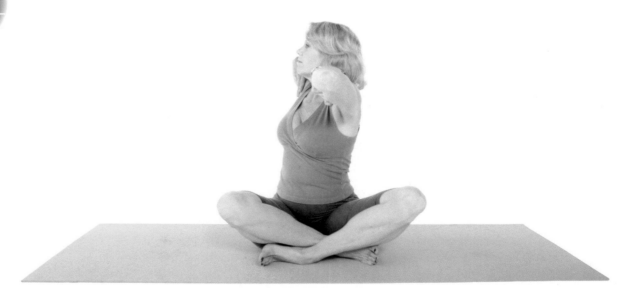

chakra four ▲

Chakra Five

1. Interlace your fingers under your chin, elbows down.

2. Inhale, lifting your elbows while keeping your fingers interlaced and your head level (position A).

3. Exhale, making a sound.

4. As you exhale, lift your chin and bend your head to the back while drawing your elbows toward each other (position B).

5. Repeat sixteen times, once for each petal of this chakra.

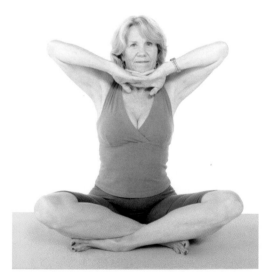

chakra five ▲
position a

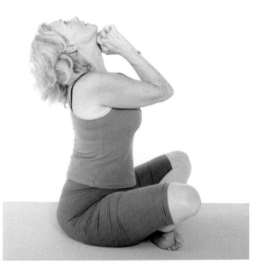

chakra five ▲
position b

Chakra Six

Now the breath becomes more subtle as you move toward the upper chakras. With this breath, imagine you are opening the curtains of a window in the morning and drinking in the light.

1. Inhale and reach your hands forward, opening your eyes wide (position A). Widen your arms as if opening the drapes, and drink in any light or color that you can see (position B).

2. Exhale, close your eyes, and bring the memory of that light or color into your inner world as you bring your hands to your eyes.

3. Repeat 10–12 times.

4. End with eyes shut, quietly breathing, and imagine your inner world flooded with light, color, and beauty.

4

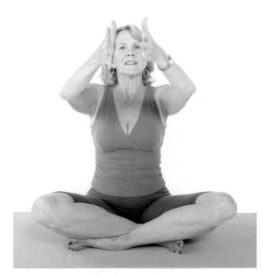

chakra six ▲
position a

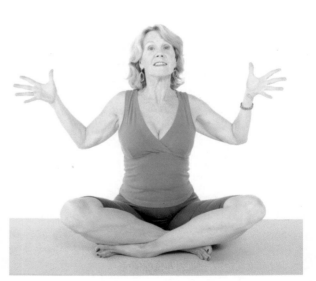

chakra six ▲
position b

Chakra Seven

1. Bring your palms together in anjali mudra, or simple prayer position, over the heart.

2. While keeping your palms together, inhale and raise your arms up overhead (position A).

3. As you exhale, separate your hands and bring them outward like a blossoming lotus flower (position B).

4. Repeat 10–20 times, then rest quietly and feel the effects.

5. When you are finished, mentally scan the inside of your body and notice which parts feel energized. If necessary, repeat the breathing for any chakra that feels like it is not holding the energy sufficiently.

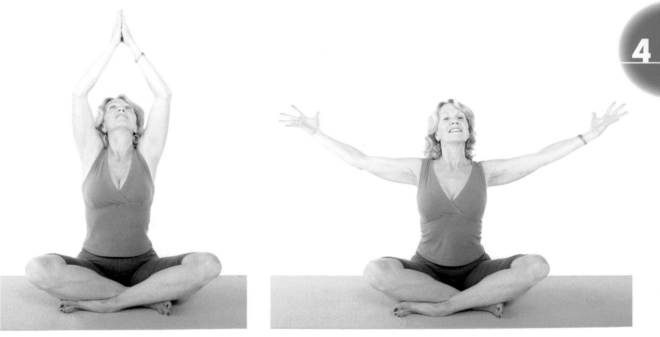

chakra seven ▲
position a

chakra seven ▲
position b

Clearing the Nadis

I find this breath to be a powerful way of clearing the subtle body and creating a deeper sense of presence. Use it carefully, as it is very potent. This breath is contraindicated for migraines or high blood pressure.

1. Sit in a comfortable cross-legged position with your back straight but not rigid. Remember: roots down, crown up.

2. Begin with a round of Kapalabhati, the rapid diaphragmatic breathing discussed in chakra three (page 187). One round should be about forty snaps of the diaphragm, but it can be up to eighty or more for more experienced practitioners.

3. After your forty to eighty snaps, take a deep inhalation and hold the breath two-thirds full. Simultaneously practice Mula bandha (root lock; see page 56) and Jalandhara bandha (chin lock; see page 327) while pulling on your knees with your hands to pull the sternum forward and the shoulder blades down the back. Imagine directing the energy into your heart chakra, and feel the increase of prana into that area.

4. When you are ready to exhale, let your breath out with one big swoosh, rounding the back.

5. Then straighten your spine again and wait a few moments, allowing your breath to do whatever it will naturally.

Guidelines

• Release the breath about two-thirds of the way into your full capacity of holding. Don't push it to the maximum, as it can be dangerous. Feel when your body cues you to release.

• You may feel a wave of dizziness, a tingling, or the sense of a breeze going through the inside of your body. Simply sit still until that wave passes. Either keep your eyes closed or focus your gaze on something particular, like a statue on your altar or a beautiful picture or a candle flame. When the dizziness passes, you will feel more present in the room.

- You can repeat this a few times, but this breath is so powerful you won't want to do too many; three to five rounds is plenty. What is important is to wait after each round until your body normalizes and to feel the shift. It can produce a profound state of consciousness.

- **Warning:** this breath practice has the potential—if you hold your breath too long before releasing—for you to pass out and fall over. For that reason, as stated previously, do not hold your breath to your full capacity. Always do it in a sitting position in a safe place where you won't hurt yourself if you happen to hold your breath too long.

Fourth Chakra Practice and Postures

Standing Yoga Mudra

The nice thing about this pose is that you can do it anytime, anywhere—on or off your mat. If you sit at a desk, it is a simple counterstretch to the rounded spine that comes from hunching over a computer and should be done every twenty or thirty minutes throughout the day. It opens the chest, shoulders, and throat, stimulating both fourth and fifth chakras. Bending forward brings blood to the brain.

1. Begin in Tadasana, Standing Mountain Pose. Align your core from heaven to earth. Anchor into your lower chakras by pressing down through the feet, rooting your tailbone, hollowing out your groin area, and lifting your ribs.

2. Interlace your fingers behind your back. Draw your elbows toward each other, straightening your arms, while simultaneously rolling your shoulders toward your back body (position A).

3. Inhale and lift the heart, expanding the chest. Tilt your head back slightly, being careful not to compress your neck or inhibit your breathing.

4. As you exhale, bow forward at the hips, keeping your hands clasped behind you and your legs straight (positions B and C).

5. Fold fully forward and allow your hands to move away from your spine.

6. Inhale to come out of the pose, returning to position A,
   then release the hands and stand tall in Tadasana.

Guidelines

- Lift your sternum upward while rooting down into the legs.

- Deepen the standing pose by drawing the wrists away from the spine.

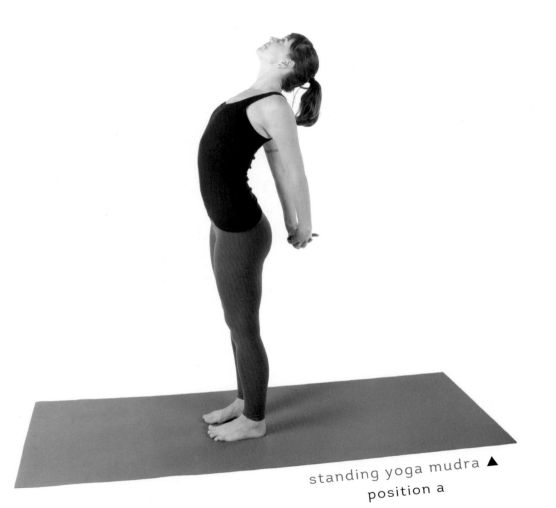

standing yoga mudra ▲
position a

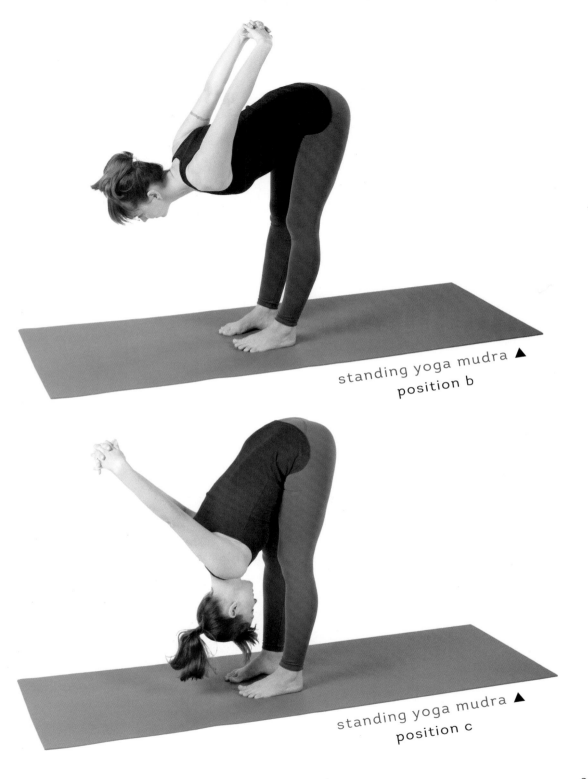

standing yoga mudra ▲
position b

standing yoga mudra ▲
position c

4

- When bowing forward, allow the natural weight of the arms to pry open the upper back.

- Rotate your inner thighs toward the back, widening the back of the sacrum.

- Gently shake your head to make sure your neck is loose.

- Lift up halfway toward a flat back and expand the heart by drawing the chest forward away from the hips (position B).

- Use a strap if you have difficulty joining your hands.

Benefits

- Opens shoulders and stretches the upper back

- Brings blood to the brain

- Relaxes the neck

- Stimulates the heart

- Opens the lungs—good for asthma

- Stretches hamstrings

- Good for a contracted or deficient heart chakra

Avoid or Use Caution

- Headaches—keep your head higher than your hips

- Shoulder injuries

- High blood pressure

Belt Stretch

This practice is wonderful to do in the morning to open the chest. Use your towel when you are getting out of the shower or use your belt or scarf when you are getting dressed. In addition, it is good to do after a long period of sitting in order to combat the hunching over that tends to happen when we work on computers, bow our head to read, or slouch when watching TV. And, of course, it is a good warm-up for backbends, as it stretches the pectoral muscles on the front of the chest and opens the shoulders. This exercise came from Selene Vega in our book *The Sevenfold Journey*.

1. Place your hands on a belt or strap with your fingers wrapped around it.

2. On an inhalation, lift your arms up overhead, elbows straight (position A).

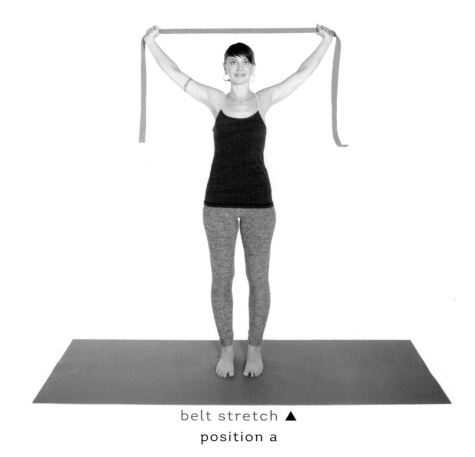

belt stretch ▲
position a

3. As you exhale, bring your arms behind you, keeping
   the elbows straight and the chest lifted and open while
   rooting down into your legs (position B).

4. Bend side to side, opening the ribs. Allow yourself to
   release by making sounds with your exhalations.

Guidelines

- Your hands should be far enough apart for you to bring your arms to
  the back while keeping your elbows straight. Your hands should be
  close enough together for you to feel a stretch in your pectoral muscles
  (front of the chest) as you do so. If moving your arms behind you is

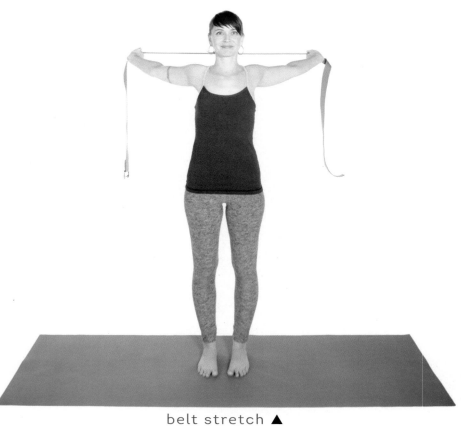

belt stretch ▲
position b

too easy, move your hands closer together. If it is too difficult or you have to bend your elbows, move your hands farther apart. For most people, the appropriate distance is approximately 30–36 inches.

Benefits

- Opens the shoulders and chest

- Promotes deeper breathing

- Strengthens the arms

- Expands the heart

Avoid or Use Caution

- Shoulder injuries

Gomukhasana: Cow Face Pose

Traditionally this pose is done with knees crossed over each other in a seated position, but I like to follow Belt Stretch with this pose by remaining standing and draping the strap over the shoulder as an aid.

1. Begin in Tadasana, Standing Mountain Pose.

2. Raise your right arm up overhead, bringing it alongside your right ear. Bend your right elbow, pointing your fingers downward.

3. Bring your left arm behind your body and bend your elbow with your fingers pointed upward.

4. Reach your hands toward each other and clasp your fingers together (position A).

5. If, like most people, your hands do not reach each other, clasp them onto the strap draped over your shoulder. Then walk your hands toward each other until you reach your edge (position B).

6. Breathe!

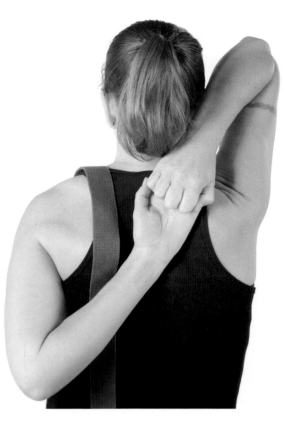

gomukhasana ▲
cow face pose,
position a

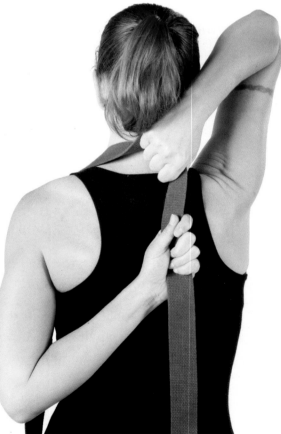

gomukhasana ▶
cow face pose,
position b

Guidelines

- The palm will face outward in the lower hand and inward on the upper hand.

- Outwardly rotate your upper arms while inwardly rotating your bottom arm.

- Keep your spine straight. Do not lean to the left or right.

- Keep your head centered over your base.

- Draw your elbows toward the midline of your spine and open the chest forward.

- For advanced deepening of the pose, move your hands away from the back of your torso.

Benefits

- Opens the chest and shoulders

- Promotes deeper breathing

- Softens the heart

Avoid or Use Caution

- Shoulder injuries

Marjaryasana: Cat Pose and Bitilasana: Cow Pose

This exercise promotes fluidity and flexibility of the spine and is always a good warm-up. It opens the heart through the process of expansion and contraction, much like we opened up our hand chakras by opening and closing our palms. Ride on the breath as you arch and flex your spine, letting the breath lead and complete each movement.

1. Begin in Table Pose.

2. Inhale, lifting your head and the tip of your tailbone while arching the rest of the spine. This is Cow Pose, as it resembles the back of a cow (position A).

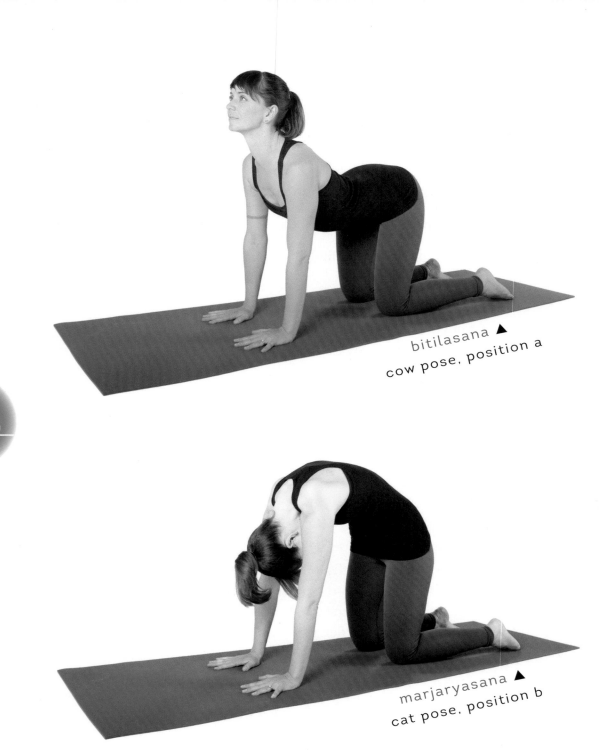

bitilasana ▲
cow pose, position a

marjaryasana ▲
cat pose, position b

4

3. Exhale and tuck your tailbone, rounding the spine in the opposite direction, head following the movement that begins in the tailbone (position B). This is Cat Pose, resembling a cat when it wakes from a nap.

4. Repeat slowly, each move coordinated with the breath, going back and forth between Cat and Cow.

5. After several rounds, end with your spine in a neutral position. Soften the heart and feel the effects of the practice.

Guidelines

• Let the breath begin each movement. Inhale, then start the movement of opening the chest, complete the movement, then complete the inhalation. Begin your exhalation, then start the rounding of the back, complete that movement, then finish the exhalation. Let the breath move your body.

• Begin the movement from the tailbone, and let the rest of the spine follow.

• Outwardly rotate the upper arms in Cow Pose.

• Energetically draw the hands toward the knees as you inhale and arch to accentuate opening the chest. Push the hands away from the knees as you exhale and round.

Benefits

• Promotes flexibility in the spine

• Deepens the breath

• Opens the heart

Avoid or Use Caution

• If knees are sensitive, place a blanket underneath

4

Anahatasana: Extended Puppy Pose

How wonderful to have a pose named after the heart chakra itself! This is a deeply peaceful posture of surrender and heart opening. You can literally melt your heart to the earth.

1. From Table Pose, walk your hands forward on the mat, keeping your wrists in line with your shoulders. Beginners may spread the wrists wider.

2. Be sure to keep the hips directly above the knees as your hands move forward. The thighs should be straight up and down, perpendicular to the floor, knees hip-width apart.

3. When you have stretched your arms forward as far as possible without lowering your hips, lower your forehead or chin toward the floor, using a small cushion or rolled blanket if necessary.

4. Soften the body and melt the heart, allowing your exhalations to become longer with each breath.

5. To come out of the pose, inhale, lift the head, and walk the hands back until they are under the shoulders once again.

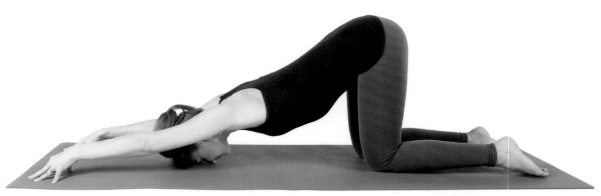

anahatasana ▲
extended puppy pose

Guidelines

- Take time in this pose to release all effort and just be. Find a place of peace and stillness.

- If you feel a pinch in your upper back or shoulders, try taking the arms farther apart. If extending the arms is still too uncomfortable, fold the hands underneath the forehead or place the forehead on a bolster or folded blanket.

- Press your fingertips in the floor like claws to better tone the arms and lift the armpits.

- Make sure the hips stay directly above the knees, with the thighs perpendicular to the floor.

- Let gravity do the work. Allow your sacrum to fall away from your hips.

- Allow each breath to bring more surrender. As long as you are anxious to move out of the pose, you haven't found your way to the heart of it yet, which is stillness.

- Melt the area between the shoulder blades. If assisting someone in this pose, it is nice to feel a loving touch behind the heart chakra.

Benefits

- Promotes deep peace

- Melts the heart

- Softens the back

- Opens the shoulders

Avoid or Use Caution

- Shoulder injuries

- Migraines

4

Thread the Needle Twist

Twisting poses compress the internal organs, release toxins, and cleanse the body. While most twists are more third chakra oriented, this one gives a nice opening to the upper back. It creates a very slight inversion, bringing prana from the hips to the heart.

1. Begin in Table Pose with a neutral spine.

2. Place your left hand on the midline of the mat at shoulder level.

3. Inhale and lift your right arm up to the ceiling. Push down through your left arm and up into your right arm, expanding the chest (position A).

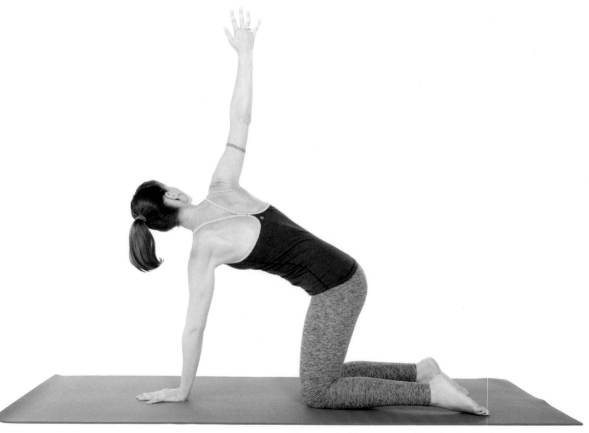

thread the needle twist ▲
position a

4. Exhale and bend the right elbow. "Thread the needle" by passing the right arm through the space between your knees and your left wrist (position B).

5. Take your right shoulder down to the floor as close to the midline of the mat as possible. Then lift the left arm up toward the ceiling, twisting the upper back (position C).

6. Relax into the pose here or take your left arm overhead, alongside your left ear (position D).

7. To come out of the pose, return to Table Pose.

8. Repeat the twist on the other side.

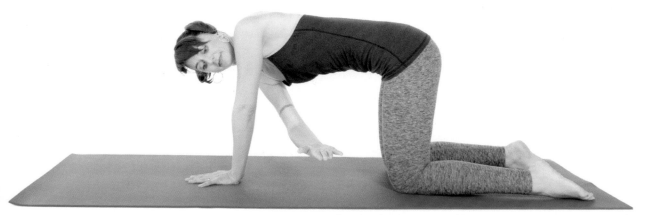

thread the needle twist ▲
position b

Guidelines

- Try to keep your hips square to the back of the mat and your spine aligned with the midline of your mat. Encourage the hip on the side of your upraised arm to move toward the back of the mat.

- Use the back of the arm that is against the floor to deepen the twist by pressing it more firmly into the floor.

Benefits

- Deeply relaxing

- Stretches ribs and shoulders

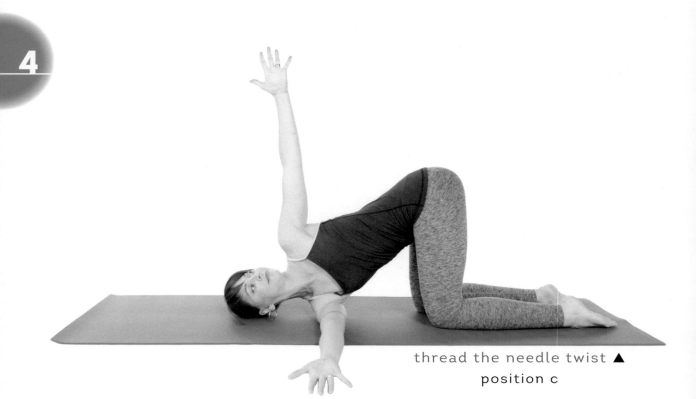

thread the needle twist ▲
position c

- Promotes spinal flexibility

- Opens the upper back

Avoid or Use Caution

- Shoulder injuries

- Headaches

- High blood pressure

- Advanced pregnancy

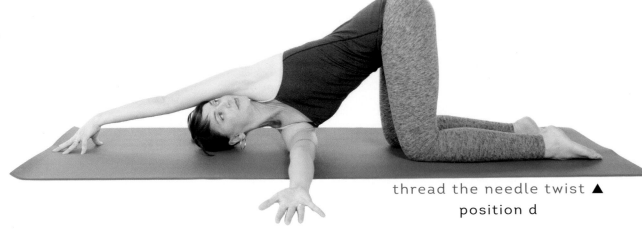

thread the needle twist ▲
position d

Parighasana 2: Half Circle Pose

We encountered Parighasana 1, Gate Pose, in the third chakra. This pose incorporates a slight backbend as well as a side stretch and is good for creating expansion in the heart chakra. Let yourself be radiant and joyful in this pose, supported by your stability in the lower chakras.

1. Begin in a kneeling position with your knees hip-distance apart. Lift your chest and crown, bringing your shoulders back and lengthening your spine.

2. Stretch your right leg out to the right side, knee straight, rotating your leg so that the knee points upward and the toes are pointed outward, moving down toward the mat. If desired, you can roll a blanket underneath your toes. Some variations do this pose with a flexed foot as well.

3. Extend the arms out to each side at shoulder height. Stretch across the heart by pressing the arms wide. Inhale.

4. Place your left hand on the floor slightly behind and to the left of your bent knee.

5. Inhaling, lift your right arm up and over your ear, drawing the upper shoulder back and extending the chest and hips forward.

6. Take a few breaths here, finding the surrender in the pose, then inhale to come back out.

7. Repeat on the other side.

Guidelines

• Keep your legs active, especially the straight one. Notice how structure and firmness in your lower body and support from your lower arm create the freedom to expand.

• Press the upper hip and shoulder forward, creating a slight backbend.

• Allow your throat to open without straining the neck.

Benefits

- Opens the heart and distributes prana through the whole body

- Opens the shoulders

- Relaxes the neck

Avoid or Use Caution

- Shoulder injuries

- Place a folded blanket under your knees if they are sensitive

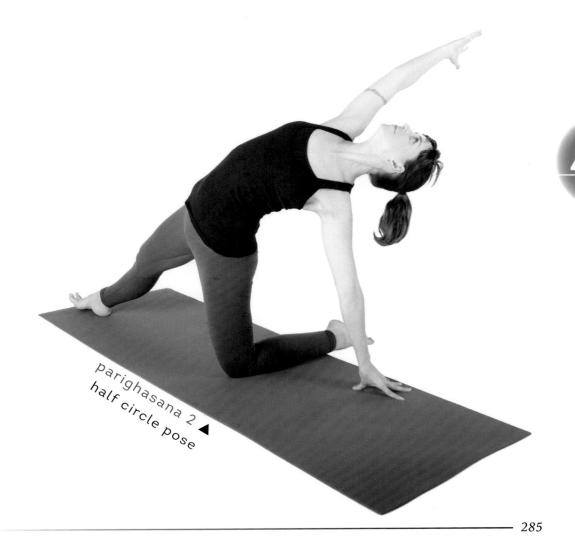

parighasana 2 ◀
half circle pose

Matsyasana: Fish Pose

The nice thing about Fish Pose is that it can usually be held without strain for longer than other backbends, allowing the chronic contraction of the heart chakra time to release. It's a good pose for beginners to start opening the upper back. If the head does not touch the floor, place a folded blanket under the back of the head to avoid straining the neck. Alternately, a folded blanket or cushion under the back can be a more passive way of experiencing the pose.

1. Lie on your back, arms by your sides, with your legs drawn together and knees straight. (For an easier version of this pose, you may bend your knees and place your feet hip-width apart.)

2. Slide your hands underneath your buttocks, thumbs up.

3. Inhale and lift your head and upper body enough to slide the heels of your hands onto the backside of your hips, bending your elbows close into your side and pressing them into the mat. Your torso will be at an angle to the floor. Exhale.

4. Inhale again and lift your chest upward, externally rotate your shoulders, and firm up your belly. You are now arching your back.

5. Press your elbows into the mat and draw your tailbone simultaneously down to the mat and up toward your shoulders.

6. Gently tilt your head back, and, if possible, touch the top of your head to the floor.

7. To come out of the pose, inhale and lift your head first, then slide your spine back down to the floor.

Guidelines

• Press your tailbone toward the back body and draw it energetically toward your elbows, curving the sacrum. Allow the curve to continue up the spine, pressing the chest upward.

• Keep your thighs active if your legs are out straight. Draw your legs together as one.

4

- Be careful not to crunch the neck. Use a folded blanket if your head cannot reach the floor.

- Press your palms into the floor to help move your spine forward.

- Breathe deeply. Use your inhalations to expand the chest. Beginners may wish to use a bolster, block, or rolled-up mat underneath their chest for more support in the pose.

- To develop core strength, lift the legs to a 45-degree angle.

- To increase the challenge and deepen this pose, slide your hands out from underneath your buttocks and bring them into prayer position over your heart.

- The full expression of this pose is with legs folded in Padmasana, Full Lotus (not shown).

Benefits

- Opens and softens the heart

- Promotes deeper breathing

- Improves posture

- Aids digestion

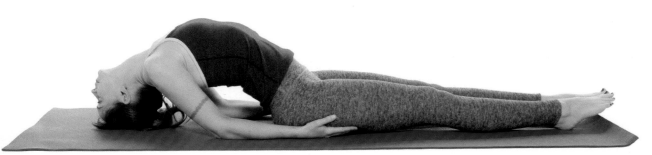

matsyasana ▲
fish pose

Avoid or Use Caution

- Neck injury

- Headaches or migraines

- High or low blood pressure

Ustrasana: Camel Pose

This is a wonderful pose for opening the chest, stretching the front of the body, and preparing for deeper backbends. It opens the groins, strengthens the thighs and buttocks, and stimulates the third chakra kidneys and adrenal glands, as well as expands the breathing by opening the ribs and letting the heart shine out. It also opens the throat chakra and expands the shoulders. It is especially good for addressing the collapsed chest of a deficient heart chakra and for relieving rigidity in the upper spine.

1. Begin in a kneeling position, knees hip-distance apart.

2. Place your hands on your low back, fingers pointing downward. If you are a beginner, you will want to keep your hands on your hips.

3. Ground down into your knees. They become the roots and foundation of this pose.

4. Hollow out the front of your groins by slightly tucking the tailbone and lifting the hip bones. Firm up the second chakra area by drawing the front and back of the second chakra toward each other.

5. Lift the sternum, outwardly rotating the upper arms and taking the head of the armbones toward the back. Inhale deeply.

6. Exhale and arch your back, pressing the hips forward and maintaining a lift in the chest. Extend the neck but keep it somewhat loose, opening across the front of the shoulders (position A).

4

7. If you are comfortable here and want to deepen the pose, bring your hands to your heels. The heels can be lifted by coming up onto your toes to make them easier to reach (position B), or your feet can be flat on the floor for the full pose (position C). There is also the option of using blocks beside your heels to place your hands higher.

8. Breathe deeply and find the surrender in the pose.

9. Come out of the pose on an inhalation, supporting your pelvis by using the buttock muscles.

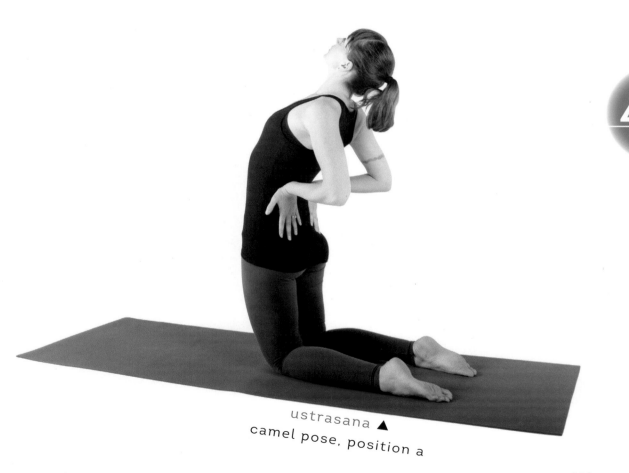

ustrasana ▲
camel pose, position a

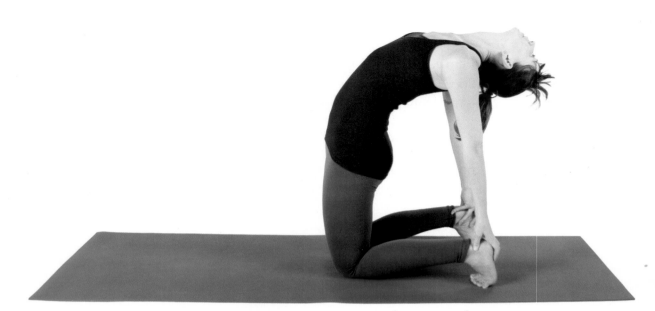

ustrasana ▲

camel pose, position b

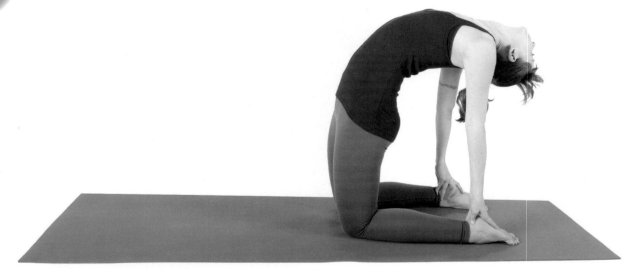

ustrasana ▲

camel pose, position c

Guidelines

- Your thighs and shins should be parallel with each other.

- Move the elbows toward one another when your hands are on your low back until the upper armbones are parallel to each other.

- Squeeze your thighs together as you enter the backbend. They will not touch, as your knees should stay hip-width apart, but the action of drawing into the center will stabilize the lower body and support your back.

- Lift your ribs and sternum before arching back. The greater the length in your spine, the easier the backbend will be.

- Be mindful of your lower back and lighten up on the backbend if you feel any discomfort.

Benefits

- Opens the heart, shoulders, and chest

- Stretches the entire front of the body

- Strengthens the legs

- Increases circulation

- Aids spinal flexibility

- Reduces anxiety

- Energizing

Avoid or Use Caution

- Low back issues

- Low blood pressure

- Neck injuries

4

Bhujangasana: Cobra Pose

This pose was first mentioned in chakra one, but it's also a classic heart chakra opener. In chakra one, the focus was on hugging the legs into the core, strengthening the back muscles, and pushing the floor away through the hands and arms.

In the heart chakra, the focus is now on the outward rotation of the upper arms, the openness and surrender in the chest, and expanding the chest. Draw your elbows into your sides and energetically draw the arms toward your hips to allow the heart to blossom.

1. Begin facedown on your belly, with elbows bent and hands placed alongside your shoulders, fingertips in line with the tops of the shoulders.

2. Draw your legs together and firm up your belly, pulling the abdominal muscles inward. Hug into your core.

3. Inhale and lift the head and chest off the floor, rolling the shoulders back. For Baby Cobra, use your back muscles only, lifting your hands off the floor a few inches. For Full Cobra, extend your arms and push the floor away to rise higher.

4. Hold for several breaths.

5. Come out of the pose on an exhalation. Turn your head to one side, place your arms by your sides, and relax.

Guidelines

• From your root chakra, extend through the core of your pelvis, up through the heart, and to the top of your crown.

• Outwardly rotate the upper arms and keep the elbows in close to the sides.

• Press your shoulder blades toward each other, pointing the tips of the shoulder blades down the back. Lower your shoulders away from your ears.

4

- Go up and down a few times, coordinating the movement with your breath and exercising the muscles of the back.

- If you cannot keep your shoulders down as you straighten your arms, bend the arms a little more and soften the pose.

- Use the resistance of the ground to deepen the pose by drawing the heels of your hands toward your hips.

Benefits

- Opens the heart

- Clears the mind

- Increases spinal flexibility

- Grounds the pelvis

- Stimulates circulatory and lymphatic systems

Avoid or Use Caution

- Pregnancy

- Spinal injury

bhujangasana ▲
cobra pose

Adho Mukha Vrksasana: Handstand

Inversions turn the entire chakra system upside down. While drawing energy up the spine occurs through effort and will when you are right-side up, the prana naturally flows into the upper body when you are inverted. Inversions also create upper body strength. By elevating the legs above the heart, inversions improve circulation, lymph drainage, and digestion. Being upside down brings energy into the head and improves mental clarity. A handstand develops arm and shoulder strength and fills the chest with energy. It also promotes blood flow to the neck and brain, so it is good for all the upper chakras. Whether you stay up just a moment or learn to hold a handstand for longer, the mere effort will energize your upper body. For finding your centerline, there is nothing like balancing upside down.

Inversions can also be disorienting. Here we start with a handstand preparation pose to get used to managing yourself upside down. If you are new to handstand, it's best to get someone to spot you the first few times.

Handstand Prep

1. Sit with your buttocks firmly against a wall and your legs out straight. Notice where your heels touch the floor in front of you, and mark that spot with your mind or with a block or strap. This measures the length of your legs and tells you where you will place your hands.

2. Place your palms on the floor, shoulder width apart, at the spot you just marked by the length of your legs, with fingers pointing away from the wall.

3. Walk your feet back to the wall, creating a Downward Dog position by placing your heels against the base of the wall.

4. Spread your fingers wide and firm up your arms by pushing through the core of each arm into the floor. Keep your arms straight and your shoulders hugging into your back. Claw the earth with your fingertips.

5. Continue to push into the floor as you begin to walk your feet up the wall behind you, step by step, making sure your arms have the strength to hold you.

4

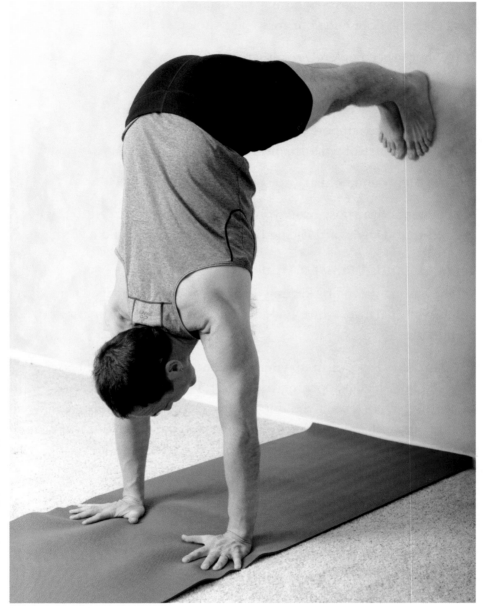

adho mukha vrksasana

▶ handstand prep, position a

6. Keep your shoulders over your wrists. Do not allow your shoulders to come forward beyond your wrists. Press your chest toward the wall.

7. Stop when your legs are parallel to the floor. Do not go higher. Your body now makes a right-angle L shape, with your legs parallel to the floor and your torso perpendicular (position A).

8. Bring your legs completely together and squeeze them toward the midline.

9. This is a good way to see if your arms and shoulders are strong enough to support your weight in a handstand and to get a sense of what the inversion feels like.

10. Breathe deeply and hold as you stabilize.

11. To come out of the pose, walk your feet back down the wall to the floor and return to Downward Facing Dog Pose or rest in Child's Pose.

Full Handstand Against a Wall

Develop your handstand by kicking up against a wall or a friend's hands, which can support your balance, while you develop the necessary strength in your arms and shoulders.

1. Begin in Table Pose. Firm up your arms and soften the place between your shoulder blades, opening your heart. Place your hands 8–12 inches away from a wall, shoulder-width apart. Rotate your upper arms slightly outward and push down into the web between your thumb and forefinger. Pull your belly in slightly to activate and firm up your core.

2. Push your hips up into Downward Facing Dog Pose, but walk your feet a little farther forward than you might in your normal Dog pose. If possible, walk forward until your shoulders are over your wrists.

3. Firm your shoulders, lift your shoulder blades up toward your hips, activate your hands and fingers, and take a deep breath.

4

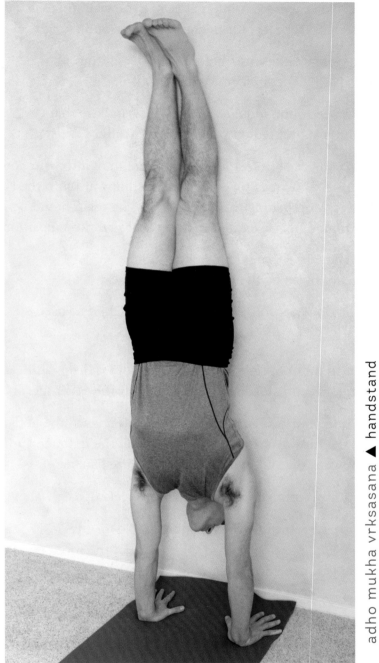

adho mukha vrksasana ▲ handstand

4

4. Bend your left knee and bring it closer to the wall, then kick up with a straight right leg. Keep your arms firm and straight.

5. Practice a few smaller kicks before you kick all the way up, to see if you are comfortable.

6. Be sure to keep your shoulders over your hands so that the weight is supported on your arms vertically.

7. Once you can get both feet against the wall, hug into your core, press your feet and legs together, and push upward into the balls of your feet, lengthening the whole body. The toes should be neither pointed nor flexed but halfway between these positions.

8. Hold for a few breaths, then take the right leg down, followed by the left leg.

9. Breathe in Downward Dog or take a rest in Child's Pose.

Guidelines

- You can also lift one leg horizontally and hold it firm; while an assistant holds and steadies that leg, you lift the other leg.

- Push up into your pelvis. Be careful not to "banana" the body but keep the hips over the shoulders. Taking the tailbone and belly in toward the core will help alleviate the banana.

- Keep your arms straight and stretch your heels up the wall.

- Gazing toward your fingertips is more stable for the shoulders, while gazing toward the middle of the room is more freeing for the neck area (and more advanced).

- Practice kicking up with each leg so you don't get in the habit of favoring one side. Keep the top leg straight and avoid twisting the pelvis while kicking up.

Benefits

- Energizing for the whole body

- Upper chakra stimulation

- Drains lymph and blood, then replenishes

- Strengthens the arms and shoulders

- Accentuates core

Avoid or Use Caution

- Shoulder or neck injury

- High blood pressure

- Headaches

- Menstruation

- Pregnancy

- Glaucoma

- Heart conditions

Urdvha Dhanurasana: Upward Facing Bow or Wheel Pose

This is an advanced pose that should only be done when the body is thoroughly warmed up, using smaller backbends such as Cat/Cow, Cobra, Camel, or Bridge to prepare the spine for this full extension. If you have never done this pose before, you are safer working with an instructor the first few times. There are many variations your teacher can suggest—such as using the wall, a chair, blocks, a strap, or holding on to someone's ankles—that can help you ease into the pose until your back is flexible enough to do it on your own.

Be patient. Gaining the flexibility for this pose takes time. The benefits are both strength and flexibility, including stimulating the frontal opening of all the chakras. It is deeply energizing yet calming at the same time.

1. Lie on your back with your knees bent, hip-width apart or slightly wider. Bring your heels as close to your sitting bones as possible.

2. Bend your elbows and place your palms on the floor just above your shoulders, fingertips pointing downward, toward the shoulders (position A). Pull the tops of your upper arms in toward their sockets, hollowing the armpits, and firm your shoulder blades into your back so that they press into the floor.

3. As you firm up your shoulder blades, simultaneously soften your heart and take a deep breath.

4. Exhale as you press your feet into the floor, especially rooting down the insides of the feet. Push your hips up into the air.

5. Next, press your hands into the floor and come up onto your head (position B). This is a momentary resting place to make any adjustments in your alignment.

6. Inhale deeply. Then, on the next exhalation, push into your arms to lift your head off the floor, pushing through the core of each arm and straightening your elbows if possible (position C).

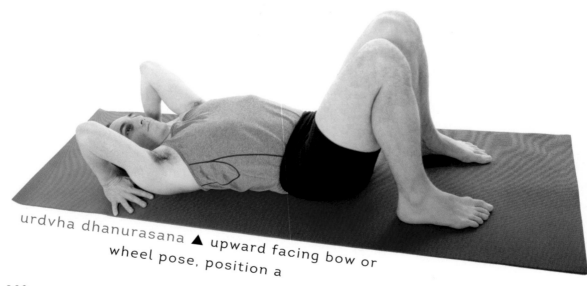

urdvha dhanurasana ▲ upward facing bow or wheel pose, position a

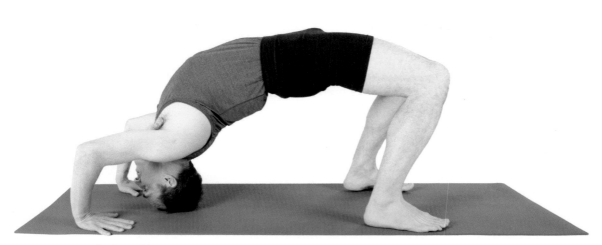

urdvha dhanurasana ▲ upward facing bow or
wheel pose, position b

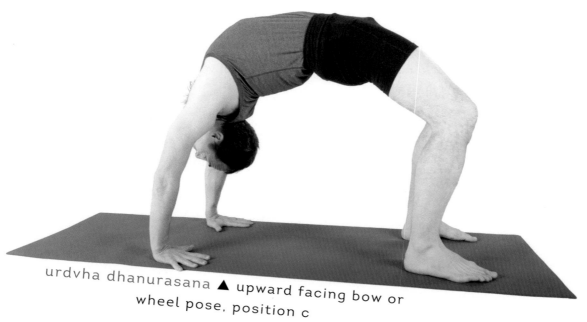

urdvha dhanurasana ▲ upward facing bow or
wheel pose, position c

7. To come out of the pose, slowly bend the elbows and knees, tuck the chin toward the chest, and lower your spine to the earth. Try to avoid the urge to draw your knees into your chest directly following this deep backbend. It's best to give the lumbar discs a moment to readjust before spinal flexion.

8. Take a few moments in Savasana to feel the wonderful effects of your backbend.

Guidelines

- The feet and legs tend to splay out on their own, so try to keep the feet parallel and the thighs rotated inward—it makes for less compression in the lower back and sacroiliac joints. Pressing the inside edges of your feet is helpful for this.

- Lengthen the tailbone toward the back of the knees.

- Firm the shoulder blades into the back, hugging your elbows into the core and rotating the upper armbones outward.

- Lengthen the neck and let the head hang with gravity, softening the throat.

- Take a few deep breaths and widen across the front of your chest while pushing through the core of your legs and arms, letting your heart radiate.

- To take the pose deeper, straighten your legs or walk your feet toward your hands.

- See if you can find at least a tiny bit of surrender!

Benefits

- Strengthens the whole body, especially the arms and legs

- Promotes spinal flexibility

- Increases breathing and lung capacity

- Promotes circulation

- Aids digestion

- Opens the heart

- Energizes

- Relieves stress

- Stimulates lymph and blood flow

- Fun!

Avoid or Use Caution

- Tricky pose—not for beginners and not without sufficient warm-up

- Back, shoulder, or wrist injuries

- Carpal tunnel syndrome

- Abnormal high or low blood pressure

- Headaches or migraines

- Pregnancy

Makarasana: Crocodile Pose

Often what blocks the heart chakra is fear of exposure and vulnerability. In response to this fear, we protect the heart. In this pose, the elbows and arms protect the heart, which allows the back to release. This allows you to arch your spine without effort or strain. The result is an effortless restorative pose that truly softens the heart.

1. Lie on your belly, legs out behind you.

2. Lift your head and bring the heels of your hands beneath your chin, elbows out in front of you, resting the weight of your head on your hands.

3. Allow the back and chest to relax.

4. For variations, widen your legs, with your toes turned outward, or bend your knees.

5. For an even more restful posture, fold your forearms over each other, turn your head to the side, and rest your head on your wrists.

Benefits

- Restful for the heart

- Eases back pain

- Relaxing

- Softening

- Good for asthma

- Helps realign the vertebrae

Avoid or Use Caution

- Pregnancy

4

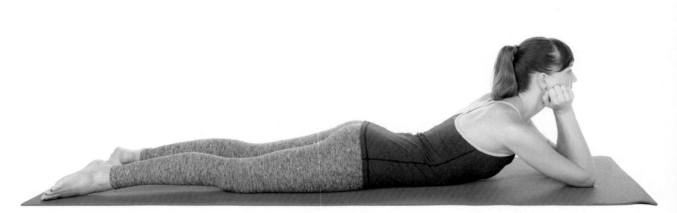

makarasana ▲
crocodile pose

Partner Poses

Since the heart chakra is about connection with another, partner poses not only give you a chance to stretch further, but they greatly enhance the opening of the heart. Of course they make you more vulnerable, but that is part of the heart chakra's opening! This is a small sampling of poses that make dynamic contact with another being.[8] Smile, enjoy, and have compassion for yourself and your partner. Let this be a playful connection, one in which your partner's presence helps you open more deeply.

Stand and Connect

1. Facing your partner, stand with eyes closed and find your inner core from base to crown. Place your left hand over your own heart and connect within.

2. When connected inside, each person opens their eyes to look eye to eye with the partner in front of them while staying centered within their own alignment.

3. Each person places their right hand on the back of their partner's left hand, which is already over their own heart.

4. Coordinate your breathing, inhaling and exhaling together. Feel the connection.

4

---

8 For more partner poses, see the book *Contact: The Yoga of Relationship* by Tara Lynda Guber and Anodea Judith.

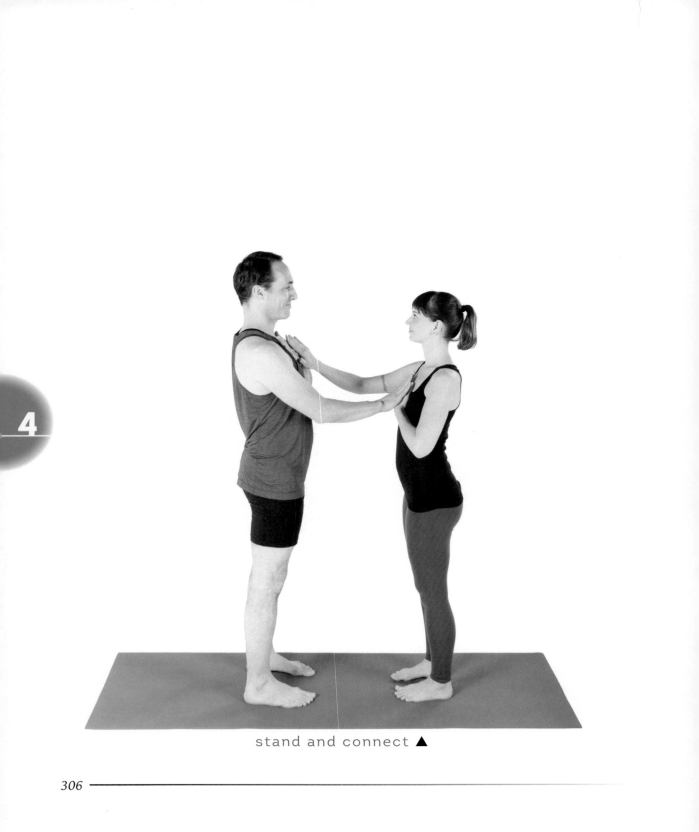

stand and connect ▲

Part A

1. While still standing, reach out with both hands to your partner's shoulders and begin massaging the tops of the shoulders.

2. Latch on firmly to each other's shoulders, bend at the hips, and walk your feet away from each other until you have a flat back (position A). Don't let go!

3. With both partners holding on to each other's shoulders, pull your hips away from each other. Lift your head to meet your partner's open eyes. Feel the spine lengthening. Breathe and smile.

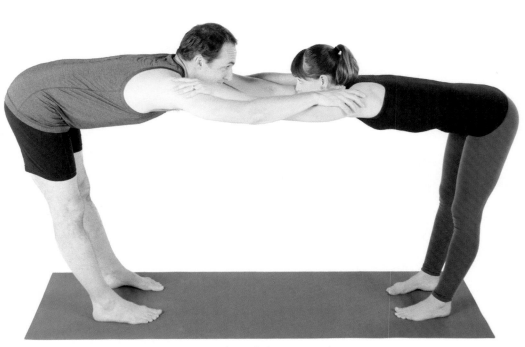

massage shoulders and arms ▲
position a

Part B: Hold Wrist to Wrist

1. Next, massage down the arms as you take baby steps away from each other. Continue to bend at the hips.

2. Hold on to each other wrist to wrist, meaning each person's palm is wrapped around the other person's wrist, as shown. (This gives you a firmer grip than just holding hands, which can get sweaty and slippery.)

3. Hold tightly as each person pulls their hips back. Allow the weight of your hips to create space between your ribs and lengthen your spine. Lift your head enough to maintain eye contact.

4. Smile and open your heart.

Benefits

- Loosens the shoulders

- Lengthens the back

- Stretches hamstrings

Avoid or Use Caution

- Shoulder injuries

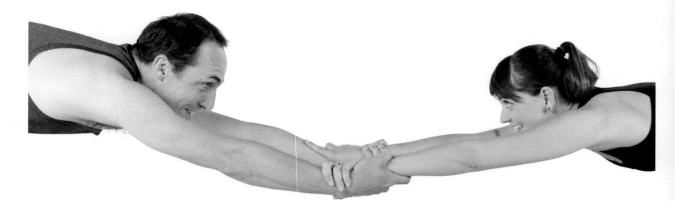

wrist to wrist ▲

Double Arch

1. Continue to hold each other's wrists, as above, and walk your feet toward each other.

2. Ground into your legs, lift the sternum, and roll the upper arms back as you would in Cobra Pose, arching the upper back.

3. Allow your arms to straighten, and let gravity take your shoulders and head into a mini backbend. This requires trust!

4. Continue to lift the heart and breathe.

Benefits

• Opens the chest and stretches the neck

• Promotes trust

Avoid or Use Caution

• Shoulder or back injuries

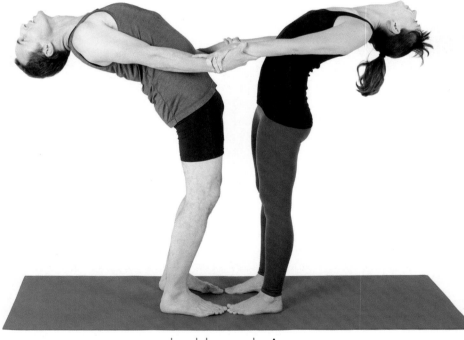

double arch ▲

Pyramid

1. Raise your hands overhead, shoulder-distance apart, and bring your palms to touch your partner's palms, also lifted overhead.

2. Bow forward, stepping back as necessary so that your legs are straight up and down and your chest can extend forward. Make sure you keep your hands 12–18 inches higher than your head and shoulder-distance apart. (Tight shoulders can move their hands a little wider or take them even higher above the head.)

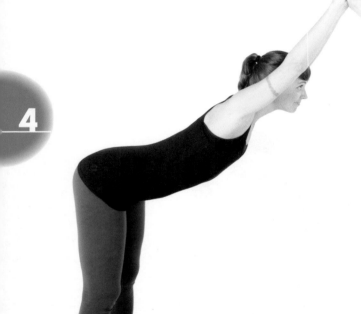

▲ pyramid ▶

3. Keep your head lifted and look eye to eye with your partner. Let gravity do the work of softening the heart.

Benefits

- Opens and softens the heart

- Promotes connection and vulnerability

- Stretches the shoulders

- Promotes spinal flexibility

Avoid or Use Caution

- Shoulder injuries

Restorative Savasana: Lying Over a Bolster

The heart chakra focus in Savasana is dissolving into the breath and feeling the embrace of universal love enveloping you. Discover the nourishment of deep surrender into the breath and the heart of love.

1. Place a bolster lengthwise on the top half of your mat, along the center line.

2. Take a flat, rectangular folded blanket and fold it again, but only two-thirds of the way. Place it on the back end of a bolster, as shown. This "stair step" fold creates an excellent support for the head and neck. The lower one-third fold goes under the upper shoulders while the base of the neck and head are lifted by the higher roll of the blanket.

3. Allow your arms to open to the side, palms upward, and relax. Soften, surrender, and expand.

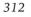

restorative savasana ▲

Fourth Chakra Posture Flow

Six Warm-Ups:

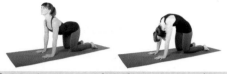

1) Marjaryasana/Bitilasana: Cat/Cow

2) Adho Muhka Svanasana: Downward Facing Dog

3) Uttanasana: Standing Forward Fold

4) Virabhadrasana: Warrior I

5) Anjaneyasana: Deep Lunge

6) Phalakasana: Plank

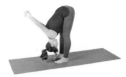

Standing Yoga Mudra

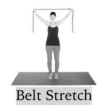

Belt Stretch

Gomukhasana: Cow Face

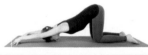

Anahatasana: Extended Puppy Pose

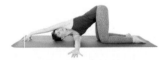

Thread the Needle Twist

Parighasana 2: Half Circle Pose

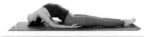

Matsyasana: Fish Pose

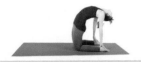

Ustrasana: Camel Pose

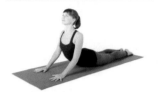

Bhujangasana: Cobra Pose

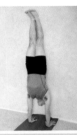

Adho Mukha Vrksasana: Handstand

4

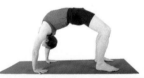

Urdvha Dhanurasana: Wheel Pose

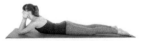

Makarasana: Crocodile Pose

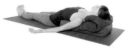

Restorative Savasana

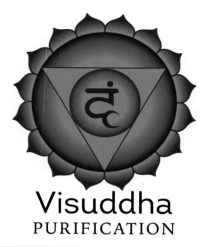

Visuddha
PURIFICATION

Elements	Sound, ether
Principle	Sympathetic vibration
Purposes	Communication, purification, refinement
Properties	Harmony, creativity, resonance, coherence, truth
Body parts	Shoulders, neck, throat, tongue, mouth, ears
Practices	Opening the throat and shoulders, chanting and sounding, vibrating
Actions	Refining vibrations, kriyas, shoulders back, shoulder blades down, head lifted
Poses	Shoulder openers, shoulder stands, headstands, handstands
Masculine	Creating order, distinctions, commanding
Feminine	Listening, creativity, harmonizing
Deficient	Shy, quiet, constricted voice
Excessive	Talks too much, loud, scattered
Balanced	Truth, coherence

chakra five

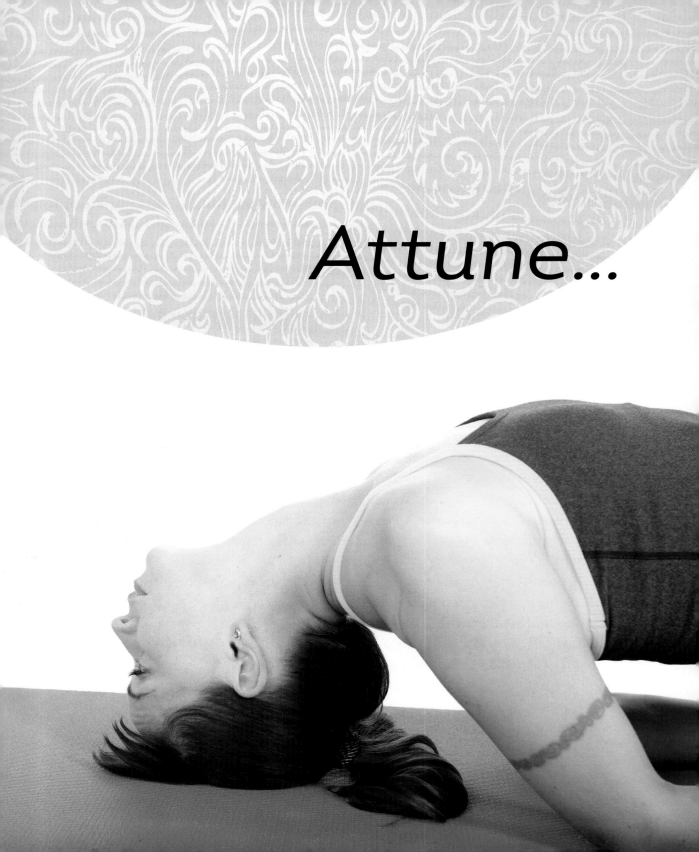

Attune...

Our body is an instrument played by divine breath. It is our job to keep the instrument well tuned and to listen to the voice of truth moving through us. ~ ANODEA JUDITH

Listen. Can you hear it now? Can you sense the subtle pulsation of your heart, the rhythmic movement of your breath, the gentle murmur of your thoughts? Can you hear the chorus of life all around you in the sound of the wind, the laughter of children, the cascade of birdsong as it announces the sunrise?

Sound and rhythm are everywhere, within you and around you. All prana is vibrating, oscillating back and forth, flickering with the steady beat of existence. You need only listen deeply to become part of this chorus of life singing the symphony of creation. You are part of this creation, and your note is needed too. But like any musician who plays in an orchestra, you must first tune your instrument.

The key to unlocking the fifth chakra is attunement. Its first step is listening.

Listening isn't just about words or sounds. It is also about listening to your body, listening to subtle cues of movement and blockages. It is about listening to your feelings, to your intuition, to inner guidance. Listening is quieting the chatter within you long enough to hear a deeper truth.

In your journey up the chakra column, you have now passed the halfway point of the heart chakra. You have entered and aligned your inner temple, you have activated the energy within it, then you have softened and expanded into the air of the heart. Now you are ready to begin refining the raw energy you have generated for the higher consciousness of the upper chakras. You do this by listening to the subtle vibrations within and attuning the etheric field of the energy body.

Imagine that your central axis—the sushumna—is a cord strung between heaven and earth like a guitar string, anchored at each end. You would want to tune the string to be just right so that its note is sweet and accurate—too tight and the string can break; too loose and the sound is lost.

When you pluck a string it vibrates the air molecules around it, which eventually dance upon your ear drum and make a sound. The vibration lasts until the impact upon the string is neutralized; then it returns to quiet and stillness again. If you hit the string harder, the sound will last longer before it is neutralized. If you hit it softly, it will barely make a sound at all.

In the same way, life will pluck the cord of your sushumna with people and events that move your soul. Positive or negative, these impacts cause a vibration at the core level of your being. If you are able to allow that vibration to echo through your body and express itself back out again, you discharge the impact and everything returns to normal. A simple example of this is uttering a spontaneous "Ow!" when someone bumps your arm or needing to talk to someone at the end of the day about something that happened to you at work. When you get these things "off your chest," you tend to feel lighter and freer. As vibrating beings who are instruments of God, this is quite normal.

But what happens when you can't vibrate the impact of something back out again? What happens when you can't say "Ow!" or when you can't talk about something or when you have to pretend that you weren't really impacted when, in fact, you were? What happens when you can't tell your truth or when nobody listens to you or when you are ridiculed for what comes out of your mouth? Then you have to shut down your throat chakra to keep the body from expressing its innate truth.

In guitar playing this is called deadening a string. The player lightly holds the string so that it doesn't vibrate, even as his other hand may strike it. When we do this to ourselves by preventing the expression of something that has impacted us, we deaden our tissue. We block the natural vibrations that result from life in general and from potent experiences in particular. Then the prana doesn't flow as easily and the tissue becomes dense. We may even put on weight, stiffen our muscles, or lose flexibility.

Because the vibration of the soul most naturally expresses itself as sound, we especially block around the throat chakra when this happens. We hold the muscles of the jaw tightly, we tense the shoulders, and the neck no longer holds the head and body in proper alignment with each other. Our self-expression no longer

5

flows easily but is halted and uncertain. We no longer trust ourselves to be spontaneous. Creativity is curtailed.

Then we need to do some work on the throat chakra and free up the body so it can dance once again to the rhythm of life. If the body is the instrument that God plays, then the task of the fifth chakra is to allow the music of life to express itself through us in harmony.

Yoga and Sound

The associated element of this chakra in the ancient texts is ether. The ethereal world is a realm of subtle vibrations emanating through space. Sound is also a result of vibration. In fact, ethereal vibrations and audible sounds are on a continuum from subtle to gross. Since the throat makes sound and is our instrument for self-expression, I equate the element of this chakra to sound.

The Sanskrit name of this chakra is Vissudha, which means purification. This implies several things. One, that we must purify ourselves of toxic substances and dissonant vibrations to go through the gateway of the fifth chakra into the higher consciousness of the chakras above. Secondly, it means that uttering sound, chanting, singing, speaking our truth—all have a purifying effect on the subtle body. We feel lighter and more coherent when we do so. And thirdly, it suggests that vibrations, when they are attuned and harmonized, have a quality of purity that puts us in touch with the essence of universal truth.

Air, the element of the heart chakra, is essential to make sound. Our mind shapes the air into words as it comes through our throat. But as any voice teacher will point out, the whole body is an instrument, not just the throat. The way we breathe and hold ourselves has a lot to do with the resonance of the sounds we make. So an open heart in the fourth chakra, along with the ability to utilize the breath, are important for an open and expressive fifth chakra.

Just as the third chakra goal was mastery, the fifth chakra goal is harmony or resonance. Our words seek resonance in the form of listening, understanding, and connection. We are also attracted to people and events with which we resonate. We read books, hear lectures, or talk about movies where some truth resonates from deep within us. Resonance puts us in harmony with deeper truths and opens us to something larger. By listening deeply and expressing our truth, we create a deeper resonance in our lives.

The deeper, more universal truths are what yoga seeks to discover. Living these truths brings us into harmony with the great chain of being. The philosophies of yoga contain descriptions of these deeper truths. The practice of yoga brings them home.

Communication is the process of sending and receiving information or consciousness from one thing to another. Our cells communicate chemically, our nervous system electrically. We communicate with each other through words and globally through the Internet. In yoga, we first learn to communicate with our inner temple through the "innernet," an elaborate inner system of neurons, muscles, breath, and sensations that tell us whether we are doing a pose correctly. The brain and body are in constant communication as we move, breathe, adjust, and come into and out of poses. Yoga is a spiritual language that we speak with the body, mind, and soul. Practicing yoga allows us to become fluent in this language and brings us into deeper communication with the Divine.

Sounding While Practicing

Chakra yoga uses the element of sound as a cleansing tool to reach the purification that the name Vissudha implies. Every sound you make vibrates throughout your body. Every sound you hear impacts your subtle energy and vibrates it as well. As you release sounds through your breath, you are "vibrating back out" unreleased impacts that may have been stored in your tissues for years. Sound unpacks the density in the body created by blocking our vibratory essence. Because it is beyond words, abstract sound lets the body do the talking in ways that are directly expressive.

I was once attending a yoga workshop in Thailand with an international student base. I distinctly remember a man from Italy, dark haired and well muscled, who practiced next to me. Whenever we did a particularly difficult pose or held a pose for a challenging length of time, I could hear him calling out, "Om namah Shivaya." It always made the rest of us laugh, but it was a lovely way to release sound while practicing.

Use sound freely when you are holding or moving into postures. Experiment with loud or soft sounds, high or low pitch, different vowels or mantras. Let them vibrate through your throat, your chest, and your belly. Express your stiff and achy places with a moan accompanied by breath. Use mantras, tones, and chants to enhance your practice, then listen for the echo of resonance in your soul. Experience how it lets you release and soften. You will feel lighter and freer.

A mantram is a spiritual formula of enormous power that has been transmitted from age to age in a religious tradition.

· · · · · · · · · · · · · ·

EKNATH EASWARAN

Tools for Fifth Chakra Practice

Sounds and the Chakras

According to Vedic mythology, the world came into being as a result of primordial sound. This is most often expressed as the familiar *om*, the sum total of all vibrations together.

In layayoga, the yoga of chakra concentration, there are four forms of sound:

Para, or supreme sound, is the power that precedes existence, welling up from the absolute source as Bindu, a focal point of concentrated power. Para precedes all creation.

Pashyanti, or radiant sound, bursts forth from Bindu and radiates outward but is only heard by yogis in concentration. Those with Kundalini experiences sometimes hear these sounds in their minds.

Madhyama is the living form of sound that creates mantra but is still not outwardly audible. This is the sound you hear when you silently intone a mantra in your head or have an inner chatter or bits of music going on in your mind. You hear it but there is still no audible sound.

Vaikhari, the fourth form, is what we know as audible sound. This includes language, music, nature sounds, artificial sounds (like trucks and airplanes), and everything that we can actually hear.

Emanating from creative essence, para is the sprout, pashyanti is the branching of the sprout into leaves, madhyama is the bud, and vaikhari is the flower of expression.

Mantra practice, the yoga of sound, has long been associated with chakra activation. Mantra, literally meaning a tool for the mind, is a vibration designed to awaken consciousness the way someone shaking your shoulder back and forth might wake you from sleep.

Mantras can be uttered as vaikhari, audible sound, which is good for connecting a group of people in a resonant field, such as the call and response group chanting at a kirtan concert or singing *om* at the start of a yoga class. Mantras can also be used in meditation as madhyama, or inward sound, which has an even deeper effect on consciousness. In this form the sounds feel as if one is carving out space inside the inner temple, shaping it like a sculptor.

At the core of each image of the chakras is a Sanskrit letter that represents a bija mantra (see figure on page 324). *Bija* means seed, so the bija mantra begins in the Absolute as para sound. Bija mantras are said to stimulate each chakra, with bija mantras classically given for chakras one through six:

Chakra	Bija mantra or stimulating sound	Resonant or clearing sound
One	Lam	Oh as in road
Two	Vam	Ooo as in pool
Three	Ram	Ah as in father
Four	Yam	Ay as in pray
Five	Ham	Eee as in speak
Six	Om or ksham	Mmm as in ommmm
Seven	Silence	Ng as in sing

In addition, when chanting with a group, such as a chakra workshop or a yoga class, I like to work with what I call resonant sounds. Resonant sounds bring a group together. They dissolve boundaries and refine energies.

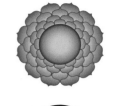

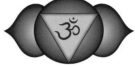

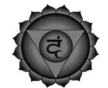

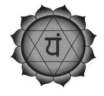

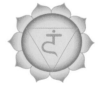

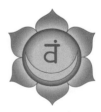

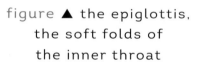

figure ▲ the epiglottis,
the soft folds of
the inner throat

figure ◄ bija mantras, starting with
chakra one (bottom) and moving
upward to chakra seven (top)

One of my Kripalu colleagues, yoga teacher and physician Jeffrey Migdow, suggested to me in a personal conversation that the resonant sounds are for clearing the chakras, while the seed sounds are for stimulating the chakras, much as hitting a bicycle wheel with a stick stimulates the wheel to spin faster.

In terms of excess and deficiency, I suggest using the resonant sounds to clear excessive chakras and the seed sounds to stimulate deficient chakras. When in doubt, use both: clear first, then stimulate.

When chanting the resonant sounds, hold them until you run out of breath, then inhale and chant some more. If chanting with a group or another person, hold until you feel the resonance take place—meaning you are singing the exact same note together and the sound is clear like a bell.

The seed sounds, however, are generally repeated rhythmically, since most of them have the "ah" sound in the middle, which makes them tend to sound alike. Instead, the seed sounds differ in their initial consonant. Feel the effects that the different consonants have on your body, and they will begin to make sense to you.

Ujjayi Pranayama: Ocean Breath

Ujjayi (pronounced *oo-jai-yee*) is a Sanskrit word meaning to conquer or be victorious. This breath is said to conquer fear and illness and to steady the mind.

Ujjayi slows down the breath through a subtle contraction in the throat, making a sound similar to that of a distant ocean—hence its name of "ocean breath." It can be practiced on its own while sitting in stillness but is often used and highly recommended while practicing postures and especially for bringing awareness to the throat chakra.

Ujjayi is a full diaphragmatic breath that begins in the lower belly (activating the first and second chakras), rises to the lower rib cage (third chakra), and finally moves into the upper chest and throat (chakras four and five).

Narrow your throat passage by constricting the epiglottis, the soft folds of the inner throat, which makes a sound similar to whispering. Breathe only through the nose, with your inhalation and exhalation equal in duration.

In his manual *Anusara Yoga*, author Doug Keller states:

The purpose of the ujjayi sound itself is to attune your awareness to each breath, putting you in immediate touch with its quality and texture while breathing more deeply. Producing the ujjayi sound does introduce some resistance, but only to encourage the diaphragm to work more efficiently. With this, you develop your ability to breathe smoothly and continuously, progressively opening each part of your torso to the breath with a smooth transition, so there is no "jerkiness" or irregularity to the breath.[9]

Fifth Chakra Subtle Energy

Sit quietly in an easy cross-legged pose. Close your eyes and go inside to your inner temple. Listen to the sounds in your body, starting with your breath. Follow the rhythm of your breath as you inhale and exhale, not forcing anything but just listening to the air flowing in and out of your nostrils.

Beneath the breath, listen for your heartbeat. Feel it as a vibrating organ at the center of your being, whose vibrations flow rhythmically throughout the body, through every artery.

Now notice the rhythm of your thoughts. Ignore their content but imagine your silent witness is listening to the cadence and tone as if it were a muffled conversation in another room.

See how your breath, heartbeat, and inner thoughts all dance to a single rhythm, each playing their individual parts. Feel the harmony of each part in concert with the others.

Now begin to listen to the sounds around you. Listen to any sounds of nature or of cars or people outside. Take your listening into the imaginal realm and imagine you can hear conversations out on the street, broadcasting on the radio or television, sounds that are occurring in schools, offices, and stores.

Imagine you can float above your city or town and listen to the chorus of the whole area as one single song. Expand your view to include your state or province, then your country, your continent, and finally the whole earth. Imagine this collective sound as one primordial *om* resonating all around you and deep within you.

When you have heard that, come back to your body and your breath. Listen for the *om* inside you, like a background buzz of your internal motor. Imagine that *om* in harmony with all that you have heard.

---

9 Doug Keller, *Anusara Yoga: Hatha Yoga in the Anusara Style*, second edition (South Riding, Virginia: Do Yoga Productions, 2001), 138.

When you can internally imagine your *om* as part of the symphony within and around you, take a breath, open your mouth, and let that sound out—softly at first, then gradually louder and louder.

Feel the sound vibrating through your body. Touch your throat and feel the subtle vibrations beneath your fingers. Feel the resonance in the bones of your head, the back of your neck, your shoulders, and down to your fingers.

Continue singing and let the sound move down your core, down to your base chakra, and out through your legs to your toes and into the earth.

Imagine your sushumna, the vertical cord of your soul, resonating with the clearest frequency in harmony with everything around you, part of the chorus of life, joyful and creative.

Then let the *om* gradually get quieter until you hear it only on the inside, in harmony with the murmur of your thoughts once again.

Finally, return to silence and simply be.

Fifth Chakra Practice and Postures

SHOULDER WARM-UPS

Jalandhara Bandha: Chin Lock

Often used in combination with mula bandha or uddiyana bandha, jalandhara bandha focuses on locking the breath at the fifth chakra level. This intensifies energy in the third and fourth chakras especially, while the practice and release of this bandha brings attention into the throat.

1. Sit in a comfortable upright position.

2. Firm your shoulder blades down your back and lift up on the sternum as you inhale.

3. Holding the breath full, lower the chin down toward the sternum. The full pose has the chin touching the top of the chest, but do not force it. This occurs through a simultaneous lifting of the chest and lowering of the chin, lengthening the back of the neck.

4. Draw the inner part of the throat (the part that intersects your midline) up toward the upper back of your skull. (You can also think of taking the upper palate and/or the hyoid bone back and slightly upward toward the occiput.)

5. Release the bandha, then release the breath.

Benefits
- Regulates the circulatory and respiratory systems

- Stimulates the thyroid

- Said to cure all diseases of the throat

Avoid or Use Caution
- High blood pressure

- Heart disease

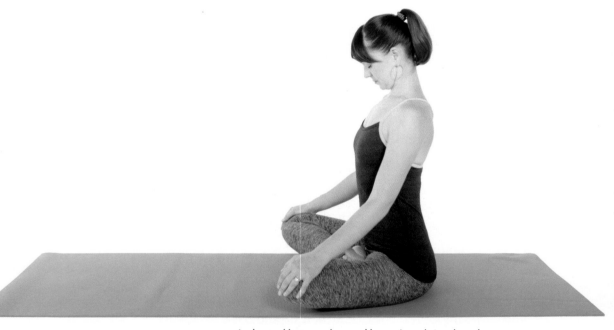

jalandhara bandha ▲ chin lock

Lateral Shoulder Stretches

1. Lift your right arm to shoulder height, directly in front you, thumb pointing upward, elbow straight.

2. Next, move your arm across your body to the left, keeping the arm parallel to the floor at shoulder height.

3. When you've moved your arm as far as possible across the body, grab your right elbow with your left hand and pull the arm in closer to your chest, keeping the elbow straight.

4. Turn your head and look out over the right shoulder.

5. Hold for several breaths, then release, and repeat on the other side.

5

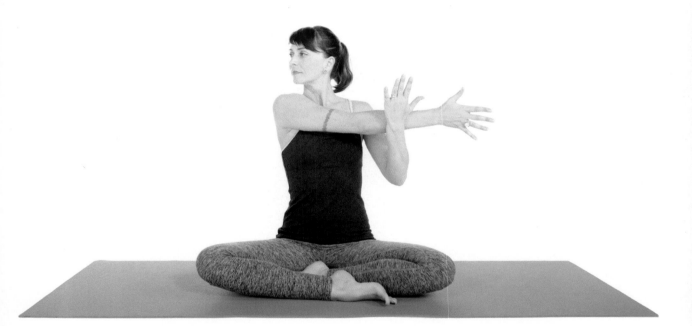

lateral shoulder stretch ▲

Shoulder Shrugs

1. On an inhalation, lift your shoulders up toward your ears.

2. Hold and tighten, then release the shoulders rapidly on an exhalation.

3. Repeat several times.

4. Make circles with your shoulders, front to back.
   Make several rotations in each direction.

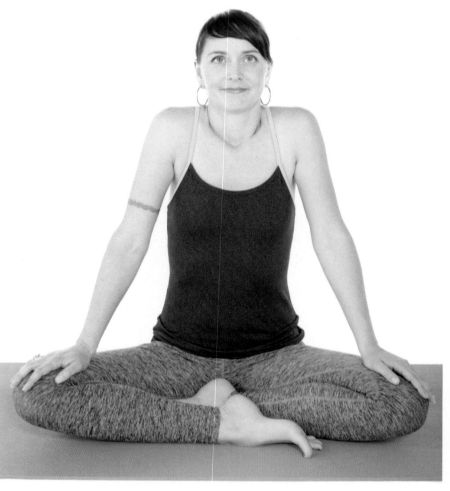

shoulder shrug ▲

Neck Stretches

1. Seated or standing, find your way to an erect spine. Ground down into your base and lift your crown. Inhale.

2. Keeping your crown lifted and your neck long, slowly bring your left ear toward your left shoulder, without lifting your shoulder. Exhale.

3. Reach around the top of your head with your left hand toward your right ear and pull the stretch deeper. Keep your chin pointed straight ahead.

4. With your right hand, you may wish to massage any tight neck muscles.

5. Inhale and lift the head back toward center.

6. Repeat on the other side.

5

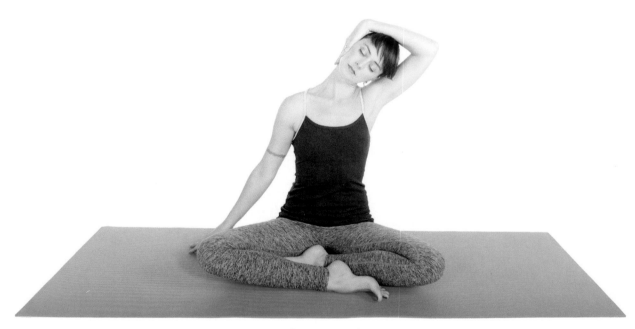

neck stretch ▲

Seated Yoga Mudra

1. Seated on your heels or in simple cross-legged pose, press your tailbone toward the back, lift your crown, and interlace your fingers behind you, drawing the heels of your hands toward each other.

2. Roll your shoulders back and straighten your elbows, allowing your shoulder blades to come toward each other and your chest to expand.

3. Lift the head high and tilt it back slightly, stretching the front of your throat (position A).

4. Inhale deeply as you lift and expand.

5. As you exhale, bow forward over your legs until you reach your edge or touch your forehead to the mat (position B).

6. Lift your arms up behind you, pressing upward into your fingers to lift your shoulders and open the upper back.

Benefits

• Opens the shoulders

• Stretches the neck

• Calms the mind

• Reduces stress

• Releases blockages in throat chakra

Avoid or Use Caution

• High or low blood pressure (don't bend forward as far)

• Pregnancy after first trimester

• Shoulder injury

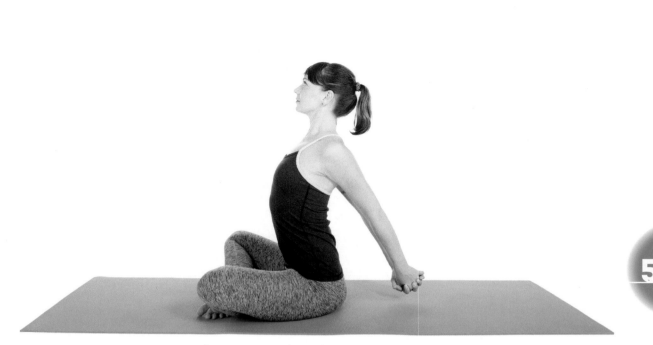

seated yoga mudra ▲ position a

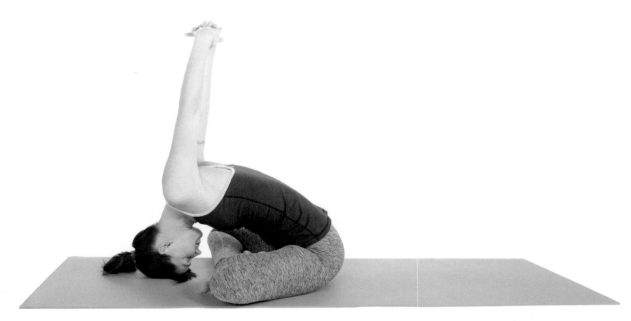

seated yoga mudra ▲ position b

Setu Bandha Sarvangasana: Bridge Pose

We first visited Bridge Pose in chakra one as we formed the foundation of our bridge with the feet and legs. The other end of the bridge is in the upper chakras, formed by the shoulders, neck, and head. This pose stimulates the thyroid gland as well as the abdominal organs of digestion, while expanding the lungs and strengthening the legs.

1. Lie on your back with your hands alongside your body, knees bent, feet hip-width apart, heels toward your fingertips.

2. Pushing through the core of each leg, press your feet into the floor, feeling how the soles of the feet make deeper contact with the mat and the solidity beneath you. Feel how your legs are energized by this action even before lifting your hips.

3. Continue pushing your legs into the floor to slowly lift your hips up off the mat.

4. Hold for as long as is comfortable, with the option of rolling your shoulders toward each other and clasping your hands beneath your body.

Guidelines

• The action in the legs, not the belly muscles, lifts the hips. Think of pressing the floor away rather than lifting the hips. Use the floor to push your hips higher.

• Press your midback toward the ceiling, your tailbone toward your knees.

• Draw the knees toward each other and rotate the thighs inward. Try holding a block between your thighs to accentuate this action.

• To press evenly into the four corners of each foot, press more deeply on the inner edges of your feet, as the feet tend to roll to the sides.

- As you press your heels down, draw them toward your shoulders to engage the hamstrings. To widen and activate the bridge, press your feet away from your shoulders. Roll slightly side to side to wiggle onto the outer edge of your upper arms, hugging your shoulder blades toward each other. Interlace your fingers with straight arms beneath your body.

- Press your arms into the floor to create more lift in the chest.

Benefits
- Strengthens the legs

- Improves shoulder flexibility

- Stimulates the nervous system

- Combats fatigue

- Aids digestion

- Stimulates thyroid and parathyroid glands

Avoid or Use Caution
- Neck or shoulder injury

- Low back injury

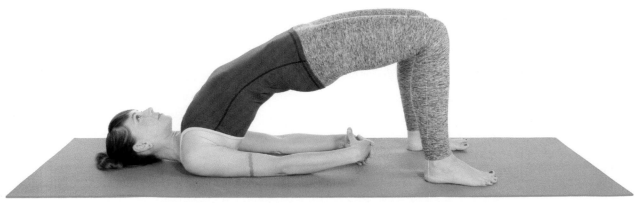

setu bandha sarvangasana ▲ bridge pose

Matsyasana: Fish Pose

Fish Pose is a nice counterstretch for the neck after doing Bridge Pose. We first visited this pose in the heart chakra, but it should be part of a fifth chakra practice as it also opens the throat and promotes flexibility in the neck.

1. Lie on your back, arms by your sides, with your legs drawn together and knees straight. (For an easier version of this pose, you may bend your knees and place your feet hip-width apart.)

2. Slide your hands underneath your buttocks, thumbs up.

3. Inhale. Lift your head and upper body enough to slide the heels of your hands onto the backside of your hips, bending your elbows close into your sides and pressing them into the mat. Your torso will be at an angle to the floor. Exhale.

4. Inhale again and lift your chest upward, externally rotate your shoulders, and firm up your belly. You are now arching your back.

5. Press your elbows into the mat and draw your tailbone simultaneously down to the mat and up toward your shoulders.

6. Gently tilt your head back, and, if possible, touch the top of your head to the floor.

7. To come out of the pose, inhale and lift your head first, then slide your spine back down to the floor.

Guidelines

• Press your tailbone toward the back body and draw it energetically toward your elbows, curving the sacrum. Allow the curve to continue up the spine, pressing the chest upward.

• Keep your thighs active if your legs are out straight. Draw your legs together as one.

• Be careful not to crunch the neck. Use a folded blanket if your head cannot reach the floor or if you feel any discomfort.

- Press your palms into the floor to help move your spine forward.

- Breathe deeply. Use your inhalations to expand the chest. Beginners may wish to use a bolster or rolled-up mat underneath their chest for a more passive pose.

- To develop core strength, lift the legs to a 45-degree angle.

- To increase the challenge and deepen this pose, slide your hands out from underneath your buttocks and bring them into prayer position over your heart.

- The full expression of this pose is with legs folded in Padmasana, Full Lotus.

Benefits
- Opens the throat

- Promotes deeper breathing

- Improves posture

- Stimulates thyroid and parathyroid

Avoid or Use Caution
- Neck injury

- Headaches

- High blood pressure

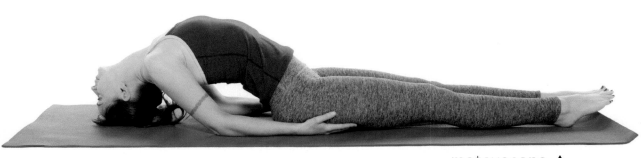

matsyasana ▲
fish pose

Parivrtta Parsvakonasana: Revolved Side Angle Pose

Your head is the last thing to rotate in a twisting pose and in many ways completes the twist. Here you line up the shoulders and twist along your core axis.

1. From Warrior I, bring your hands together over your head. With fingers interlaced, turn your palms upward (position A).

2. Press firmly into your legs, drawing your feet toward each other. Slightly rotate the back thigh inward and the front thigh outward. Establish your stability.

3. Lifting your chin and chest, gaze up at the back of your knuckles. Take a few deep breaths as you extend upward and stretch open the throat.

4. Lower your hands to your heart, pressing your palms together in prayer position. Lift your back heel and square your hips to the front edge of the mat.

5. Twist on your axis to bring your opposite elbow to the front knee. If your left leg is forward, then bring your right elbow or upper arm to your left knee, keeping your palms together (position B).

6. Stack your elbows, one above the other, as your right upper arm presses firmly into your knee or thigh.

7. Align your head and neck with the midline of your torso.

Guidelines

• Extend from your back heel to your crown.

• Try to get as much of your right upper arm across your front thigh as possible.

• Use your elbow as a fulcrum to twist deeper. Pull your lower ribs forward and your upper shoulders back.

• If turning your neck upward creates strain, simply look straight ahead in line with your chest, creating a straight line through your core and your neck.

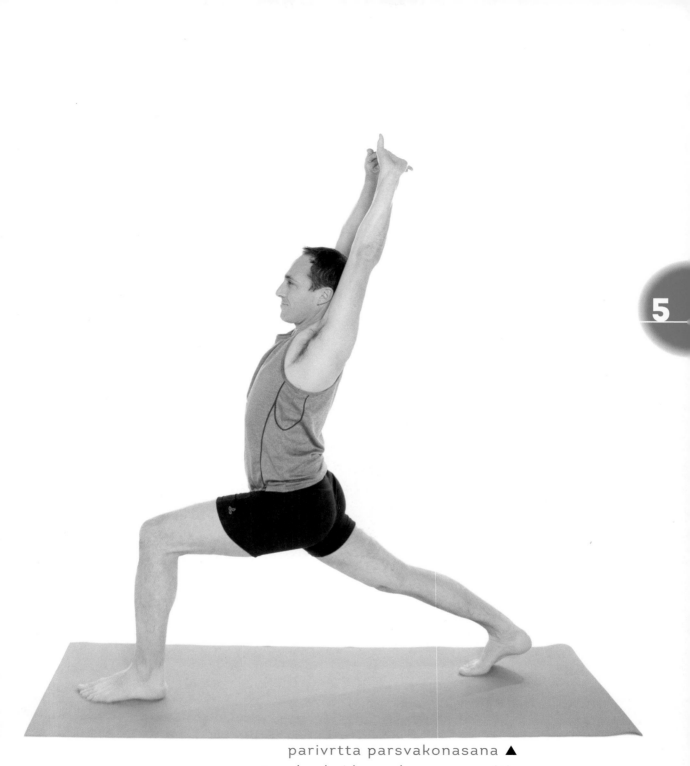

parivrtta parsvakonasana ▲
revolved side angle pose, position a

- To improve your balance, brace your back heel against a wall.

- More advanced: bring your back heel to the ground.

Variations

- Hook your right armpit over your left knee and place your lower hand on the floor or a block. Extend your upper arm straight above (position C) or extend it out over the head (position D).

- Most challenging: interlace your hands behind your back to create a bind (position E).

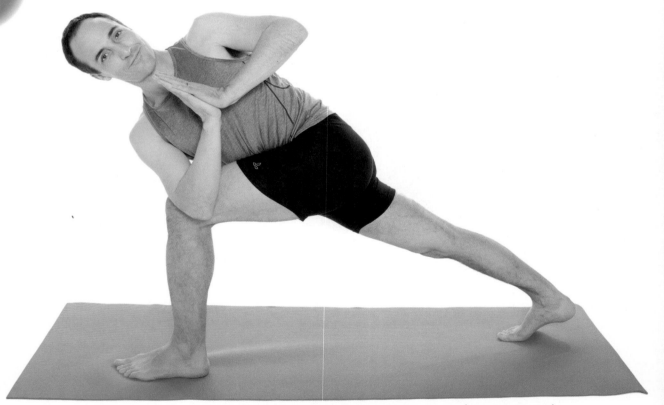

parivrtta parsvakonasana ▲
revolved side angle pose, position b

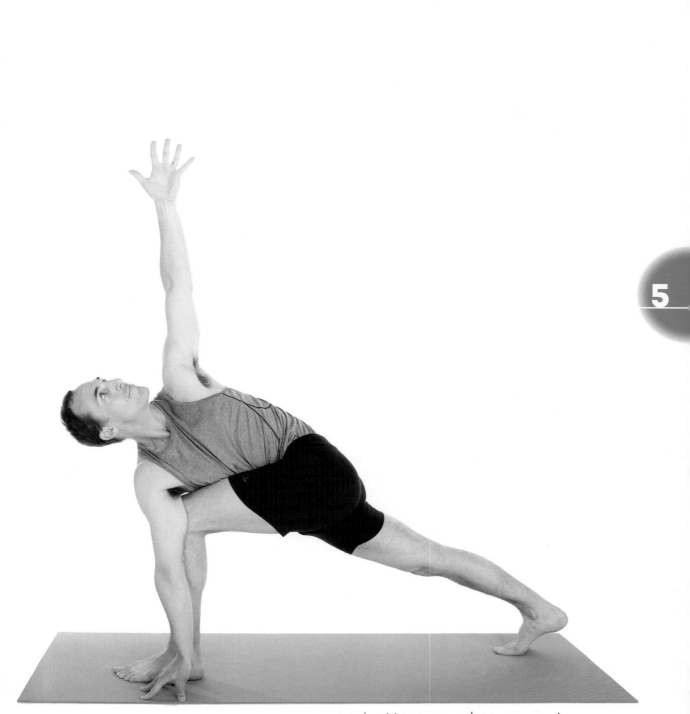

parivrtta parsvakonasana ▲
revolved side angle pose, position c

5

Benefits

- Strengthens the legs

- Twists the torso

- Stimulates digestive organs

- Opens the chest

- Increases lung capacity

- Stretches intercostal muscles of the ribs

- Strengthens the neck and shoulders

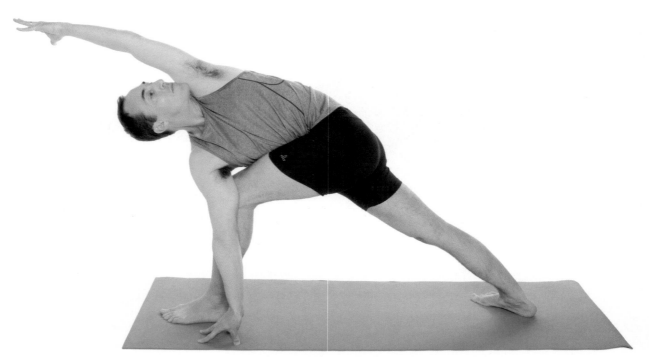

parivrtta parsvakonasana ▲
revolved side angle pose, position d

- Improves balance and concentration

- Stimulates lymphatic system

Avoid or Use Caution

- Knee injury

- Shoulder injury

- Low back injury

- Low blood pressure

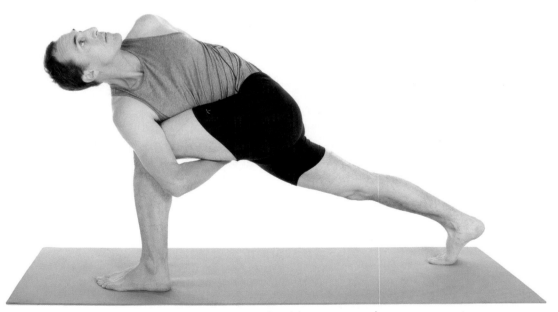

parivrtta parsvakonasana ▲
revolved side angle pose, position e

Bakasana: Crane Pose and Kakasana: Crow Pose

There is much confusion on the name of this pose, as there is a subtle distinction between Crow and Crane. Crow Pose (Kakasana) is with the arms slightly bent, resembling the shorter legs of a crow, and is a bit easier. Crane Pose (Bakasana) is with the arms straight and more advanced. However, the pose is most commonly referred to as Bakasana, or Crow Pose, since few people can get their arms straight without years of practice. Arm balances require strength and concentration in the core. This pose could be considered a good third chakra pose for that reason, yet it contains a moderate inversion and angles the neck. After doing either form of this pose, or even attempting it, sit and feel the effects on the back of your neck and shoulders. You'll see why it also stimulates the fifth chakra.

1. From Tadasana, bend your knees and squat down, placing your hands shoulder-distance apart on the floor. Spread your fingers wide and press the tips into the floor, creating a clawing action.

2. Balancing on your tiptoes, bend your elbows, bringing the inside of your knees to your upper arms, as high up as you can manage.

3. Engage your arms firmly, drawing energy up the arms from the base of the wrists to the shoulders. At the same time, draw your knees inward, pressing against your arms. Do this a few times to get the sense of drawing into your core, holding your arms strong.

4. Pick a focal point a few feet in front you and steady your gaze.

5. Slowly lean your weight forward onto your hands, coming first onto your tiptoes, then lifting your feet off the ground.

6. When balanced, gradually work toward straightening your arms (position A).

7. Hold as long as you comfortably can, increasing the time you hold the pose as you practice.

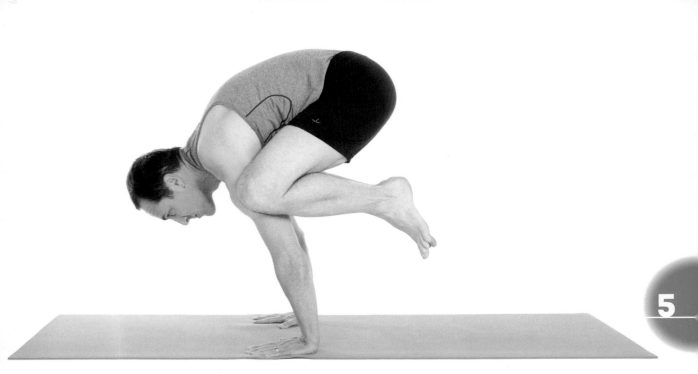

bakasana ▲ crane pose, position a

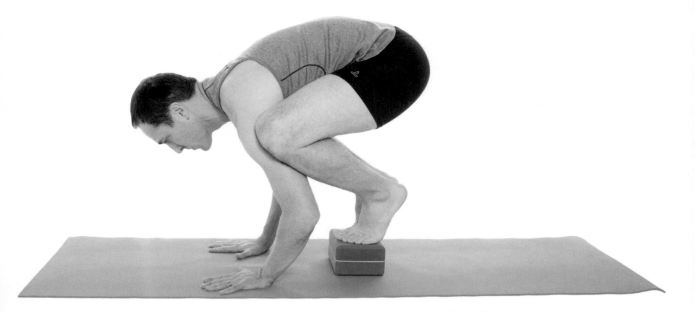

kakasana ▲ crow pose, position b

Guidelines

- For beginners, simply come onto your tiptoes or elevate your feet on a block. Practice lifting one foot at a time (positions B and C).

- Initially bend your elbows enough to make a shelf for your knees to land on.

- The more you hug into the midline, the less your knees will slide back down your arms.

- Most people lean too far back and fall out of the pose. Lean slightly forward and let the clawing of your hands keep you from falling forward. Make sure your fingers are spread nice and wide.

- Once your feet are lifted off the floor, try to press the mounds of the big toes together, then the inner edge of each foot together.

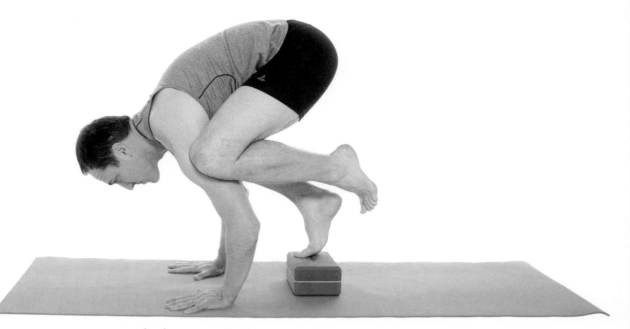

bakasana/kakasana ▲ crane/crow, position c

Benefits

- Strengthens the core

- Develops arm and shoulder strength

- Promotes digestion

- Good preparation for handstand

- Develops balance and concentration

Avoid or Use Caution

- Carpal tunnel syndrome or wrist injury

- Pregnancy

- Headaches

- High blood pressure

Sasangasana: Rabbit Pose

Rabbit Pose lengthens the entire spine and stretches the back of the neck and shoulders. It compresses the thyroid and parathyroid, which, when released, rejuvenates them. It is said to be therapeutic for colds and sinus problems. It is a deep hugging in to the self, good for inner listening.

1. Begin by sitting on your heels.

2. Bend forward and place your head as close to your knees as possible.

3. Grab onto your heels. If you cannot reach your heels, you can use a strap or fold the mat or a towel over your feet and hold on to that.

4. Press your hips up into the air, drawing your forehead toward your knees.

Guidelines

- If your knees are far from your forehead, slowly inch them forward.

- Pull on your heels (or the strap or towel) to intensify the pose.

- Press the tailbone upward, strengthening the spine.

- This is a good warm-up for plow and shoulder stand or a good substitution if inversions are not possible or appropriate.

- A folded blanket under the knees can make the pose more comfortable.

Benefits

- Lengthens the spine

- Stimulates immune system

Avoid or Use Caution

- High blood pressure

- Headaches

- Neck injury

- Knee injury

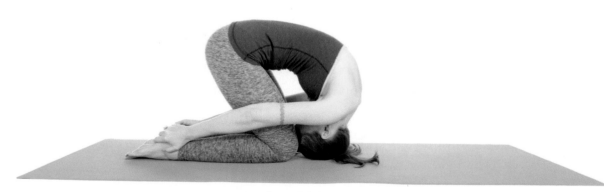

sasangasana ▲ rabbit pose

Halasana: Plow Pose and Karnapidasana: Ear Pressure Pose

The deep inward folding of Halasana and Karnapidasana allows you to come home to yourself while stretching the entire spine. And while it is relaxing, there is also an important lift occurring from the upper spine to the hips.

1. Begin by lying on your back, arms at your sides, palms down. Widen your shoulder blades with a slight inner rotation of the upper arms.

2. Inhale fully. As you exhale, press your palms into the floor and firm up your legs, drawing them together, then lift your legs upward, perpendicular to the floor.

3. Take a few ujjayi breaths here, releasing the neck and relaxing the jaw and tongue. Extend your shoulders downward, away from your ears, and press the head of the armbones toward the floor.

4. On the next inhalation, press your arms into the floor, engage your core, and lift your hips up over your shoulders.

5. Keeping your legs straight, bring your feet to the floor above your head.

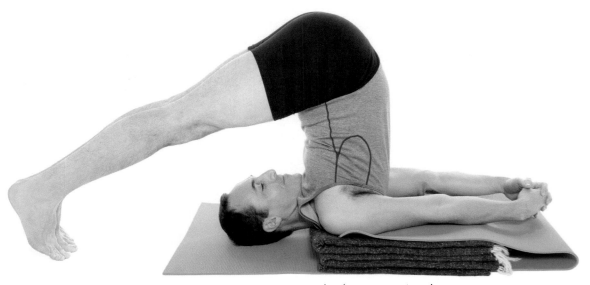

halasana ▲ plow pose

6. Wiggle side to side to bring your shoulders beneath you and your shoulder blades closer together.

7. Interlace your fingers behind your back.

8. To enter Karnapidasana (see Plow variation below), bend your knees toward your ears, squeezing in toward the midline.

Guidelines

- Press the feet into the floor and firm up the legs, pressing into the backs of the thighs.

- Press the thighs straight up toward the sky and your arms straight down into the earth to lengthen the spine.

- Engage the abdominal muscles, extend through the sitting bones, and create length in the spine.

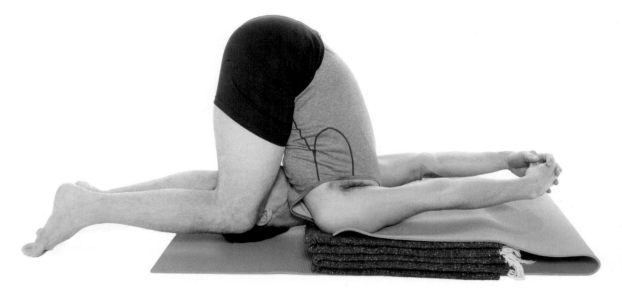

karnapidasana ▲ ear pressure pose
or plow variation

- Press the back of your head into the floor to create space between chin and chest and increase the curve in your neck.

- Pressure on the neck can be relieved by elevating the shoulders on one or two folded blankets so that the back of your head touches the mat and the neck and shoulders are slightly elevated. The cervical spine should not be pressing against anything when elevated.

Benefits
- Stimulates the fifth chakra glands of thyroid and parathyroid

- Stretches and strengthens the shoulders and neck

Avoid or Use Caution
- Menstruation (for which inversions in general are contraindicated)

- Neck or shoulder injuries

- Pregnancy

- High blood pressure

- Asthma

Salamba Sarvangasana: Shoulder Stand

1. From Plow Pose, separate your hands, bend your elbows, and bring your hands to your hips. Press your hips upward as high as you can.

2. Pressing into your pelvis, lift your legs and feet up over your hips.

3. Broaden the shoulders by drawing the elbows energetically toward each other and pressing them down to form a firm base.

4. Firm up your legs by hugging the muscles to the bones, drawing your legs together, and rotating the inner thighs toward the back.

5. Extend upward from your tailbone into the balls of your feet while flexing and spreading your toes. Half Shoulder Stand (position A) keeps the hips a little lower than Full Shoulder Stand (position B).

6. To come out of the pose, release the hands to the floor, bring the feet back down overhead into Plow, then roll back down to the floor one vertebra at a time. Keep the head back as you roll down, using the abdominal muscles to slow the descent.

Guidelines

- As in Plow Pose, you can create more ease for your neck if you elevate your shoulders slightly on a folded blanket (or two or three). This is strongly advised if you plan on holding the pose for any length of time. There should be no pressure on the cervical spine.

- As you lift your hips, your hands may work themselves toward your shoulders.

- If you are stable, you may wish to deepen the pose by interlacing your hands on the floor or pressing your palms into the floor.

- Lift the chest away from the chin.

- Press the head gently back into the floor to keep length through the cervical spine.

Benefits

- Like all inversions, brings blood and prana to the upper body

- Strengthens and stretches the back of the neck

- Opens the shoulders

- Drains the legs—good for varicose veins

- Stimulates fifth chakra glands thyroid and parathyroid

- Improves circulation

- Good for mild depression

Avoid or Use Caution

- Neck or shoulder injury

- Menstruation

- Pregrancy

- High blood pressure

- Headaches

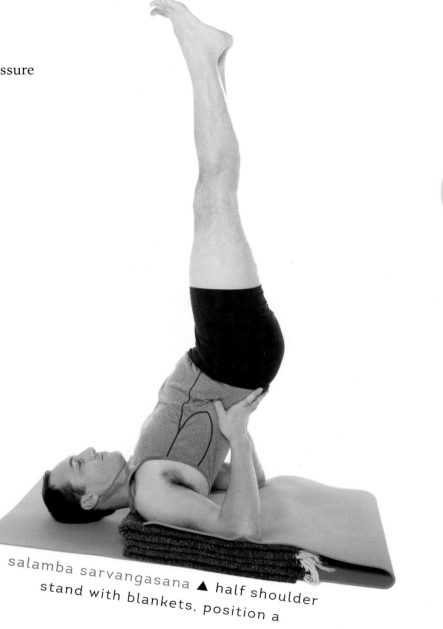

salamba sarvangasana ▲ half shoulder
stand with blankets, position a

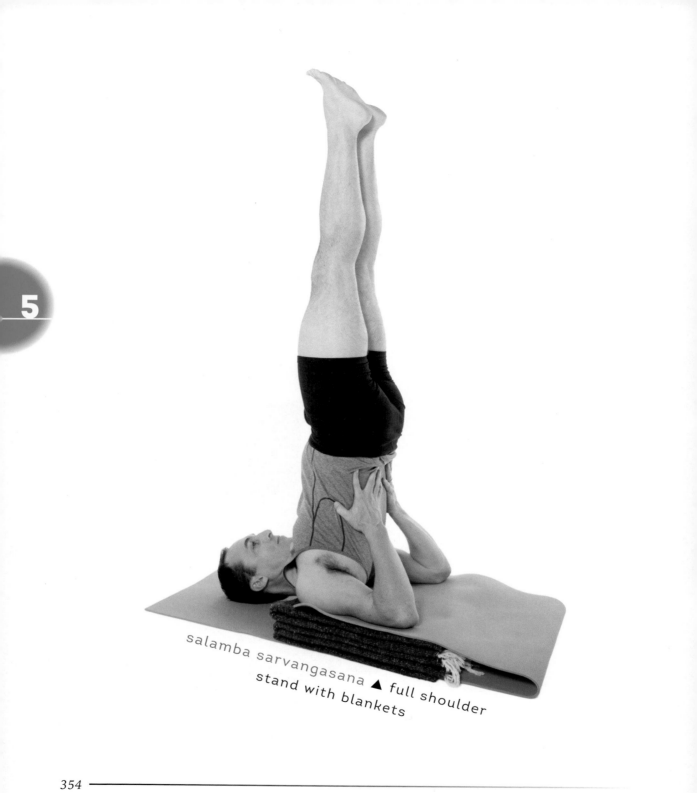

salamba sarvangasana ▲ full shoulder
stand with blankets

Nakulasana: Mongoose Pose

It is said that the mongoose is one of the few animals that can kill the cobra, so this posture is even greater for opening the neck and shoulders than Cobra Pose. It is deceptively simple and rather uncomfortable, yet it has a profound effect on the neck and shoulders. Thanks to my teacher Antonio Sausys for sharing this little-known pose with me.

1. Sit in Dandasana, Staff Pose, legs straight and feet out in front of you.

2. Slide both hands back about a foot and a half or until you reach your edge, keeping your fingers pointing forward toward your hips.

3. Allow your sternum to soften and the chest to sag toward the floor. You should feel an intense stretch in the tops of your shoulders.

4. When you have all this in place, lift your chin and slowly take your head back, allowing the weight of your head to open the throat.

5. Loosen your jaw and take several slow breaths here. Hold the pose until you feel some softening in your shoulders and neck and the discomfort begins to melt away.

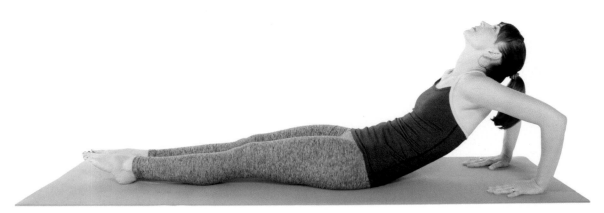

nakulasana ▲ mongoose pose

6. To come out of the pose, first lift your head, then sit up again in Dandasana.

7. Feel the openness at the back of your neck and shoulders.

8. It's nice to follow this up with a forward fold such as Paschimottanasana.

Guidelines

- In this pose I like to go back and forth between lifting my sternum and allowing the chest to sag. Each gives a different element to the stretch.

- Draw the elbows gently toward each other.

- Keep your legs relaxed.

- Move the head back slowly. Avoid causing any pain to the neck.

Benefits

- Stretches the shoulders

- Opens the throat

- Relaxes the chest

Avoid or Use Caution

- Any shoulder injuries

- Neck injuries

- Carpal tunnel syndrome

Savasana: Corpse Pose

In fifth chakra Savasana the focus is on listening to the subtle vibrations coursing throughout the whole body. If you've had a good practice, the whole body should be buzzing with a subtle hum. Allow your body to settle into its natural vibration, vibrating in harmony with all the vibrations around you. Imagine your body is an instrument, perfectly tuned, being played by a master in an orchestra, harmonizing with all the other sounds.

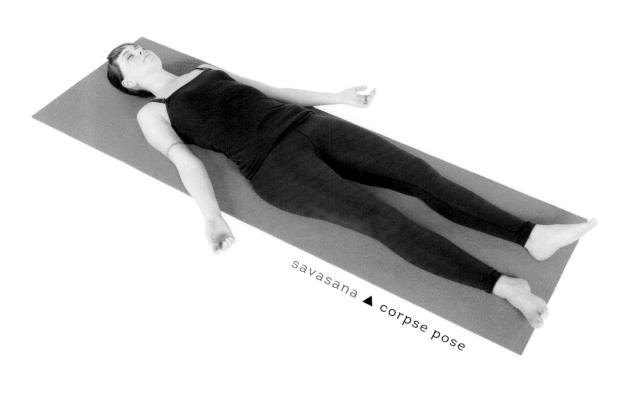

savasana ▲ corpse pose

Fifth Chakra Posture Flow

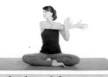

Lateral Shoulder Stretches

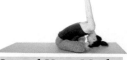

Shoulder Shrugs

Neck Stretches

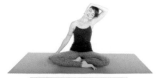

Seated Yoga Mudra

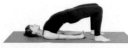

Setu Bandha Sarvangasana: Bridge Pose

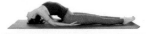

Matsyasana: Fish Pose

5

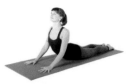

Bhujangasana: Cobra

Adho Mukha Svanasana: Down Dog

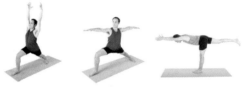

Virabhadrasana: Warrior I, II, and III

5

Trikonasana: Triangle Pose

Parivrtta Parsvakonasana: Revolved Side Angle Pose

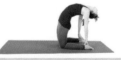

Ustrasana: Camel Pose

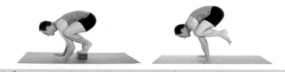

Kakasana: Crow Pose or Bakasana: Crane Pose

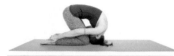

Sasangasana: Rabbit Pose

Salamba Sarvangasana: Shoulder Stand

Halasana: Plow Pose

Karnapidasana: Ear Pressure Pose

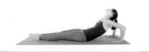

Nakulasana: Mongoose Pose

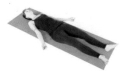

Savasana: Corpse Pose

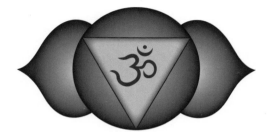

Ajña

PERCEIVE, COMMAND

Element	Light
Principles	Luminescence, illumination
Purposes	Insight, guidance, wisdom
Properties	Radiance, beauty, stillness, single-pointed focus, steadiness in core, inner light
Body parts	Eyes, forehead, pineal gland
Practices	Quieting the mind, focusing the gaze (drishti)
Actions	Centering, stillness, imagination, visualization, pratyahara
Poses	Sitting, balancing, inversions
Masculine	Illumination, revelation, penetrating insight, vision
Feminine	Beauty, intuition, radiance, perception
Deficient	Denial, cynicism, close-mindedness
Excessive	Delusion, hallucination
Balanced	Clarity, vision, wisdom

chakra six

Illuminate...

6

*Never lose an opportunity of seeing anything
that is beautiful, for beauty is God's
handwriting.* ~RALPH WALDO EMERSON

After attuning your subtle vibrations through the purification of the fifth chakra, you are ready to develop the luminous light of chakra six. Now the experience is more transcendent, taking you beyond this world and into an archetypal realm of deep wisdom and beauty. Color and form, insight and intuition spring into view as the third eye center opens wide. Here is where you find the light that will illuminate your path.

As each of the chakras represents a perspective of consciousness, the sixth chakra represents seeing, which brings you revelations about yoga, your life, and the world. By now you have enough practice in your bones that you may find yourself saying, "Oh, I see," meaning that you are beginning to see what your teachers have been pointing to and what yoga philosophers have been describing for millennia. You may be able to see your own patterns, perceive the movement of subtle energy, or have more access to your intuition. You can imagine the lines of energy within a pose and see your "light body." Your inner sight illuminates the inside of your temple, bathing it in golden iridescence.

As you enter the upper chakras, you start to move toward stillness. This is less about vigorous asana practice than about slowing down both body and mind in preparation for the stillness of meditation. The intersecting nadis of ida and pingala, which wind around the chakras like a DNA helix, are said to meet in chakra six, collapsing duality into single-pointed, non-dual consciousness. Here you begin to experience the union of body/mind, observer/observed, individual/universal that is the true meaning of yoga.

Why do we need to become still in order to see clearly?

Imagine that you are visiting the wilderness on a summer vacation, camping near a lake in the mountains. If you wake up early in the morning and sit by the lake, you see that its surface is perfectly still, reflecting the mountain behind it in total clarity, like a mirror. As the day progresses and the wind and boats stir up the surface, the choppy water no longer gives you the perfect vision of the mountain. You see bits of it but not as a whole.

Your personal life is a reflection of your consciousness. In order to see that reflection clearly, you must become as still as the lake in the morning. Clarity results when your mind no longer has a ripple or fluctuation. That clarity is ultimately about seeing who you truly are.

The first stanza of Patanjali's Yoga Sutras states the essence of yoga: "Now begins the instruction of yoga. Yoga is the cessation of the fluctuations of the mind. Then the Seer abides in its own nature."

This important verse that begins the most famous written treatise on yoga implies many things. First, that we can only see in the "now." Yoga occurs in the present moment—not as a concept but as a profound experience. Secondly, yoga is a discipline that requires instruction passed on from teacher to student. And thirdly, the goal of yoga is to cultivate a state of consciousness in which the mind is no longer distracted, agitated, or fluctuating but is calm, clear, present, and still. When this is achieved, our true nature—as a Seer—is revealed.

The name of this chakra, ajña (pronounced *ahj-nya*), means both to perceive and to command. The idea of perception is fairly obvious for a chakra that is about seeing. It is through our eyes that we see the world and through our consciousness that we perceive its meaning. But even more, it is when we truly "see" that we realize, meaning we see with real eyes, perceiving the underlying truth and luminous light within all creation. Intuition, insight, memory, and dreams all have to do with the process of consciousness perceiving something. This aspect of perception is somewhat passive. We receive insight, impressions, or dreams, often without really trying.

The translation as "command center" is the active principle of the sixth chakra. Shiva sends out lightning bolts from his third eye to destroy ignorance. We form pictures in our mind that command our reality. Those pictures are the first impression that consciousness encounters on its downward journey into manifestation, moving from the seventh chakra to the sixth chakra. No wonder the process of visualization is an important part of creating what you want!

Location, Location, Location

People rightly think of the sixth chakra as the third eye center but often misplace its location. It's often called the brow chakra because its height in the body coincides with the center of the forehead; however, its center intersects the vertical axis of the core, meaning its true location is closer to the center of the head, several inches behind the brow. Here lies a part of the brain called the Cave of Brahma, at the base of which is found the pineal gland, a light-sensitive organ of mystical significance.

Since its discovery, philosophers have made reference to the pineal gland as a site of mystic experience. In the seventeenth century René Descartes called it the seat of the soul. The pineal gland produces melatonin, a derivative of the neurotransmitter serotonin, which is produced during sleep. This tiny gland, about the size of a pea, is suspected to be a key factor in dreaming, near-death visions, and psychedelic experiences through the synthesis of dimethyltryptamine (DMT), a structure that resembles natural neurotransmitters and produces internal visions. Interestingly, children produce much more melatonin than adults, as melatonin production drops off at puberty and declines steadily in later life, which may explain why we forget these natural luminous states. Unlike most of the mammalian brain, the pineal is not insulated by the blood-brain barrier and is a blood-rich organ, second only to the kidney. In keeping with the sixth chakra's association with non-dual consciousness, the pineal gland is the only unpaired organ in the brain.

I've seen many books on the chakras that equate the sixth chakra to the pituitary and the pineal to the seventh chakra because the pineal is just slightly higher in the brain by physical location, but I strongly disagree with this association. The pituitary is a master gland, coordinating the other glands much like the seventh chakra is our "master" chakra, whereas the pineal is light sensitive and may be involved in producing visions, pointing clearly to the sixth chakra. In fact, the pineal evolves from a third eye in the embryo. What is not yet known is whether focusing on the sixth chakra area can influence the pineal gland—and, if so, how.

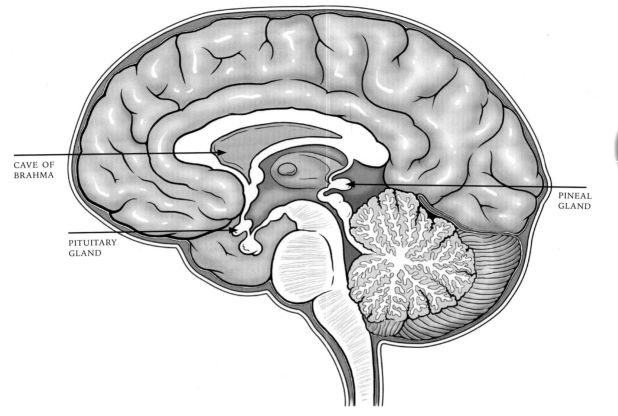

▲ the location of the pineal gland
in relation to the pituitary gland

What we do know is that advanced states of consciousness often produce the experience of mystic visions, which points to a developed sixth chakra.

Working with Your Drishti

The Sanskrit word *drishti* means gaze. What you gaze upon focuses your attention. Where your attention is focused becomes your experience. Keeping your gaze steady can help keep your postures steady, such as looking at a focal point when standing in a balancing pose.

But your gaze, or drishti, means much more than that: it is also your perspective, what you look for, what grabs or traps your attention. If you focus on what's wrong with yourself, with your practice, or with those around you, that will color your experience. If you focus on appreciating the good, your interior experience will shift. A deeper level of yoga is learning to command your perspective.

In the active sense of seeing as commanding, focusing on the good begins to command your reality in that direction. This is not to say that you engage in positive thinking to the point of denial. There is definitely a time and place to acknowledge when something is wrong and needs to be addressed. But this kind of negative seeing can become an unconscious habit. It takes effort and will to change that habit into looking for and acknowledging the good.

In studying the brain, scientists have found that "neurons that fire together wire together."[10] What you focus on and habitually associate with literally shapes the neural structure of your brain, creating habits of thinking. This, in turn, shapes your experience and attitude toward life.

Modern neuroscience tells us that the brain naturally focuses on what's wrong as an ancient survival mechanism. Our ancestors needed to notice any movement in the landscape that could be a threat so they could respond to it. Rick Hanson calls this phenomenon "experience-dependent neuroplasticity."[11] He states that the brain is like Velcro for bad experiences—which tend to stick—but Teflon for good experiences—which quickly slip away. It takes conscious effort to soak your neural network in the positive experiences and a continued redirection of your attention to reshape the habits of your brain.

Yoga is precisely that direction of your attention toward a deeper world suffused with light and meaning within everyday life. Yoga teaches you to see differently, shifting your perspective and therefore your experience. This new way of seeing—your inner gaze—illuminates the path forward.

10 Sometimes called "Hebbian Theory," this idea was first introduced by Donald Hebb in his book *The Organization of Behavior* (New York: Wiley and Sons, 1949).

11 Rick Hanson, *Hardwiring Happiness: The New Brain Science of Contentment, Calm, and Confidence* (New York: Harmony Books, 2013), 10.

Train yourself to be in awe of the subtle and
you will live in a world of beauty and ease.

• • • • • • • • • • • • • •

RODNEY YEE

Sixth Chakra Subtle Energy

Breathing Into the Midline

This is a breathing exercise that develops your inner seeing through focused visualization of the chakras. Its purpose is to settle the fluctuations of the nadis and bring you deeper into your midline. The result is a more focused consciousness, stilling the body in preparation for meditation.

There is a bit of preamble, however, to understanding just how this exercise works. Having this understanding is essential to the success of the exercise.

In the introductory chapter I talked about how chakras can become excessive or deficient through the buildup of character defenses, behaviors, and body armor. In terms of the midline of the body, excessive chakras tend to carry energy in front of the midline. The excessive energy rushes forward, ahead of the rest of the energy body. If you look at someone sideways, you may see the body forming itself around this excessive energy, throwing the spine out of alignment. Sometimes the pelvis is pushed forward, other times a rounded belly protrudes in front of the chest. Some people throw their neck out of alignment by jutting their head forward.

Deficient chakras, by contrast, tend to carry the center of the chakra a bit behind the midline. It's as if they are energetically hanging back, not too sure of themselves, not having enough energy to come fully forward or even "online." You often see this in the heart chakra with a collapsed chest and rounded shoulders.

The center of a chakra may also seem to be located slightly to the left or right of its desired location. This can be interpreted as an imbalance between masculine (right side) and feminine (left side), though such interpretations must always be made lightly and checked against one's experience.

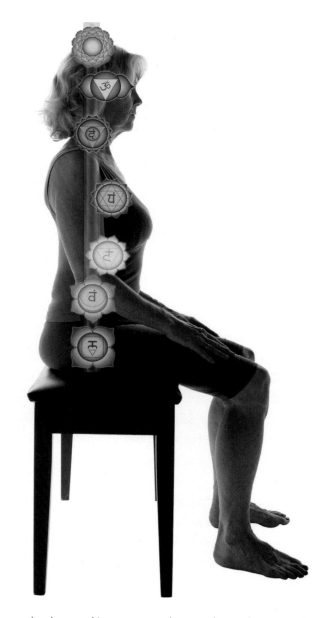

chakra alignment breath ▲ here, chakras one,
two, five, and seven are in alignment, while
chakras three, four, and six are slightly forward of
the center line and would be deemed excessive

Breathing into the midline is a chakra balancing meditation where you imagine your breath as a thick thread that moves forward and backward through the center of a particular chakra. My students affectionately call this "chakra flossing," since it resembles the way you use a thread to floss your teeth. (When you get to the upper chakras, it's "mental floss"!)

To understand how this exercise works, imagine a balloon filled with air. If you let go of the balloon without tying it off, it will fly through the air, moving in the opposite direction from the stream of air coming out of it. Another analogy is the way a jet moves forward, pushing a stream of energy behind itself.

In the same way, you can use the direction of your breath to subtly push a chakra forward or backward so that you experience its center more deeply in the midline.

As you inhale, there is a tendency to move energetically toward the direction from which you are drawing the breath. If you imagine breathing toward the front of your heart chakra, for example, there is a slight tendency to open your chest toward the front.

As you exhale, there is a tendency to move energetically away from the direction the air is moving—like the balloon. If you imagine exhaling out the front of your heart chakra, it tends to move the chakra slightly toward the back.

What if you feel your chakra is already in the middle? Great! Then simply imagine the inhalation expanding the chakra all the way around, like a sphere, and the exhalation embracing and brightening the core.

Because the top and bottom chakras define your midline, you don't breathe forward and backward through them but up and down. For the first chakra, draw the breath up from the earth on the inhalation and exhale the breath back down to the earth. For the seventh chakra, inhale the heavenly energy down into your crown chakra and exhale it upward, imagining it sprouting out like a fountain.

In this picture, the person's first, second, and fifth chakras appear to be right on the midline, whereas the third, fourth, and sixth chakras are slightly in front. To center the chakras she would breathe into the back of her third chakra, for instance, and breathe out the front, subtly shifting the chakra toward the midline. If a chakra were behind the line, she would breathe into the front and breathe out the back of the chakra to move it toward center.

Now you are ready. Begin in a meditation position with the principle of roots down, crown up, drawing the core line as straight as possible without being rigid. Ideally this should align all your chakras like beads on a string. However, due to blockages and habits, this simple technique doesn't quite do it for most of us. So as you extend your spine in opposite directions, notice which of your chakras seems to be out of alignment with the center core, focusing on one chakra at a time. If you can't tell, make your best guess or simply imagine the chakra expanding and contracting.

Begin at the base chakra, which sets your ground. Inhale, drawing earth energy up into your first chakra, hold for a few moments, then exhale and send the energy down your roots. Repeat 3–4 times or until you feel connected with your roots.

Then move to the second chakra. Assess from within whether it feels like your second chakra is situated in front or behind your midline. Inhale toward the side you want the chakra to move and exhale out the opposite side, imagining the air stream gently nudging the chakra forward or back as you intend. Take 3–4 full breaths here.

Then move to the third chakra and assess its location in your body. Take 3–4 breaths here, breathing into the front or back of the chakra and breathing out the other side, using the breath to gently nudge the chakra forward or back (or left or right).

Continue, chakra by chakra, with the same steps, taking 3–4 slow, full breaths at each chakra.

On the seventh chakra, breathe into your crown, drawing energy down from above, and breathe out the top of your head, sprouting up and out like a fountain.

When you are complete, come to a natural breath and reassess the degree to which you feel aligned along your core.

Capturing Light

Light is a necessary vitamin, as important as food, water, or love. In our indoor society we spend most of our time behind walls, and the result is a kind of light deprivation. This simple exercise can be done anywhere and takes only a few moments. It is the process of drinking in light from natural surroundings and bringing it inside to the inner temple, much like squeezing color out of a tube of paint and putting it on your palette. This exercise invites you to stop and appreciate the beauty you see. I've been doing this for years, and the result is an inner incandescence that is often present in my meditations, as well as more potent imagery in guided visualizations and dreams.

1. When you see something bright, colorful, or beautiful, such as the sun streaming through the leaves of a tree, a ruby-red rose, or simply a vision of beauty, be it natural or artistic, stop and take it in fully.

2. Open your eyes wide, drinking in the light and color as if you could inhale the light into your body.

3. When you have fully received the light, close your eyes and imagine you are depositing that imagery into your sixth chakra. Re-create the image in your mind until you can see it clearly. You can open and close your eyes, repeating the process, until you feel you can see the image clearly with your eyes closed.

4. This can also be done while meditating in a dark room with a candle flame. Gaze upon the flame, drinking in the light, then close your eyes and bring the image to your inner temple.

5. Do *not* look directly at the sun or you will damage your eyes. If you are standing in direct sun, you can actually look up at the sun with your eyes closed and still feel light coming in through your eyelids.

Sixth Chakra Practice and Postures

Yogic Eye Exercises

Seeing clearly on a physical level depends on the muscles of the eyes. As we age our muscles get weaker, and this affects the lenses of the eyes and their ability to focus. Sitting at a computer or watching TV, the eyes focus at one distance for a long period of time, and this trains the eyes to be lazy. Living in the natural world, from which we evolved, one naturally focuses both near and far throughout the day. The following practice exercises the eye muscles and is said to improve vision.

1. Sit erect in a comfortable position. Keep your head and neck as relaxed as possible. Find a fixed point for your gaze, straight in front of you. Look at it dispassionately, with a neutral mind, noticing the details. This will be your central focal point.

2. Gently move your eyes up and down ten times. The motion should be very slow, smooth, and calm, without moving the head or neck. Continue looking through your eyes as you move them, but let the contents of what you see pass by like scenery when you are driving in a car, without attachment. Keep your gaze steady.

3. Next, move your eyes very slowly from side to side, level with the horizon. Repeat ten times. As above, let your gaze be steady but dispassionate, observing from a neutral mind. You will able to move your eyes farther in each direction and more easily with practice.

4. Next take your gaze from the upper right to the lower left five times, then from the upper left to the lower right five times.

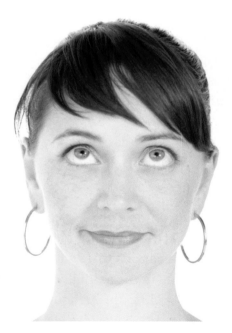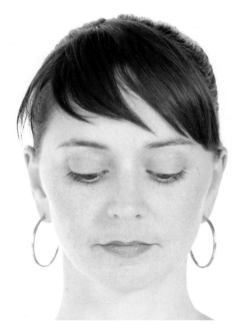

yogic eye exercises ▲

5. Finally, imagine a large circle around the field of your view. Move your eyes gently and slowly around the complete circle five times without moving your head. Rest for a few seconds, then repeat the circle five times in the other direction. Allow the movements to be slow and effortless.

6. Complete this exercise by rubbing your palms together rapidly, creating heat, then gently cup your warm palms over the eyes and let the heat sink in. Feel the nourishment of the heat and bathe your eyes in the darkness.

Benefits

- Improves vision

- Develops concentration

- Calms the mind

- Improves focus

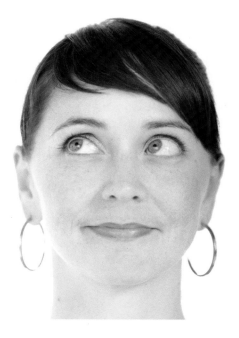 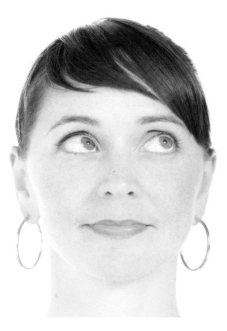

Drawing the Line in Tadasana

This slow movement from Tadasana, Standing Mountain Pose, calls your gaze upward and invites you to become still, calm, and focused.

1. Stand in Tadasana. Lift your arms overhead and interlace your fingers in a steeple position with the first fingers pointing upward.

2. With your eyes closed, imagine a laser beam of light between your fingertips that flows into you from the heavens, down through your fingertips into your crown, down through the core of all your chakras and into the earth between your feet, all the way to the center of the earth. See this laser illuminating your core fully in a white or golden light.

3. Now open your eyes and gaze upward. Direct your gaze (drishti) to the tips of your pointed fingers. Lift and lengthen your spine while rooting down into your ground.

4. Inhale, continuing to lift upward, then arch backward, imagining that you can extend your laser to draw a line backward across the ceiling, and—if your flexibility allows—partway down the back wall.

5. When you reach the limit of your flexibility, exhale, then inhale and draw the line slowly back up the wall and across the ceiling to directly above your head once again, keeping your gaze fixed on your fingertips at all times.

6. Continue exhaling as you bow forward, fingers extended. Still training your gaze on your fingertips, now draw a line forward across the ceiling and down the wall in front of you, then across the floor until your fingertips point to the spot between your feet in the middle of your first chakra square (remember that? see page 55) as you bow forward in Uttanasana, Standing Forward Fold.

7. Close your eyes, visualize your beam of light bending through your core, then once again rise up on an inhalation, slowly drawing the light across the floor, up the wall, and across the ceiling to the point directly above your head once again.

8. Once standing upright again, reimagine the laser light running through your core from above to below.

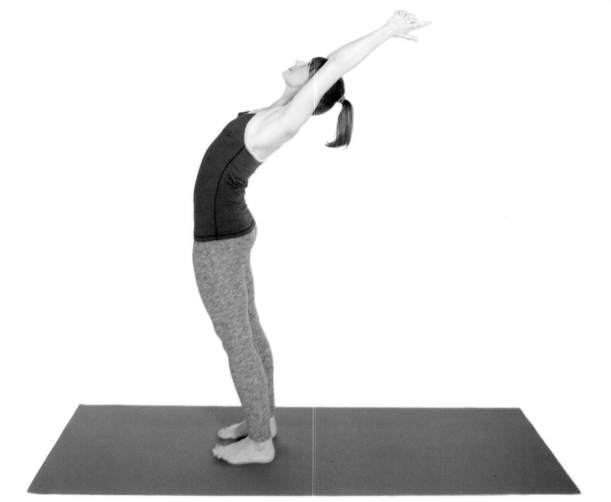

drawing the line in tadasana ▲

Guidelines

- Make your moves slow and steady, tracing an even, straight line. You might choose to practice with a small flashlight and watch the spot of light move along the wall and ceiling, trying to make as smooth a line as possible. You'll see that this isn't so easy!

- Keep your gaze focused on your fingertips or, if using a small light, on the place the light lands on the wall or ceiling.

- Continue to imagine the glowing light at your core.

- Deepen the length of the line you trace with subsequent iterations through the pose.

Benefits

- Increases spinal flexibility

- Opens the chest, increasing lung capacity

- Increases concentration and calms the mind

- Good preparation for meditation

Avoid or Use Caution

- Back injury

- Migraines

Virabhadrasana: Warrior III

Continue to focus on this glowing core as you step into Warrior III, seeing the line from fingertips to toes. This pose first appeared in chakra three.

1. Begin in Tadasana, Standing Mountain Pose. Take a step back with your right foot, placing it about two feet behind your left foot.

2. Bring your weight onto your left leg and find your core stability. Place your hands on your hips, making sure your hips are squared toward the front of your mat.

3. Extend out through your back leg as you hinge your whole torso forward, lifting your right leg parallel to the floor.

4. Root into your standing leg and find your stability, with hands on your hips. Attempt to keep the front of both hips parallel to the floor.

5. When stable, extend both arms forward, palms facing each other.

6. Fix your gaze between your hands or, if that is difficult, start with a point a few feet in front of you on the floor.

7. Hold for as long as you feel stable, though generally this pose is held for a shorter length of time. To come out of the pose, inhale and lift your arms overhead as you hinge back upright, bringing both feet together in Tadasana, with your arms by your sides.

8. Repeat on the other side.

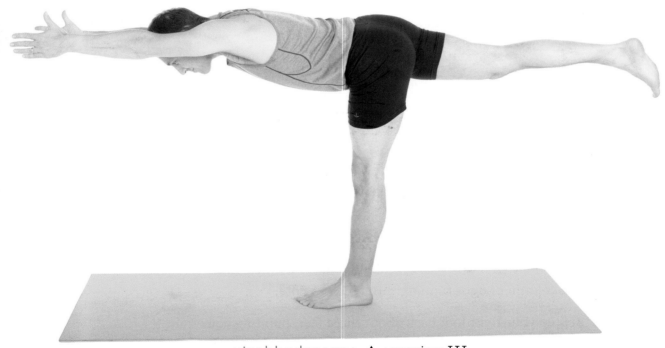

virabhadrasana ▲ warrior III

Guidelines

- Move slowly, seeking steadiness and balance at each stage. If you fall out of the pose you can always come back in, but it's easier to keep your balance as you go if you move slowly.

- Press your palms toward each other, firming your shoulder blades onto your back as you reach forward.

- Firm up your belly into your ribs.

- Attempt to bring the front of your hip bones level with each other. Ideally you could place a pencil on your back.

- Extend from the back toes to the front fingertips in one energized line.

Benefits

- Strengthens the core

- Develops balance

- Promotes concentration

- Focuses the attention, or drishti

Avoid or Use Caution

- Balance problems

Parsvottanasana: Intense Side Stretch Pose

Connect more deeply with your core by keeping your drishti focused on your fingertips as in the Drawing the Line in Tadasana exercise, continuing to draw a straight and steady line with your fingertips as you bow forward and bring your forehead toward your knee.

1. Begin in Tadasana, Standing Mountain Pose. Imagine a column of light running through your core.

2. Step your right foot back about three feet, pointing your right toes toward the right front corner of the mat. Inhale.

3. Exhale and square your torso to the front of the mat. Rotate your back thigh slightly inward and your front thigh slightly outward.

4. Draw your legs into the core as if you were holding a block between your thighs.

5. Inhale and lift your arms up overhead, forming a steeple position with your hands. Firm up your back, hugging your shoulder blades inward and downward.

6. Keeping the length in your spine and focusing your gaze on your fingertips, exhale and bow down over your front leg, bringing your forehead toward your knee. Move slowly and steadily, keeping your gaze on your fingertips at all times.

7. To come out of the pose, inhale and press actively through your back heel as you lift up to standing, focusing your gaze on your fingertips and moving slowly and steadily.

8. Draw the feet together in Tadasana and repeat on the other side.

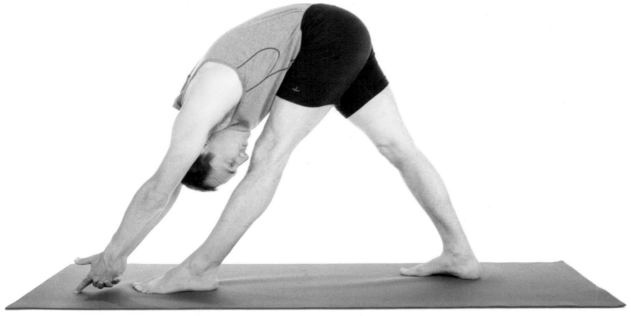

parsvottanasana ▲ intense side stretch pose

Guidelines

- You may need to separate your hands and place them on either side of your front foot or on blocks for easier balance, gradually working your hands toward each other as your balance is developed.

- Hugging into your core will help you maintain balance when your fingertips are together.

- Firm up your thighs by hugging the muscles to the bones and lifting up on your kneecaps. Elongate both legs and lift the pelvis up out of the thighs, pressing the thigh bones back into the hamstrings.

- Turn your lower belly over your front leg.

- Move your front hip slightly back and your back hip slightly forward to keep your hips square to the front of the mat.

- Energetically draw your feet toward each other.

Benefits

- Improves balance

- Develops concentration and focus in the sixth chakra

- Calms and quiets the mind

- Stretches the hamstrings and strengthens the legs

- Opens the hips

- Tones abdominal muscles

- Lengthens the spine

Avoid or Use Caution

- Abnormal blood pressure

- Pregnancy

Garudasana: Eagle Pose

Half eagle, half human, Garuda is the mount of the god Vishnu. Vedic lore credits Garuda as the personification of courage who stole the ambrosia of immortality. When flying, his wings are said to chant the Vedas. Garuda is associated with snakes and often wrapped in serpents, much like the pose below wraps you up like a serpent. This pose accentuates hugging into the core by squeezing everything like a wet washcloth. Keep your gaze focused and steady on a point in front of you.

1. Begin in Tadasana. Affirm your center line as you root down and lift your crown. See your core as a column of light.

2. From your third eye, fix your gaze upon a focal point a few feet in front of you.

3. Inhale your arms up overhead, then exhale and swing them downward, wrapping the right elbow under the left elbow.

4. Draw your forearms together so that your palms are facing each other as much as possible. If that is not possible, you may want to work with a strap.

5. If possible, place the thumb of your right hand on the surface of your third eye and point your hands straight up so that your right and left eye can see forward on either side of your hands. Squeeze your arms together.

6. Bend both knees as if going into Utkatasana, Awkward Chair Pose.

7. Lift your right leg and wrap it around over your left thigh, balancing on your left leg, with both knees bent.

8. If possible, tuck the toes of your right foot around the left calf.

9. Hold until your balance becomes firm and your breathing is steady.

10. To come out of the pose, unwrap your legs, followed by your arms; lift your arms overhead, then bring them down to your sides or wrap them up again for the other side, with the left elbow under the right.

11. To repeat on the other side, wrap the left leg up and around the right.

Guidelines

• Keep all four corners of the standing foot rooted into the ground.

• There is a strong tendency to lean forward. Pull your shoulders up and back, lifting into your crown chakra. Reestablish your core from crown to base after you wrap your legs and arms.

• Hug into your core by wrapping your arms and legs even more tightly. Imagine you are squeezing a washcloth to get the water out. This pushes toxins out of your body.

• Deepen the pose by bending the knees more.

• Work the shoulders by raising and lowering the elbows.

• If your hands cannot reach each other, use a strap.

• If balance is difficult, work up to it by using a block beneath the raised foot.

• Breathe into the broadness of the upper back.

Benefits

• Detoxifying

• Develops focus on the third eye

• Develops balance and concentration

• Strengthens the legs

• Improves circulation

• Promotes digestion

- Develops willpower

- Increases clarity

Avoid or Use Caution
- Shoulder inury

- Knee injury

- Low blood pressure

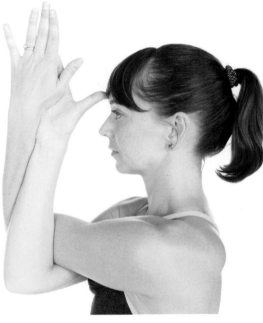

garudasana ▲ close-up of arms
and hands in front of sixth chakra

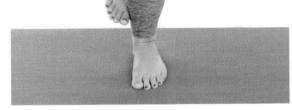

garudasana ▲ eagle pose

Makarasana II: Dolphin Pose

1. From Table Pose, bend your arms so that your forearms come down to the floor, keeping your elbows shoulder-distance apart.

2. Bring your palms together and interlace your fingers, gripping firmly.

3. Curl your toes under your feet, then lift your knees and hips upward into a modified Downward Facing Dog Pose.

4. To come out of the pose, bend your knees and return to Table or press upward into Downward Facing Dog.

Guidelines

- You may bend the knees to make the pose easier and gradually work to straighten the legs and get the heels down.

- Beginners may wish to elevate their elbows on a blanket or rolled-up mat.

- Press the forearms actively into the floor.

- Draw the core of each leg up into the hips.

- Lift the sitting bones up toward the ceiling.

- Widen your shoulder blades and point them toward your tailbone.

- Lift your heart chakra and shoulder blades away from the floor.

- To deepen, walk the feet forward and move the heart toward the thighs.

Benefits

- Strengthens the arms and shoulders

- Good preparation for inversions

- Stimulates the brain

- Focuses concentration

Avoid or Use Caution

- Shoulder injuries

- Glaucoma

- High blood pressure

- Head injuries

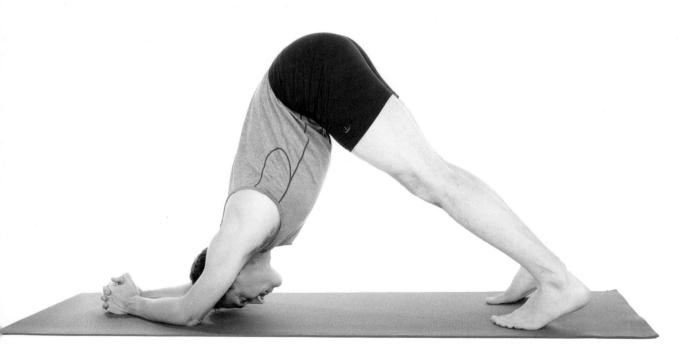

makarasana II ▲ dolphin pose

Adho Mukha Vrksasana: Handstand

We spoke about how inversions turn the entire chakra system upside down and force the attention into the core. Here, the drishti aimed between your hands helps to steady your pose.

- **Note:** See chakra four, page 294, for handstand prep.

It is good to develop your handstand by kicking up against a wall or a friend's hands, which can support your balance while you develop the necessary strength in your arms and shoulders.

1. Begin in Table Pose. Firm up your arms and soften the place between your shoulder blades, opening your heart. Place your hands 8–12 inches away from a wall, shoulder-width apart. Rotate your upper arms slightly outward and push down into the web between your thumb and forefinger. Pull your belly in slightly to activate your core.

2. Push up into Downward Facing Dog but walk your feet a little farther forward than you might in your normal Dog pose. If possible, walk forward until your shoulders are over your wrists.

3. Firm your shoulders, lift your shoulder blades up toward your hips, activate your hands and fingers, and take a deep breath.

4. Bend your left knee and bring it closer to the wall, then kick up with a straight right leg. Keep your arms firm and straight.

5. Practice a few smaller kicks before you kick all the way up, to see if you are comfortable.

6. Be sure to keep your shoulders over your hands so that the weight is supported on your arms vertically.

7. Once you can get both feet against the wall, hug into your core, press your feet and legs together, and push upward into the balls of your feet, lengthening the whole body. The toes should be neither pointed nor flexed but halfway between these positions.

8. Hold for a few breaths,
   then take the right
   leg down, followed
   by the left leg.

9. Breathe in Downward
   Dog or take a rest
   in Child's Pose.

Guidelines

• You can also lift one leg
  horizontally and hold it
  firm; while an assistant
  holds and steadies that
  leg, you lift the other leg.

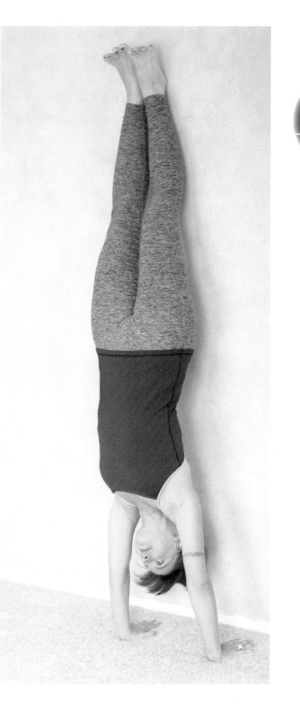

adho mukha vrksasana ▶ handstand

- Push up into your pelvis. Be careful not to "banana" the body but keep the hips over the shoulders. Taking the tailbone and belly in toward the core will help alleviate the banana.

- Keep your arms straight and stretch your heels up the wall.

- Gazing toward your fingertips is more stable in the shoulders, while gazing toward the middle of room is more freeing in the neck area (and more advanced).

- Practice kicking up with each leg so you don't get the habit of favoring one side. Keep the top leg straight and avoid twisting the pelvis while kicking up.

Benefits
- Energizing for the whole body

- Upper chakra stimulation

- Drains lymph and blood, then replenishes

- Strengthens the arms and shoulders

- Accentuates core

Avoid or Use Caution
- Shoulder or neck injury

- High blood pressure

- Headaches

- Menstruation

- Pregnancy

- Glaucoma

- Heart conditions

Pincha Mayurasana: Feathered Peacock Pose

Practicing Dolphin Pose will strengthen your shoulders and prepare you for Feathered Peacock, a more advanced pose. This is a great one for opening the shoulders and expanding the rib cage and is actually easier to balance than a handstand. Begin at the wall until you can comfortably hold the pose on your own for twenty seconds or more.

1. Begin in Table Pose, facing a wall, with the option of the front of your mat folded to create a cushion for your elbows.

2. Place your forearms parallel to each other on the floor, shoulder-width apart. You may choose to set a block between your hands or wrap a strap around your arms just above your elbows to keep your hands and elbows at the proper distance, as shown below.

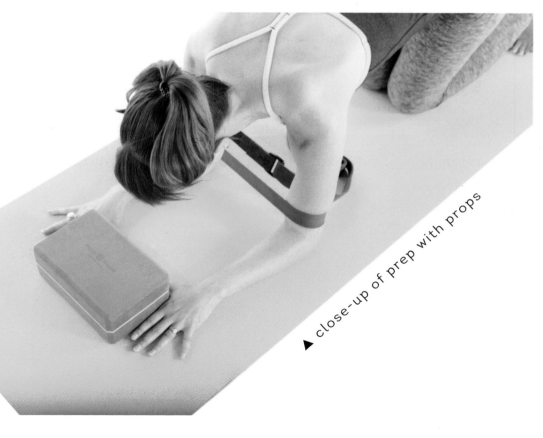

▶ close-up of prep with props

3. From here, slowly walk your feet toward your hands until you are in a modified Dolphin Pose, keeping your shoulders firm and hugging the head of your upper arms into the sockets. Walk your feet forward until your shoulders are over your elbows.

4. Take a few breaths here, find your core, and stabilize. If you have pain in your shoulders at this point, do not progress any further.

5. If you feel ready, lift one leg off the ground with the knee straight, then bend the other leg and try a few practice kicks, testing your strength. Keep the top leg straight and avoid twisting while kicking up.

6. If ready, kick up as if going into a handstand, lifting your hips over your shoulders and bringing your heels against the wall.

7. Once here, pull your upper arms into the core, pushing downward into your elbows. Lift your head toward the corner of the wall or higher. Draw the feet and legs together and push the heels upward toward the ceiling. Point your feet and flex your toes, spreading them wide.

8. Hold until you feel steady, then settle into the pose as long as you can hold that steadiness comfortably. You may try and practice moving your feet slightly away from the wall to see if you can balance on your own.

9. Come out of the pose by bringing one foot to the floor, then the other.

10. Rest in Child's Pose and feel the effects.

Guidelines

- Rotate your upper arms outward to keep the shoulder blades broad.

- Use the strap and block to stabilize your base in the pose.

- Press the center of your forearms down and lift your shoulder blades up.

- With or without the strap, hug your forearms inward, as they tend to splay outward once your weight is on them. Press down through the inner edges of the palms.

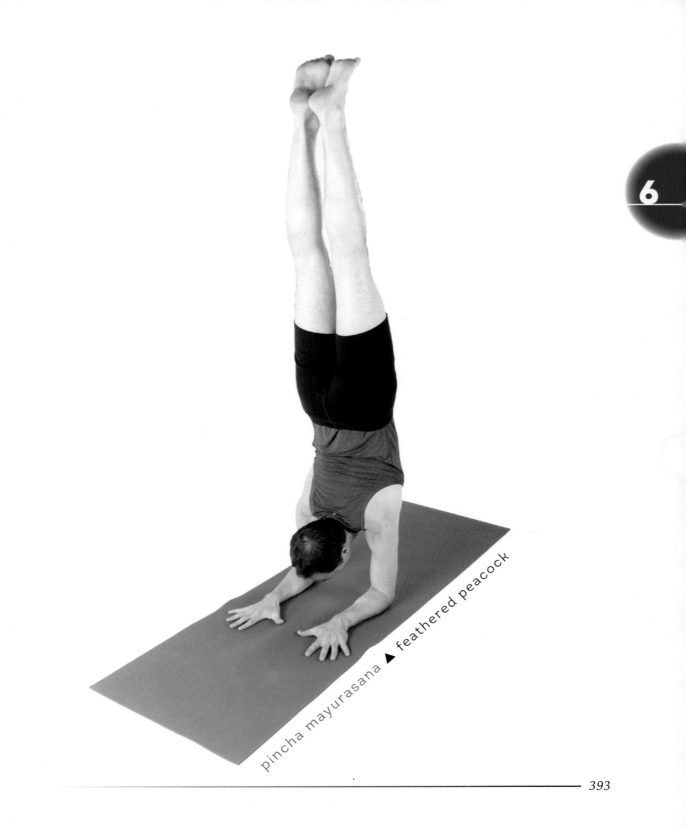

pincha mayurasana ▶ feathered peacock

- Keep the tailbone in and firm the belly to keep from collapsing into your lower back.

- Downward Facing Dog, Dolphin, and Plank are good buildups to this pose.

Benefits
- Strengthens shoulders, arms, and back

- Develops balance

- Develops focus and concentration

- Stimulates the upper chakras

- Relieves stress and depression

Avoid or Use Caution
- Back, shoulder, or neck injury

- Headaches

- High blood pressure

- Menstruation

- Pregnancy

- Heart condition

Savasana: Corpse Pose

As you surrender into Savasana, draw your attention up to your sixth chakra. Imagine you can look down into your inner temple and see all the prana within your body glowing with light. Imagine you can see the nadis as rivers of light, flowing through the chakras as glowing jewels of rainbow colors. Bask in this inner light. Dissolve your physical body into your light body.

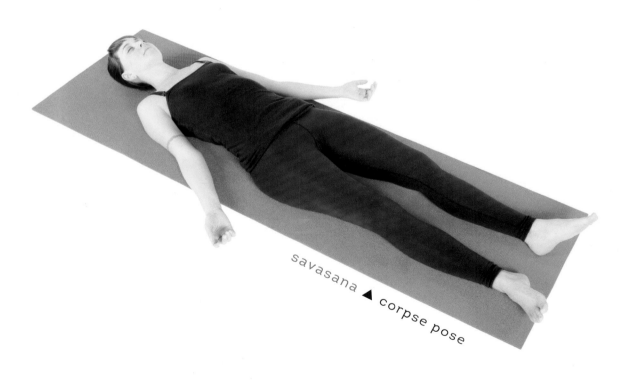

savasana ▲ corpse pose

Sixth Chakra Posture Flow

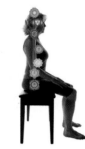

Chakra Alignment Breath

Yoga Eye Exercises

Drawing the Line in Tadasana

Vrksasana: Tree Pose

Garudasana: Eagle Pose

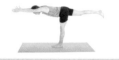

Virabhadrasana: Warrior III

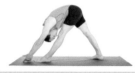

Parsvottanasana: Intense Side Stretch Pose

Anahatasana: Extended Puppy

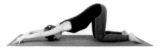

Adho Mukha Svanasana: Down Dog

Anjaneyasana: Deep Lunge

Parivrtta Parsvakonasana: Revolved Side Angle Pose

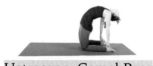

Ustrasana: Camel Pose

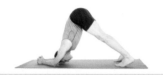

Makarasana II: Dolphin Pose

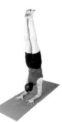

Pincha Mayurasana: Feathered Peacock Pose

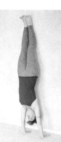

Adho Mukha Vrksasana: Handstand

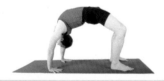

Urdhva Dhanurasana: Wheel Pose

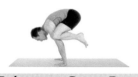

Bakasana: Crane Pose

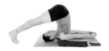

Halasana: Plow Pose

Savasana: Corpse Pose

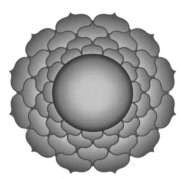

Sahasrara
THOUSANDFOLD LOTUS

Elements	Consciousness, thought
Principles	Omnipresence, omniscience, sat-chit-ananda (truth, consciousness, bliss)
Purpose	Awareness, unity with the Divine
Properties	Stillness, emptiness, presence, intelligence, awareness, knowledge, understanding, grace
Body parts	Head, brain, nervous system in general
Practices	Meditation, meditation, meditation
Actions	Drawing inward and upward, dharana, dhyana, samadhi
Poses	Sitting still, Savasana, headstand, inversions in general
Masculine	Knowledge, order, emptiness
Feminine	Wisdom, unity, fullness
Deficient	Materialistic, disconnected, cynical
Excessive	Overly intellectual, spiritual addiction, spaciness
Balanced	Realization, grace, enlightenment, bliss

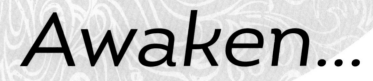

Awaken...

The supreme adventure in a man's life is his journey back to his Creator. To reach the goal he needs well-developed and coordinated functioning of his body, senses, mind, reason, and Self. ~B.K.S. IYENGAR

Yoga is a philosophy, a practice, and a set of principles for awakening the divine nature of the soul. In the true meaning of the word, yoga is union with the Divine through the realization of ultimate truth, consciousness, and bliss.

This awakening is not a sudden moment of enlightenment that overtakes you during meditation one bright morning, though elements of it may occur that way. Nor is it an awakening that happens inside your head or alone on your mat in isolation to everything else. Rather, it is a gradual process—a little awakening that takes place each day. Your body awakens as you develop strength and gain flexibility. Inner spaciousness awakens as you expand your breath. Clarity awakens as you still your mind. Wisdom awakens as you study and grow. Joy awakens as you come into harmony with yourself and your surroundings.

Awakening is a gradual realization of an integrated wholeness in everything, a deeper access to who you really are, and a persistent presence of grace. Ultimately the Divine is experienced everywhere, at every moment, in every thing.

As your inner world transforms, your life changes as well. A quiet contentment begins to grow through the presence of an eternal inner peace. As you spend more time in your inner temple, things that used to bother you seem less significant. Slowly, the distinctions between inner and outer worlds begin to fade as you realize there is no separation. What is within shapes what is without, and vice versa. You discover that the keys you now have to the inner temple unlock the outer temple as well.

We are here to awaken the Divine within, to experience union with the Divine without, and to see that they are one. This is what the journey is all about, just as it has always been. Yoga is a royal road on this journey. The chakra system is the map to its treasure.

You have now explored six of the seven keys to the inner temple. There is one key left to awakening the Divine who resides within the temple. This key is an elusive mystery, yet it is always present. It is simultaneously everywhere and nowhere. You hold that key at every moment, but you cannot see it. It is not a thing. It cannot be measured or quantified. It is an experience. Ask yourself who holds that key, and the answer is the key itself: consciousness.

There is a consciousness that is deeply intelligent and ancient as time, and it forms the underlying unity of the cosmos. It is not created by our minds or brains, as some scientists suggest; rather, our brains are tools for perceiving that consciousness: our minds are the repositories of it and our bodies are the processors of it. Just as the Internet is a vast field of virtual information, accessed by our attention through our personal computers, life is a vast field of consciousness from which we download a tiny portion through our own awareness. And just like the browsers on our computers, what we download depends on where our consciousness is directed.

Attention!

The capacity to direct consciousness is called attention. It is the facet of consciousness we are most familiar with yet least able to master. The root of the word is from the Latin *tendare*, to stretch toward something. Attention stretches consciousness toward an object.

When you put your attention on something, you have an experience. If I put my attention on my feelings, I have an experience of joy or sadness, worry or excitement. If I put my attention on my inner alignment, I have a deeper connection to grace. If I put my attention on universal truths, beauty, or love, I begin to experience the underlying source of everything.

Learning to command your attention is one of the goals and by-products of yoga. Your focus gets sharper; you become aware of subtler levels of reality.

You can concentrate better, and your perception deepens. Now you are ready to explore subtler levels of attention itself.

The eight limbs of yoga that form the backbone of Patanjali's Yoga Sutras, listed below, describe a path toward awakening, as do the chakras themselves. Almost every book on yoga philosophy discusses these principles in detail, so we will just touch on them briefly to see how they form a structure for building up to the upper chakra awareness we are seeking.

The Eight Limbs of Patanjali's Ashtanga Yoga

1. Yama	Universal morality
2. Niyama	Personal observances
3. Asanas	Body postures
4. Pranayama	Breathing exercises
5. Pratyahara	Withdrawal of the senses
6. Dharana	Concentration
7. Dhyana	Deep meditation
8. Samadhi	Absorption into union with the Divine

We begin with the yamas—guidelines on how to behave toward others. The yamas advise us to refrain from violence, lying, stealing, greed, and unmoderated sexuality. Then the niyamas turn our attention toward how we treat ourselves. They advise us to develop purity, contentment, discipline, self-study, and devotion to the Divine. The yamas and niyamas form a foundation for life that happens off the mat in our daily interactions. They form a platform for the third and fourth limb, the practice of postures, or asanas, whose effects are heightened by the breathing practices of pranayama. Most of this book has been about the third and fourth limbs. The fifth limb is pratyahara, withdrawing the senses from the outer world in order to bring our attention more deeply inside, to the inner temple.

In the upper chakras we turn our attention toward the last three limbs, which direct our attention toward the true meaning of yoga as union. Through dharana we develop the ability to concentrate our mind. This directs attention to a single focus in order to cultivate stillness and concentration. Most meditation techniques highlight the principle of dharana, such as focusing on a mantra, an image, a candle flame, or counting your breaths. When attention can be unified in one direction it becomes like a laser beam, able to pierce illusion and illuminate anything. I think of dharana as a sixth-chakra process. You might say it's a highly focused I-It relationship between subject and object.[12]

Something profound happens when attention is focused in the concentration of dharana. We slip into the next stage of meditation, which is dhyana. Here we become aware not only of the object of our attention but of the source of it. We become aware of the infinite nature of consciousness itself—not only our own but the universal field in which we are enveloped. Our focus deepens, unwavering. Our I-It relationship shifts to an I-Thou as we contemplate the Divine. As our contemplation deepens we become fully absorbed, losing the distinct "I-ness" of individuality.

That absorption brings us to the final stage, samadhi, which is union with the Divine through the gradual dissolution between seer and seen. Yet even to talk about this union is to imply a separation. Instead, samadhi is the realization that it was never separate to begin with. There is no I and Thou; there is only one immense unified consciousness. In that way it is an awakening to a fundamental reality, an experience of being, rather than something we do or have. The mind and intellect have ceased their fluctuations, and we become the essence of yoga itself: complete union. This is the ultimate seventh-chakra experience. It is beyond words, since words exist within the realm of the intellect and are by nature part of dual consciousness.

All wisdom traditions point to an ineffable divine presence that permeates everything. Religious beliefs and practices are all about how to make contact with that divine Source—how to eliminate the clutter and illusion that keep us separate. Yoga is a way to yoke with the Divine. But its goal is to experience a state where there is no separation, nothing to yoke—where we *are* the Divine. This is the shift from sixth chakra to seventh, as the last three limbs take us from beholding to becoming to being.

12 For more on the I-Thou and We process, see Anodea Judith's *The Global Heart Awakens: Humanity's Rite of Passage from the Love of Power to the Power of Love* (San Rafael, CA: Shift Books, 2013).

Ordinary Consciousness

The state described above is a realization of the ultimate nature of reality, yet few people are able to access this state, let alone stay there. The rest of us may touch it briefly in a good meditation or a peak experience, but we spend most of our time in more mundane states of consciousness. What are we doing then? We're busy thinking, analyzing, interpreting, extracting meaning, and making beliefs.

Our thinking mind is largely concerned with finding order and meaning. Through the functions of the lower chakras—seeing and hearing, connecting, doing and feeling—we draw meaning from our experiences. As a child we might experience our father's anger and make up a meaning that we are bad. As an adult we have good or bad experiences, and we create meaning from them that will hopefully guide us to more positive experiences and less negative ones. We create a belief that doing this action brings rewards, while doing something else is dangerous. Our beliefs govern how we eat, dress, interact with others, and what goals we pursue or avoid.

As we derive meaning from our interpretations, we heap these meanings together over time to create beliefs.

If the mind is like software and the body its hardware, with the life force energy correlating to the electricity running through the system, then the seventh chakra is analogous to the operating system. The meaning we derive and the beliefs we create tell us how to operate in the world. If you practice yoga, it's because you believe it is a good thing to do. If you eat a certain way or treat people well, it is because that behavior is in accordance with your beliefs. If you've read this far in this book, you believe the chakra system is worth learning about.

However, our beliefs, like any operating system, need to be upgraded every so often. We need to let go of outdated beliefs that were formed in childhood, when we had very little understanding. We need to examine our beliefs and let go of those that limit us or negate us, such as believing that we are flawed or unlovable, or that life is hard, unfair, or dangerous. Not that we can't find evidence for those beliefs—that's the easy part. Anyone can point to their less-desirable traits or cite the long list of ills in the world to support negative beliefs.

What requires a greater order of consciousness is to fully examine our beliefs, actively deconstruct old beliefs, and consciously create new ones. The process of constructing new beliefs—or upgrading our operating system—begins with disengaging from our old ways of thinking. In computer terms, we delete one program before installing a new one. This requires allowing the mind to empty out now and then, "defragmenting the hard drive of consciousness," and coming to a more coherent state of awareness.[13] For this we go to the practice of meditation, the quintessential seventh-chakra practice.

*The paradox of meditation is that when you are
losing yourself, you are finding meditation.*

. . . .

ANODEA JUDITH

Meditation

If you get on your mat every day—even doing the most advanced asanas and pranayama—and you do not meditate, I would venture to say that you have not truly begun to practice yoga. While asana practice can be its own meditation, there is nothing like the simple practice of sitting still and doing nothing to understand the true secrets and purpose of yoga. From this elegantly basic experience, all else emerges.

Why is this simple practice—that costs nothing, requires no equipment, and can be done anytime and anywhere—so elusive in our culture? Even I, a regular meditator for over forty years, find some days too busy or other activities too engaging to sit down in silence and commune with grace as often as I would like to. Yet every time I engage in meditation, I am reminded of its wonders, like a balm to the soul, providing rest and renewal, inspiration, and guidance. Indeed, as I get older, I find I desire less asana practice and more meditation. Cultivating a meditative state enhances everything I do.

When the mind is no longer engaged in lower chakra activity—feeling and doing, loving and speaking, seeing and interpreting—it is free to frolic in the infinite. This is the opposite pole of the body, which is finite and singular. The

---

13 For more information on deconstructing beliefs, see Judith and Goodman, *Creating On Purpose* (Boulder, CO: Sounds True, 2012). Also check out Lion Goodman's e-book on transforming beliefs at http://www.transformyourbeliefs.com.

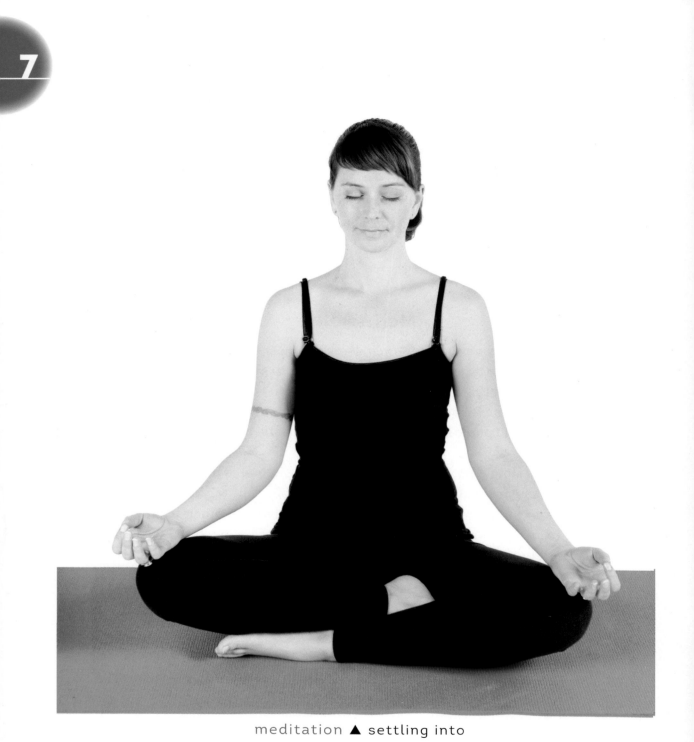

meditation ▲ settling into
your upright core

infinite takes us into the universal, the Supreme, the undifferentiated pool of primordial Source from which all things emerge. We have moved from Prakriti to Purusha, from Shakti to Shiva.

Meditation is a foray into emptiness, cleansing the mind for clear perception the way a shower cleanses your body. Meditation is communion with the Divine, a penetration by an infinitely loving presence and intelligence. Meditation is deep rest and renewal, a source for everything you do.

In meditation you may find a direct download of information for a problem you are working on. You may find a change in perspective. You may find detachment from something that created an upset. You may find compassion and understanding, a place to abide in that guides you through your day and becomes ever more present over time. You may find the key to the treasure that unlocks all of the chakras; indeed, we only see, hear, love, act, and feel because there is a consciousness within us that is doing all that.

So how do you do this thing that is basically doing nothing?

Books and courses abound that talk about meditation. You can go to a ten-day silent Vipassana retreat or engage in a ten-minute Savasana. You can take a quiet walk through the woods or sit still and focus on your breath. You can internally chant a mantra or you can gaze at a candle flame or image of a deity. You can contemplate a Zen koan or you can ask your own question. You can sit at the feet of your favorite deity or recite scripture from your favorite sacred text. You can imagine running energy through your system or you can focus on the moments between your thoughts.

The means of meditation are dharana, and they are all tools for taking you to the same place. What is important is that you pick one and stick with it. It takes time for a practice to be incorporated into your nervous system. It takes time for the neuroplasticity of your brain to adjust. It takes time to become adept at using your tools.

Settling into your upright core, where the body can breathe with ease and grace, is meditation's first step. This requires getting inside your temple and arranging your body so that it can be comfortable, upright, and still. This one step could take months or years of fine-tuning, yet its benefits are instantaneous every time you attempt it. Hatha yoga—the practice of postures—is said to have been designed to prepare the body for meditation. Meditation is by far the older form of yoga, with postures coming much later.

The next step is to withdraw your attention from the outside world and bring it into your inner temple. It is here you can set an intention to stretch inside. You might ask a question you have been pondering, say a prayer to a particular deity, visualize a thousand-petaled lotus infinitely opening, or log on to your "inner-net" with a secret password. Keeping your attention inside takes practice, and it is advised to choose a regular time for meditation, where distractions are minimized. That becomes your special time to enter your sacred center.

After a while, you will start getting lost in your meditation. Time will go by without measure. Twenty minutes can seem like five. An hour can seem like a full night's sleep. The inner commentator of the sports game of your life becomes blessedly silent, yet the observer is keenly awake. You lose track of your mantra, you forget your intention, and you find that you go through moments without any thoughts at all.

When you get to this place of getting lost, you are finding meditation. At first it happens in brief instants. You notice it after the fact—"Oh, I was there for a moment!"—but as soon as you have that thought, you are no longer there; you are back in dual consciousness. Gradually, the instants become longer and more frequent. You start to long for those states, and they begin to creep into your waking life. You notice your mind is silent while listening to a friend or you are wide open to a sunset without internal chatter.

More about meditation I cannot tell you. It is your own treasure to discover. What I can say is that meditation is the sparkling jewel of the lotus, the ineffable experience of surrender, and the greatest love affair you will ever have.

Seventh Chakra Subtle Energy

Find your way to a comfortable upright posture—one you can hold easily for at least 20–30 minutes. Use any props necessary to make this vertical sitting effortless.

Close your eyes and go inside to your inner temple. You should know the way well by now. Take a few slow breaths here, settling into your body with each breath, going more deeply inward. Let your body become more still with each breath, settling into place, consolidating into finer and finer stillness.

When your mind begins to quiet, listen to the emptiness. Direct your attention more to the spaces between your thoughts rather than to the thoughts themselves. Allow the thoughts to become like a distant mumble as you move further and further away from them. Simply observe without comment as the emptiness grows larger and the thoughts begin to wane.

Then allow yourself to become aware of your body. From the inside, with your eyes still closed, feel its weight and breadth, the presence of your body taking up space.

What is it that is now aware of your body? Shift your attention to that awareness and draw it back from the body and up to the crown.

Now become aware of any emotions or urges. Perhaps you are restless, hungry, sad, or impatient. Allow your awareness to keenly observe the sensations that produce those feelings and bring your attention to your awareness rather than the sensations. Who is it that is feeling these things? Bring your attention to that awareness.

Next, become aware of any part of you that is worried about doing things correctly. Be amused at yourself; relax your effort and smile. Connect with the awareness inside and let go of all effort.

Now bring your attention to your breath. Imagine each breath as a loving entity that is filling you as you inhale and cleansing you as you exhale, like a loving caress. Who is it that is watching the breath? With what are you able to sense the breath? Withdraw your awareness from the breath, knowing it will continue, and draw your attention up to the crown.

Notice any inner dialog that is going on—the subtle murmur of commentary in your head that we call thinking. Detach yourself from that commentary as if it were a conversation in another language. Become aware of the person that is hearing these thoughts.

Next, imagine that you can see your subtle body as a light body. All the nadis are sparkling with light, with each of the chakras shining like jewels in their rainbow colors. See the beauty of the prana within you.

Who is it that is seeing this beauty? Who is looking? With what faculty are you able to imagine and see?

Bring your awareness now to the part of you that is aware. Feel your awareness becoming aware of itself—and becoming aware of the part that is aware of that—and aware of that. Notice how this inquiry is infinite and pause for a long time here.

Finally, imagine there is a greater awareness above and around you that is completely aware of you as you sit in meditation. Imagine you are this awareness, calmly and dispassionately holding your consciousness in this awareness. Allow the space of that awareness to get emptier and emptier, imagining that you are piercing the space between the stars and moving out beyond the galaxy, even beyond the universe itself.

See the whole universe as a pulsating state of awareness that is ever-present, eternal, and intelligent. Bask here in the miracle of cosmic consciousness and pause for a long time here.

Allow your universal awareness to become aware of your tiny body sitting in meditation down here on this planet we call Earth. Imagine a direct flow of love and grace from that universal awareness to your individual self. Allow that flow to be like a cloak of love wrapped around your temple, holding you in perfect stillness and understanding.

Return your awareness to your heart as you receive this divine love and grace. When you are filled up, say thank you and slowly open your eyes.

Seventh Chakra Practice and Postures

In general, there are fewer poses that focus on the seventh chakra specifically. Yet any posture can have a seventh-chakra aspect if one uses the pose to lift the crown upward, refine the awareness toward a meditative state, and direct the prana toward surrender, exaltation, and worship of the Divine.

What follows are a few poses I would use in a seventh-chakra yoga class for an intermediate-level yoga student. At the end of the chapter I offer a suggestion for how to use poses previously introduced in the lower chakras to build up to these poses.

Natarajasana: Dancer Pose

The god Shiva is often shown in an ecstatic state of dance, with his left foot raised and his right foot dancing on the body of ignorance. When doing this pose, I like to think of my extended hand as offering a lotus flower to Shiva. I consider it a crown chakra pose because the base is very small (one foot) while the raised foot, head, and hand are lifted upward, reflecting your reach for the highest grace and the blessings of the gods. Pushing down into matter and rising up into the heavens reflects the eternal dance between Shiva and Shakti, with Shakti being the force of creation that enlivens Shiva from his meditative stillness.

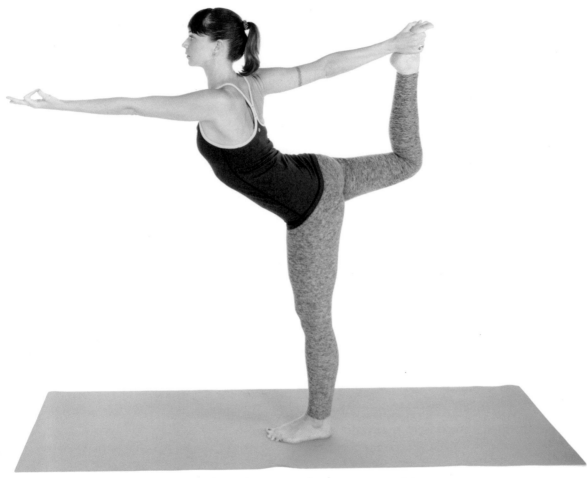

natarajasana ▲ dancer pose

1. Begin standing in Tadasana, Standing Mountain Pose, and find your midline. Extend your roots down and draw your crown upward.

2. Bend your right elbow in toward your waist with your forearm out to the side, forming a right angle. Lift your left arm up high overhead. Imagine reaching for the highest flower on a tree to pick your offering.

3. Bend your right knee and reach back with your right hand to grab your right ankle from the inside, fingertips pointing outward, thumb toward the back. Regain your balance and steadiness by drawing your thighs together, rooting your tailbone downward, and reestablishing your upright core.

4. Lengthen from root to crown as you tip your torso forward, pressing your back foot into your hand and lifting your back leg as high as you can without losing your stability. Move slowly and steadily.

5. Extend your left arm forward and slightly upward, holding the imaginary flower between your thumb and first finger, your other three fingers outstretched.

6. Lift your crown, your back foot, and your outstretched hand.

7. To come out of the pose, lift your torso upright again and release your back foot to the ground. Stand in Tadasana, then repeat on the other side.

Guidelines

- Beginners may wish to use a strap to connect the hand to the foot.

- Move slowly, establishing your balance at each step.

- Hug into the midline as you extend forward.

- Pick a focal point for your gaze a few feet in front of you to help maintain balance.

- Lift as you hinge forward, pressing your lifted leg more firmly into your hand.

- Root down into the standing leg, hugging the muscles to the bones, and feel how pushing down allows you to lift up.

- Endeavor to keep your hips level to the ground, both shoulders square to the front of the mat.

- Smile as you imagine the deity accepting your offering!

Benefits

- Strengthens core

- Develops balance and concentration

- Opens the chest and shoulders

- Increases lung capacity

- Reduces stress

- Promotes mental clarity

- Promotes a feeling of expansion

- Strengthens the legs

Avoid or Use Caution

- High blood pressure

- Shoulder injury

- Dizziness

- Balance problems

Sirsasana: Headstand

Headstand is one of the few poses that puts direct pressure on the top of the head. It forces you deeply into your core, as that is the only way you will balance. Like all inversions, learning to do Headstand requires hugging into the midline, activating your core, and strengthening your arms, neck, and shoulders.

1. Begin by folding a mat or blanket to create some extra cushioning for your arms and head. Beginners should place the edge of their folded mat against a wall.

2. Kneel on the floor in Table Pose. Place your forearms on the mat, with each hand grasping the opposite elbow. This will give you the correct distance between your elbows.

3. Now that you have measured the space between your elbows, keep them directly below your shoulders while you swing your forearms forward, interlacing your fingers to form a small rounded pocket with your hands. Ideally your forearms and the distance between your elbows form an equilateral triangle (position A).

4. Lengthen through your torso and soften the back of the heart.

5. Lower the crown of your head and place it on the mat, nestling the back of your skull into the cuplike shape made with your hands. Keep your arms just as you established them in step 3.

6. Make sure the very top of your head is against the floor. Tilting the skull forward or backward puts undue strain on the neck. The cervical spine should maintain its natural curvature.

7. The movement that supports Headstand and minimizes pressure on the neck is through the shoulders. They need to be lifted away from the floor by pushing down through your upper arms and pulling your shoulders away from your ears. Try this a few times before lifting your torso.

8. Keeping the lift in the shoulders, tuck your toes into the floor and slowly walk your feet toward your head until your hips are over your shoulders (position B). This leaves only the weight of the legs to lift, rather than the whole torso. This is a good place to stay and develop strength if you are new to the pose. You should certainly stop here if you feel any discomfort in your neck or shoulders.

9. To rise up, bend both knees and use the strength of your core to slowly lift both legs with bent knees. This may also be a stopping place while you stabilize your balance.

10. Straighten your legs as you find your stability. If the muscles of your core are strong, you can lift both legs directly from position B.

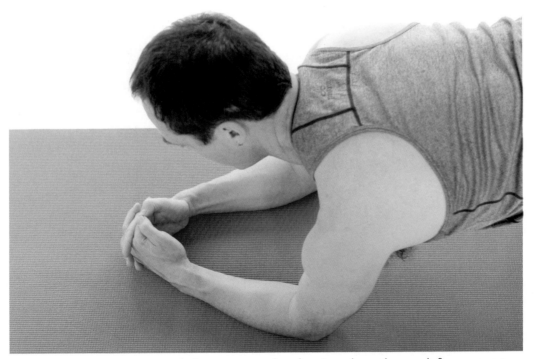

sirsasana ▲ placing hands and forearms for headstand base, position a

11. Once you are upright, hug your legs firmly together and imagine your core running from your crown to the point between your feet. Lengthen your tailbone toward your feet (position C).

12. To come out of the pose, bend your knees and lower your feet to the floor. Try to move slowly so as not to disrupt the prana.

13. Rest a few moments in Child's Pose before sitting up.

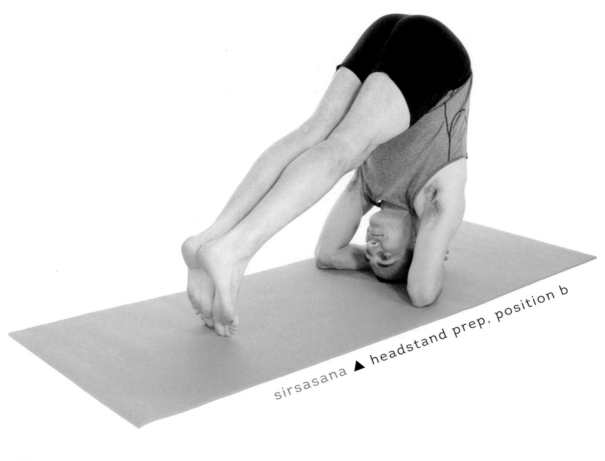

sirsasana ▲ *headstand prep, position b*

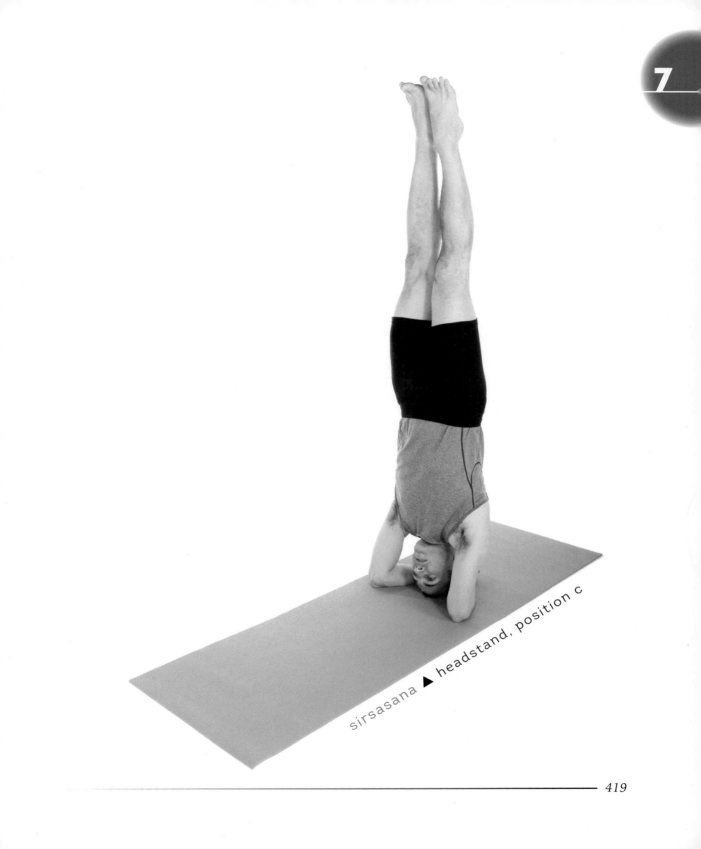

sirsasana ▶ headstand, position c

Guidelines

- Put a strap around your arms just above your elbows if your arms tend to move wider than your original placement of forearms shoulder-width apart.

- Maintain the lift in the shoulders at all times. If you feel too much weight on your head, you are not working your shoulders enough. Continue to press your forearms actively into the ground and lift the shoulders up.

- Move slowly from step to step, finding your stability in each step before proceeding to the next one.

- Draw your abdominals inward and firm up the buttocks by hugging your tailbone.

- Pull your legs together as if you had only one leg. Hug them into the core and push into the balls of your feet, spreading your toes wide.

Benefits

- Accentuates the core

- Develops balance

- Stimulates the upper chakras

- Improves circulation and digestion

- Strengthens the spine, arms, legs, and core

- Drains legs—good for varicose veins

- Calms and focuses the mind

Avoid or Use Caution

- Absolutely contraindicated for any injury or misalignment in the neck

- Shoulder injuries

- Migraines

- High blood pressure

- Menstruation

- Pregnancy

- Glaucoma

- Heart condition

Urdhva Dhanurasana: Upward Facing Bow or Wheel Pose

Also called Chakrasana, as the word *chakra* literally means wheel, this pose pops open all your chakras. It requires considerable warm up with smaller backbends such as Cobra, Camel, or Upward Bow as well as poses that strengthen the shoulders such as Dolphin, Handstand, and Headstand. This pose requires a flexible spine as well as openness in the groins and shoulders. It is not a beginner's pose and is best learned from a live teacher, as your first time getting up into Wheel can be disorienting. Work up to the pose in successive stages.

- **Note:** See chakra 4, pages 299–303, for more detailed instruction on this pose.

Stage 1

1. Lie on your back and bend your knees in the setup for Bridge Pose: feet hip-width apart and parallel to each other, heels within a foot of your buttocks.

2. Bend your elbows and place your palms on the mat just above your shoulders, fingertips pointing toward your feet. Take a breath or two here and pull the head of your armbones down toward the ground, hollowing out the armpits and firming your shoulder blades onto your back. Soften your heart as you firm up your back.

3. Inhale, then exhale as you press the core of each leg into the floor (especially the insides of the feet) to lift your hips upward as in Bridge Pose. Pause here and take another breath. **Note:** if you cannot lift your hips at least as high as your knees, you are not ready to push up into a full Wheel. Continue to work on Bridge Pose until your groins are more flexible.

Stage 2

4. Open your groins by pressing your tailbone down and drawing your knees toward each other. Orient to your core.

5. Next, press your hands into the floor and come onto the crown of your head, making a triangle between your head and two hands. Take a breath here and acclimatize. Make sure you are ready to go further. Make sure your fingertips are not turning inward but remain pointed toward your feet.

Stage 3

6. Press your hands into the floor and straighten your arms, lifting your shoulders off the ground. Lift up from the base of your heart.

7. Lift your heels up off the mat, and, if possible, walk your feet a little closer to your hands.

8. Hold for as long as you can be stable and breathe easily or until you get the cue to come down.

Stage 4

9. To come out of the pose, slowly bend the elbows and knees, tuck the chin into the chest, and then lower your spine from the top down.

10. Rest and breathe, feeling the powerful effects of your backbend. Avoid the urge to bring the knees to the chest in an immediate counterpose. It's best to give the lumbar discs a moment to readjust before spinal flexion.

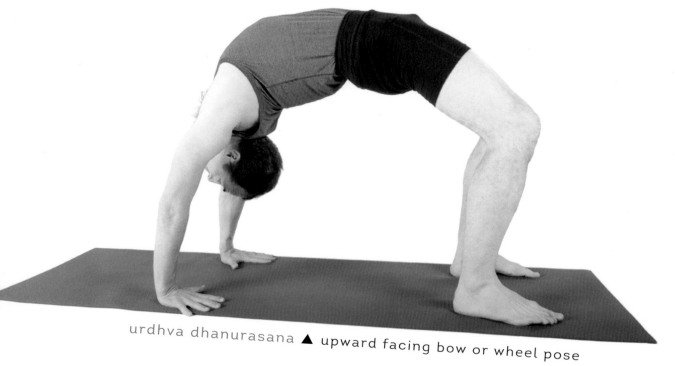

Guidelines

- For beginners or those with tight shoulders, having your hands higher than the floor can help. This can be done by using a wall, putting your hands on blocks, or grabbing onto someone's ankles. In any case, as you attempt this pose it is wise to have someone with you to spot you and give you proper instruction. If you feel any pain, come down or go to a previous stage.

- Beginners can also work Stage 1 or Stage 2 without going to later stages until developing the strength and flexibility the full pose requires.

- The knees and feet tend to splay outward. Draw the legs toward each other and put more pressure on the inner edges of the feet. This will take pressure off your lumbar spine.

urdhva dhanurasana ▲ upward facing bow or wheel pose

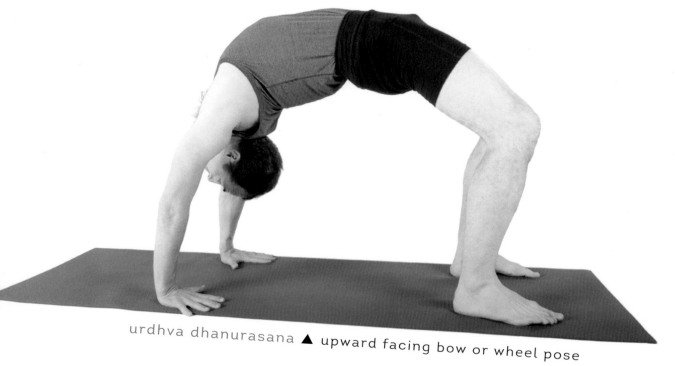

- Make sure fingertips are pointing straight back toward feet or slightly turned out.

- Externally rotate the shoulders and upper arms.

- There should be an evenness in the curve of the back. Ideally your navel wants to be the highest point in this pose (not that you can tell when you're upside down)!

- Move your spine deeply into your core. Imagine lengthening through the entire spine as you arch. The bigger the circle of your body, the more room there is for the vertebrae to arch back. Press your entire spine up into the front side of your body.

- The downward push through the hands and feet helps you lift higher.

- Press your shoulder blades into the back of your heart.

- Keep your head and neck relaxed. Look toward the fingers and lift the chest.

- If you can't hold the pose for very long, come out of the pose, then try again. Each time you try, you will be a little more flexible, and it will get a little easier. Get used to pushing up and coming down several times.

Variations
- Lift one leg straight up into the air, then switch legs (variation A).

- Bend your elbows and interlace your fingers for a deeper stretch in the chest and shoulders (variation B).

Benefits
- Strengthens the whole body, especially the arms and legs

- Promotes spinal flexibility

- Increases breathing and lung capacity

- Promotes circulation

- Aids digestion

- Opens the heart

- Energizes

- Relieves stress

- Stimulates lymph
  and blood flow

- Fun!

urdhva dhanurasana ▲ upward facing bow
or wheel pose, variation a

Avoid or Use Caution

- Tricky pose—not for beginners and not without sufficient warm-up

- Back, shoulder, or wrist injuries

- Carpal tunnel syndrome

- Abnormal high or low blood pressure

- Headaches or migraines

- Pregnancy

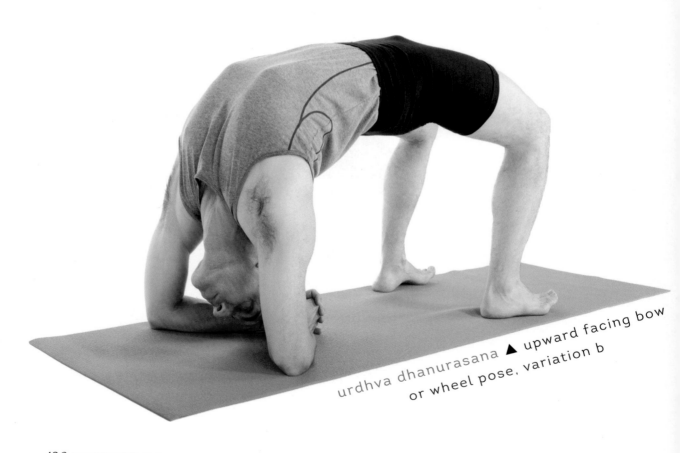

urdhva dhanurasana ▲ upward facing bow or wheel pose, variation b

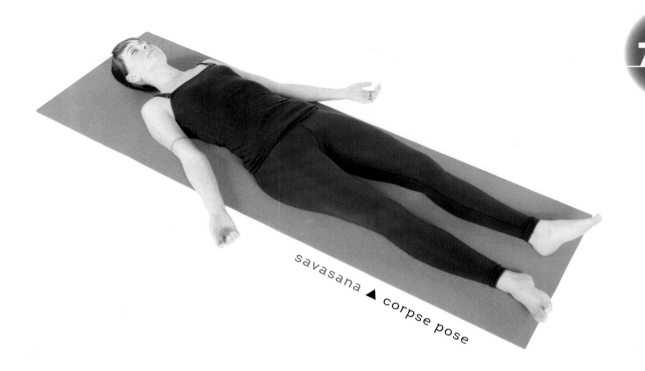

savasana ▲ corpse pose

Savasana: Corpse Pose

Savasana is the ultimate seventh chakra state of awareness and emptiness, presence and non-doing, allowing and sensing. Far from the easiest pose, true Savasana may be one of the most difficult. Can you keep your mind from wandering? Can you relax completely and not fall asleep? Can you enter deep stillness and let go of all urges to move and fidget? Can you remain present in your body as you let go of your body?

Through each of the chakras, we have focused our Savasana on different aspects: chakra one focused on the density of the body, chakra two on the internal flow of prana, chakra three on the energy body, chakra four on the breath, chakra five on the subtle vibration, chakra six on the inner light. Now, in chakra seven we focus on dissolving awareness of everything except awareness itself.

Align all your chakras as you lay down for Savasana. Extend your tailbone down toward your feet, point your feet upward, extend into your heels, then relax your legs and allow your feet to fall outward. Draw the front and back of your second chakra toward the midline and imagine widening your hips. Soften your ribs and deepen your breath, especially through the belly. Expand the heart and take your shoulder blades beneath you, rotating the head of the armbones toward the floor. Relax your jaw and face, close your eyes, and bask in the infinite. See if you can find meditation by losing yourself.

When coming out from this intense inner focus, there is a tendency to jump right back into outer consciousness, perhaps rolling up your mat and clearing out for the next class. Instead, try to maintain a dual focus: one part of your awareness still dwelling within while another part calmly and contentedly looks out from within. Allow rolling up your mat, putting your props away, and even getting in your car to be a meditation.

Eventually life itself will be a meditation in which the Divine within constantly frolics and brings you joy and bliss.

Namaste!

Seventh Chakra Posture Flow

Since there are far fewer poses that directly influence the seventh chakra, yet all poses do so to some degree, this sequence includes lower chakra poses sequenced for building from base to crown, chakra by chakra.

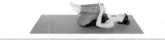

Apanasana: Knees to Chest Pose

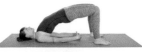

Setu Bandha Sarvangasana: Bridge Pose

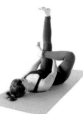

Sucirandhrasana: Eye of the Needle Pose

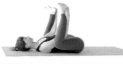

Ananda Balasana: Happy Baby Pose

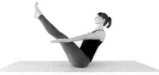

Paripurna Navasana: Boat Pose

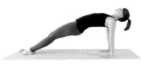

Purvottanasana: Inclined Plane Pose

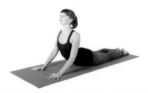

Bhujangasana: Cobra Pose

Adho Mukha Svanasana: Downward Facing Dog Pose

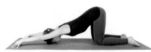

Anahatasana: Extended Puppy Pose

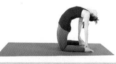

Ustrasana: Camel Pose

Salamba Sarvangasana: Shoulder Stand

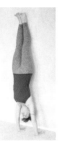

Bakasana: Crane Pose

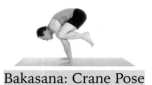

Adho Mukha Vrksasana: Handstand

Sirsasana: Headstand

Natarajasana: Dancer Pose

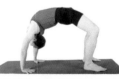

Urdhva Dhanurasana: Wheel Pose

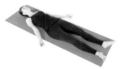

Savasana: Corpse Pose

Integrate

*It is through your body that
you realize you are a spark
of divinity.* ~B.K.S. IYENGAR

Fairy tales abound about a king and a queen who have a baby but, for some reason, cannot raise the child in the kingdom. Perhaps the child was illegitimate, strangely marked in some way, or cursed by an ancient spell that ends their life on their sixteenth birthday. Whatever the reason, the child is wrapped up in a blanket, put under a bush, sent down the river, or exposed to the elements. The child's fate is left to chance. It is now up to the gods.

Of course, the child does not die. Instead the child is found and raised in a humble environment, fostered by a farmer or peasant and raised in nature, far from the lights and splendor of the kingdom.

But something always happens in these stories as the child grows up. Sometime around adolescence the budding young adult hears or sees something out of the ordinary. They are attracted to something beyond the awareness of the people around them. They cannot explain it—perhaps no one understands it—and they might even be ridiculed. But the call has been heard; they feel compelled to explore its mystery.

Eventually, their exploration leads to a series of coincidences in which the grown child finds their way back to the original kingdom and discovers who they really are: a prince or a princess—a future king or queen. They are accepted back into the kingdom, to their rightful place, and resume their development into these exalted roles.

This mirrors the journey to divine awakening. We are born of a divine source, but we were separated at such a young age that we forget who we are, or perhaps we never knew. We are raised by humble, well-meaning parents, who did the best they could with their wounding and the tools they had yet were ignorant about the glorious kingdom that rules the territory. Outside of the kingdom, our more humble origins, along with our exposure to the elements of nature, ground us into the earth, water, fire, and air—elements of the first four chakras.

Once we resonate with deeper truths and glimpse the illumination that pierces illusion, we are on a path to something greater. We are on a path back to our divine origins and the realization of our divine nature. We realize who our parents really are: the divine mother and father, god and goddess, Shiva and Shakti, heaven and earth.

Through this journey, we awaken to who we really are: a spark of the Divine seeking expression and manifestation. We remember. With our humble beginnings and our divine realization, we can at last be fully integrated. We become the divine child whose destiny is the healing of our world.

From that realization of the Divine within ourselves, we then recognize it in others and in all life around us. This is the true meaning of the word that is the ultimate salute to our divine nature: *Namaste!*

From Theory to Practice

At the end of my workshops, students always want to know how to apply what they have learned. Often people want some kind of prescribed formula: *do this for seven days and do that for fifteen minutes on alternate Thursdays.*

Unfortunately, it is not so easy, and frankly, I refuse to give out such formulas. For one thing, we are not all the same. Some people need to work on grounding (most of us!) while others need to develop their power. Some have open hearts and some do not, and some live in their heads while others are barely scratching the surface of higher consciousness. There is no one size fits all.

Ultimately yoga and chakra work is designed to put you more in touch with yourself. It is from within your own temple that you will find your own answers. What I've given you in these pages is some understanding of the chakra system and some tools to use for working with it. But feeling your way from within is what is required to find out how those tools best work for you—to discover which ones you need most and which are less useful.

Here are some general guidelines: when in doubt, follow the path of the chakras in their liberating current from bottom to top. Start with centering and grounding (chakra one), then get things moving (chakra two), lubricating the hips and joints. That will warm you up and generate energy (chakra three) that you can direct and expand as you soften with the breath (chakra four), using postures to open the chest and upper body. Then attune your energies to finer vibrations (chakra five), perhaps with some chanting or sounding; focus your attention on something beautiful (chakra six) and go deeper within the nature of your own consciousness (chakra seven), ending with meditation. This basic formula is described by the chakra map, but you have to figure out how to work it into your life. It might be a daily routine that incorporates all seven chakras or a weekly routine that focuses on one chakra each day. You might even spend one month focusing primarily on each chakra, as Selene Vega and I did for many years in our monthly Chakra Intensives.

If you need more grounding on a particular day or need lots of it due to past issues, then focus on that until it gets in your bones. If you flow too much or not enough, then balance your second chakra accordingly. If your energy is lethargic and you need to get going, work on your third chakra. But if you are already a strong-willed person who is constantly busy doing this and doing that, then lay back for awhile, choose some more restorative poses, and see what happens. If you want more spaciousness, work with pranayama or meditation.

I can only give you the map; I cannot tell you where to go. Ultimately you are the one who holds the seven keys and will decide what to do with them. Trust yourself, listen deeply to your inner guidance, and practice, practice, practice. Divine intelligence is embedded within you. It is there to guide you and only awaits your discovery.

Why are you here? Why have you come to earth?
Why are you here? Why have you taken birth?
To love, serve, and remember.

· · · · · · · · · · · · ·

ANONYMOUS

From Inner to Outer: On and Off the Mat

The chakras are chambers in the inner temple and portals between the inner and outer worlds. We open these gates to discover the inner temple, and we clean up the chambers to better embody the Divine.

But then what?

In the dissolution between inner and outer that gradually occurs, we realize that sitting on our mats and counting our breaths is only the tool; the question is what do we build with that tool? Asanas and pranayama are the alphabet of a spiritual language, but the real yoga has to do with what we say and do with that language—what we take out into the world around us.

Our world today is seriously threatened—something that was never the case in the previous eras in which our ancient religions were developed. Environmental degradation that threatens the future of human life was never an issue in those days. A global network armed with the tools of mass communication did not exist; in fact, only a tiny minority of privileged scholars even knew how to read or write. We now live in very different times.

The crises and awakenings that are occurring everywhere are asking us to step up fully to becoming something greater than ordinary beings, not just for our own ego gratification or to preen our postures into perfection on our mat each day but to become better servants to the planet's evolution. Yoga is the path through which we evolve, but ultimately we have to take our yoga beyond ourselves in service and right action.

The elements of the chakras that dwell within us—earth, water, fire, air, sound, light, and consciousness—exist outside of us as well. The earth is threatened through millennia of philosophies that told us the material world wasn't real or didn't matter. (Then why do we call it matter?) The waters of emotions and sexuality have been dammed for centuries, and now the waters of our world are out of balance, with floods and droughts creating problems everywhere. The fires of power have been corrupted and our personal power usurped by domination and aggression. Now the fire element is out of control and overheating the climate. The air is polluted with carbon and chemicals. The sound waves are full of lies and distractions. We are starved for the natural light of day, while beauty is a forgotten spiritual value. The world itself has forgotten its divine nature.

As we use these seven keys to awaken the inner temple, we find that these same keys can restore the outer temple. As we clean up our first chakras, we see that the world needs to come to terms with its collective first chakra and heal the ailments of financial, environmental, and health crises. As we reclaim the waters of our soul, releasing them to flow once again, perhaps the waters of the planet will begin to balance. As we find our power, we can use that power in service of right action. As we open our hearts, we create space to breathe, a new way of connecting to each other, a culture of compassion. As we learn to communicate, we can speak out into the airwaves. As we imagine a better world, we create a guiding vision. And as we become better informed, we start to see the bigger picture and understand what needs to be done.

These actions in the outer world don't happen by themselves. Getting grounded is a good start, but it alone will not protect the rainforest from devastation or keep the topsoil from washing down the river. Having a good cry is not going to save the four thousand children in India from dying each day from lack of clean water. Taking a deep breath does not clean up the air pollution, though it may make us more aware of it.

These things require that we stand in our ground, engage our passion, utilize our power, open our hearts, speak our truth, tell-a-vision, and bring higher consciousness to the world around us. They require that we get involved, take action, donate money, become informed, and take on the leadership that our era requires.

This is the initiation into the simultaneously inconvenient and glorious truths of the world we live in. As the general population is becoming more enlightened every day through access to information and teachings, we are being asked to step into something we have never been before: gods and goddesses in training. For as I stated in the beginning of my book *The Global Heart Awakens*, "Evolution is the gods' way of making more gods." The path of evolution proceeds with greater awareness, intelligence, complexity, power, and creativity—all powers of the Divine.

The chakra system is a rainbow bridge that reconnects heaven and earth through the core of our very selves and reconnects ourselves to the glorious world we have inherited, complete with all its challenges so perfectly designed for our awakening. There are many walking this path, and more and more climb on board each day.

We need a good map to guide us along the way. We need a map for our own journey and a map for humanity to navigate this rite of passage from our adolescence to our planetary adulthood. It is the time of the greatest mass awakening humanity has ever experienced, and you are an essential part of it.

The chakra system is that map. It embraces everything that we are and everything that is and always has been. It shows us how inside and outside are intimately connected—indeed, never even separate. It leads us to divine realization while reclaiming our rights to pleasure, power, creativity, and love. It contains the keys to our awakening—if we dare to use those keys.

May you use them often and wisely. May you walk the rainbow bridge and connect with others along the way, and may the long-lost connection between heaven and earth be restored so that we can finally begin to create heaven right here on earth.

Namaste!

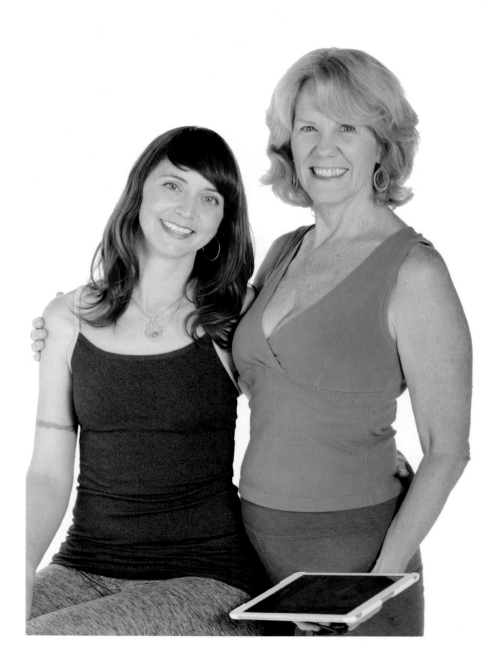

Glossary of Sanskrit Terms

Abhyasa: Effort or consistent spiritual practice over a long period of time.

Adho Mukha Svanasana: Downward Facing Dog Pose

Adho Mukha Vrksasana: Handstand

Agni Sara: The action of pumping the belly muscles in and out while holding the breath empty in uddiyana bandha.

Agnistambhasana: Fire Log or Double Pigeon Pose

Ajña: (ahj-nee-uh) The name of the sixth chakra, located in the center of the head at brow level, meaning command center.

Anahata: (ah-nah-huh-tah, accent on second syllable) The name of the fourth chakra, located in the heart area, meaning unstruck.

Anahatasana: Extended Puppy Pose

Ananda Balasana: Happy Baby Pose

Anjaneyasana: Deep Lunge Pose

Anuloma krama: A pranayama practice that utilizes short inhales and a long exhale and brings energy up the chakras.

Apanasana: Knees to Chest Pose

Apana Vayu: Downward wind current, one of the five basic vayus, or pranic winds.

Ardha Chandra Chapasana: Sugar Cane Pose

Ardha Chandrasana: Standing Half Moon Pose

Ardha Hanumanasana: Reverse Lunge

Ardha Matsyendrasana: Half Lord of the Fishes Pose or Seated Twist

Asana: Hatha yoga posture. The word originally meant a sitting position used for meditation but has come to mean any yoga posture. The third limb of Ashtanga yoga, which Patanjali describes as "to be seated in a position that is firm but relaxed."[14]

Baddha Konasana: Bound Angle or Cobbler Pose

Bakasana: Crane Pose

14 Verse 46, chapter II; for translation refer to *Patanjali Yoga Sutras* by Swami Prabhavananda, published by the Sri Ramakrishna Math, ISBN 81-7120-221-7, page 111.

Bandha: A lock, as in a channel lock found in a waterway. Bandhas are a way to retain or direct prana in a particular part of the body.

Bharmanasana: Table Pose

Bhujangasana: Cobra Pose

Bija: (bee-juh) Literally "seed." Bija is usually used in conjunction with mantras for the chakras. The bija mantras are represented by the symbols inside the chakras as illustrated in the old texts. Chanting the bija mantras is said to stimulate the chakras. There are only six bija mantras given. From first chakra to sixth, they are *lam, vam, ram, yam, ham,* and *om,* though some esoteric texts give mantras for subtler chakras.

Bindu: A dimensional focal point of concentration, symbolizing the point from which all creation emerges and into which it dissolves. The red dot often placed on the forehead represents the supreme bindu of consciousness.

Brahmana: To expand. Pranayama practice that tonifies, nourishes, heats, and builds energy. Often emphasizes the inhalation.

Chakra: (chuck-ruh, with a hard *ch* as in church) Literally "wheel." A center of organization located in the subtle body for receiving, assimilating, and expressing life force energy, or prana.

Dandasana: Staff Pose

Dhanurasana: Bow Pulling Pose

Dharana: Focused concentration. The beginning stage of meditation, which focuses the mind on an object such as the breath, a mantra, a candle flame, or an image of a deity. The sixth limb of Ashtanga yoga.

Dharma: One's own duty, often expressed through work or right action. The way to balance one's karma, or the effects of action and ignorance.

Dhyana: Deep meditation, producing an awareness of the unity in all things without being identified with it. The seventh limb of Ashtanga yoga.

Drishti: Gaze. In holding a yoga pose, especially a balancing pose, your drishti focuses your gaze on an unmoving point, which is helpful for balance and concentration. It also reflects your perspective, what grabs your attention, and what you are looking at.

Eka Pada Kapotasana: Pigeon Pose

Garudasana: Eagle Pose

Gomukhasana: Cow Face Pose

Gunas: Qualities. The three gunas represent qualities that exist in everything: *tamas* (matter), *rajas* (energy), and *sattvas* (consciousness).

Halasana: Plow Pose

Glossary of Sanskrit Terms

Ida nadi: One of the primary channels of prana moving around and between the chakras. Ida represents the moon, the color white, the feminine and coolness, and is associated with the Ganges River.

Jalandara bandha: Chin lock

Janu Sirsasana: Head to Knee Forward Bend

Jathara Parivartanasana: Knee Down Twist

Kakasana: Crow Pose

Kapalabhati: Literally "shining skull." A rapid diaphragmatic breathing technique that utilizes a passive inhalation and an active exhalation. Also known as the Breath of Fire.

Karma: The inevitable debt incurred by the needs of life and our actions.

Karnapidasana: Ear Pressure Pose

Kirtan: A call and response musical concert in which the performers play and chant devotional songs while the audience sings back each phrase repeatedly. Kirtans are a kind of group devotional practice that is said to "clean the dust off the mirror of the heart."

Kleshas: Afflictions. There are five basic kleshas: *avidya*, or ignorance; *asmita*, or ego; *raga*, or attachment; *dvesha*, or aversion; and *abhinivesha*, or clinging to life.

Krama: Literally a step. Kramas are a type of breathing exercise in which the breath is inhaled or exhaled in small sips, or steps.

Kriya: Involuntary physical movements as a result of subtle energy, prana, or Kundalini moving through the body.

Kumbhaka: Breath retention

Kundala: Coiled

Kundalini: A potent force of concentrated prana that moves through the body to pierce through blockages and awaken the chakras. Also the name of a serpent goddess who represents this awakening force, whose full name is Kundalini-Shakti.

Langhana: To fast. Pranayama used for relaxation, contraction, purification, cooling, and conservation of energy.

Madhyama: Inward sound. The sound you hear in your head with the silent intoning of a mantra or even listening to the chatter of your thoughts.

Makarasana: Crocodile Pose

Makarasana II: Dolphin Pose

Manipura: (mah-nee-poo-ruh) The name of the third chakra, located in the solar plexus, meaning lustrous gem.

Mantra: Literally "tool for the mind." A mantra is a sound, phrase, or vibration designed to wake you up the way someone shaking your shoulder can wake you from sleep. Mantras are used to steady the mind in meditation, to activate the chakras, and to honor various deities.

Marjaryasana/Bitilasana: Cat/Cow Pose

Matsyasana: Fish Pose

Mula bandha: Root lock

Muladhara: (moo-luh-dah-ruh) The name of the first chakra, located at the base of the spine, meaning root support or foundation.

Nadi(s): Subtle channels or rivers of prana in the body.

Nadi Shodhana: Alternate Nostril Breathing

Nakulasana: Mongoose Pose

Namaste: A common greeting in India offered with hands in prayer position, meaning to bow to or honor the Divine in yourself, in another, and in all life.

Natarajasana: Dancer Pose

Niyamas: The second limb of Ashtanga yoga, which advises conduct and care of the self. There are five niyamas: *sauça*, or purity and cleanliness of mind and body; *santosha*, contentment; *tapas*, heat or spiritual fire created from practices; *svadyaya*, study of self and of scriptures and text; and *isvara pranidhana*, devotion or surrender to the Divine.

Para: Supreme sound, the power that precedes existence, raw potential.

Parighasana: Gate Pose

Parighasana II: Half Circle Pose

Paripurna Navasana: Boat Pose

Parivrtta Parsvakonasana: Revolved Side Angle Pose

Parsvottanasana: Intense Side Stretch Pose

Paschimottanasana: Seated Forward Bend

Pashyanti: Radiant sound, which bursts through the bindu point and radiates outward, only heard by yogis in concentration.

Phalakasana: Plank Pose

Pincha Mayurasana: Feathered Peacock Pose

Pingala nadi: One of the primary channels of prana moving around and between the chakras. Pingala represents the sun, the masculine channel, the color red, warmth, and is associated with the Yamuna River.

Prakriti: Primordial substance, as matter and energy, from which everything is made. Counterpart to Purusha (spirit or consciousness) from Samkhya philosophy.

Glossary of Sanskrit Terms

Prana: Literally "first unit." Prana is the vital life force found in everything.

Pranayama: Breathing practices designed to enhance the flow of prana. The fourth limb of Ashtanga yoga.

Pratiloma krama: A pranayama practice that involves short inhalations and short exhalations. A good technique for beginning meditators to slow down the mind and balance the breath.

Pratyahara: Withdrawal of the senses from the outside world to focus on the inner world. The fifth limb of Patanjali's Ashtanga yoga, which prepares the yoga practitioner for meditation.

Purusha: Pure consciousness, transcendent self, the unmanifest. Counterpart to Prakriti from Samkhya philosophy.

Purvottanasana: Inclined Plane Pose

Rajas: The active guna, or quality, of fire, energy, or movement.

Sahasrara: (sah-huss-rah-ruh) The name of the crown chakra, located at the top of the head, meaning thousandfold lotus. The number 1,000 is not literal but denotes the concept of infinity.

Salabhasana: Locust Pose

Salamba Sarvangasana: Shoulder Stand

Samadhi: The final stage of absorption that leads to bliss and enlightenment. The eighth limb of Ashtanga yoga, which results from years of cultivating the other seven limbs, especially those of concentration and deep meditation.

Sasangasana: Rabbit Pose

Sat-chit-ananda: Literally "truth, consciousness, and bliss"; the nature of ultimate reality.

Sattvas: The guna, or quality, of consciousness, awareness, and stillness.

Savasana: Corpse Pose

Setu Bandha Sarvangasana: Bridge Pose

Shakti: The living goddess of the life force energy that moves through the body and enlivens us. Counterpart to Shiva.

Shaktipat: The spontaneous awakening of Kundalini, brought about by contact with a guru or master who has already awakened this energy in themselves. Transmission of spiritual awakening.

Shiva: The masculine god representing supreme consciousness, counterpart to Shakti.

Shiva lingam: A symbol representing the male organ, depicted within the square of the first chakra, which signifies the rising energy of the masculine. Shiva lingams are also large conical stones that can be found in India, as representations of the god himself.

Siddhasana: Baby Cradle Pose

Sirsasana: Headstand

Spanda: Pulsation—the basic expansion and contraction of all life.

Sucirandhrasana: Eye of the Needle Pose

Supta Baddha Konasana: Reclined Bound Angle or Butterfly Pose

Supta Padangusthasana: Reclining Hand to Big Toe Pose

Supta Virasana: Reclining Hero Pose

Surya Namaskar: Salutation to the sun. A series of linked postures or vinyasa practice that is often used in yoga classes as a way to warm up the body. This practice originated in India as a worship of the solar deity Surya. There are many variations of these sun salutes.

Sushumna nadi: The central nadi moving up and down the core, or midline, of the body, through which the chakras are arranged like beads on a string. Associated with the Saraswati River.

Svadhisthana: (svah-dee-stah-nuh) The name of the second chakra, located in the sacral area, meaning one's own place.

Tadasana: Standing Mountain Pose

Tamas: The guna, or quality, of earth, inertia at rest, solidity, and heaviness.

Tapas: Internal spiritual fire built through disciplines, austerities, and practices.

Trikonasana: Triangle Pose

Uddiyana bandha: Upward abdominal lock

Ujjayi: Literally "to conquer or be victorious." Sometimes called the ocean breath, ujjayi is a pranayama practice that creates a subtle contraction of the epiglottis in the throat, which slows down the movement of the breath and creates a sound like the ocean while also strengthening the diaphragm.

Upavistha Konasana: Open Leg Forward Fold

Urdvha Dhanurasana: Upward Facing Bow or Wheel Pose

Ustrasana: Camel Pose

Utkata Konasana: Goddess Squat

Utkatasana: Awkward Chair Pose

Uttanasana: Standing Forward Fold

Uttan Pristhasana: Lizard Pose or Humble Warrior Pose

Utthita Hasta Padangusthasana:
Extended Hand to Toe Pose

Vaikhari: Audible sound. The
fourth level of sound, which can
be uttered by the voice, made
by machinery and instruments,
or found in nature.

Vairagya: Detachment,
dispassion, or renunciation.

Vasisthasana: Side Plank Pose

Vayus: Literally "winds," the five vayus
refer to movements of prana within
the body. The five vayus are *apana,*
samana, prana, udana, and *vyana.*

Viloma Krama: A pranayama practice
that involves a long inhalation
and several short exhalations.
Said to bring energy downward.

Vinyasa: The literal translation of
this word is connection, or linking.
A generic meaning of this word
is flow, and it relates to linking
various postures together in a way
that flows logically from one to
the other. Often describes a type
of yoga class that flows quickly
through a series of postures,
such as Sun Salutations.

Virabhadrasana I: Warrior I Pose

Virabhadrasana II: Warrior II Pose

Virabhadrasana III: Warrior III Pose

Virasana: Seated Hero Pose

Vissudha: (vi-shoo-duh) The name
of the fifth chakra, located in the
throat, meaning purification.

Vrksasana: Tree Pose

Yamas: The first limb of Ashtanga
yoga, which advises restraints
or behavioral guidelines on how
to treat others. There are five
yamas: *ahimsa,* or nonviolence;
satya, or truthfulness; *asteya,* or
non-stealing; *brahmacharya,* or
moderate sexuality; and *aparigraha,*
or detachment and non-clinging.

Glossary of Sanskrit Terms

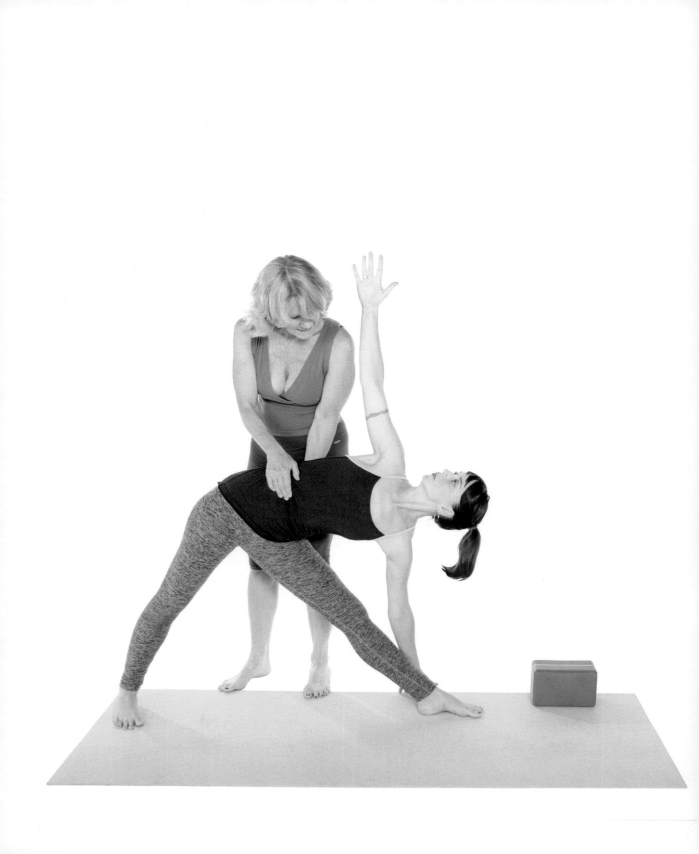

Index

GET MORE AT LLEWELLYN.COM

Visit us online to browse hundreds of our books and decks, plus sign up to receive our e-newsletters and exclusive online offers.

- Free tarot readings • Spell-a-Day • Moon phases
- Recipes, spells, and tips • Blogs • Encyclopedia
- Author interviews, articles, and upcoming events

GET SOCIAL WITH LLEWELLYN

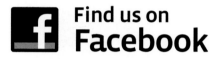
Find us on Facebook

www.Facebook.com/LlewellynBooks

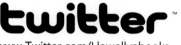
Follow us on twitter™

www.Twitter.com/Llewellynbooks

GET BOOKS AT LLEWELLYN

LLEWELLYN ORDERING INFORMATION

 Order online: Visit our website at www.llewellyn.com to select your books and place an order on our secure server.

 Order by phone:
- Call toll free within the U.S. at 1-877-NEW-WRLD (1-877-639-9753)
- Call toll free within Canada at 1-866-NEW-WRLD (1-866-639-9753)
- We accept VISA, MasterCard, and American Express

 Order by mail:
Send the full price of your order (MN residents add 6.875% sales tax) in U.S. funds, plus postage and handling, to:
Llewellyn Worldwide, 2143 Wooddale Drive, Woodbury, MN 55125-2989

POSTAGE AND HANDLING

STANDARD (U.S. & Canada):
(Please allow 12 business days)
$25.00 and under, add $4.00.
$25.01 and over, FREE SHIPPING.

INTERNATIONAL ORDERS (airmail only):
$16.00 for one book, plus $3.00 for each additional book.

Visit us online for more shipping options. Prices subject to change.

FREE CATALOG!

To order, call
1-877-NEW-WRLD
ext. 8236
or visit our
website

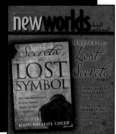

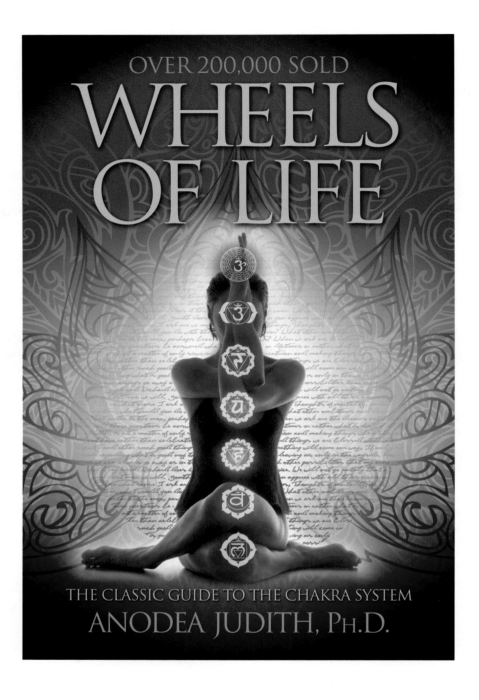

OVER 200,000 SOLD

WHEELS OF LIFE

THE CLASSIC GUIDE TO THE CHAKRA SYSTEM

ANODEA JUDITH, Ph.D.

Wheels of Life

The Classic Guide to the Chakra System

Anodea Judith

Wheels of Life is an instruction manual for owning and operating the inner gears that run the machinery of our lives. Written in a practical, down-to-earth style, this fully illustrated book will take the reader on a journey through aspects of consciousness, from the bodily instincts of survival to the processing of deep thoughts.

Discover this ancient metaphysical system under the new light of popular Western metaphors: quantum physics, Kabbalah, physical exercises, poetic meditations, and visionary art. Learn how to open these centers in yourself, then see how the chakras shed light on the present world crises we face today—and learn what you can do about it!

This book is a vital resource for meditators, yoga practitioners and teachers, healers of all types, mystics, evolutionaries, and all who are interested in spiritual growth and healing.

978-0-8754-2320-3, 528 pp., 6 x 9, illus. $21.95

To Order, Call 1-877-NEW-WRLD
PRICES SUBJECT TO CHANGE WITHOUT NOTICE
WWW.LLEWELLYN.COM

To Write to the Author

If you wish to contact the author or would like more information about this book, please write to the author in care of Llewellyn Worldwide and we will forward your request. Both the author and the publisher appreciate hearing from you and learning of your enjoyment of this book and how it has helped you. Llewellyn Worldwide cannot guarantee that every letter written to the author can be answered, but all will be forwarded. Please write to:

Anodea Judith
c/o Llewellyn Worldwide
2143 Wooddale Drive
Woodbury, MN 55125-2989

Please enclose a self-addressed stamped envelope for reply or $1.00 to cover costs. If outside the USA, enclose an international postal reply coupon.

Many of Llewellyn's authors have websites with additional information and resources. For more information, please visit our website:

WWW.LLEWELLYN.COM